T0263606

Clinical Pharmacology for Dentists

Editor

HARRY DYM

DENTAL CLINICS OF NORTH AMERICA

www.dental.theclinics.com

April 2016 • Volume 60 • Number 2

ELSEVIER

1600 John F. Kennedy Boulevard ● Suite 1800 ● Philadelphia, Pennsylvania, 19103-2899

http://www.dental.theclinics.com

DENTAL CLINICS OF NORTH AMERICA Volume 60, Number 2
April 2016 ISSN 0011-8532, ISBN: 978-0-323-41750-1

Editor: John Vassallo; j.vassallo@elsevier.com
Developmental Editor: Kristen Helm

© **2016 Elsevier Inc. All rights reserved.**

This periodical and the individual contributions contained in it are protected under copyright by Elsevier, and the following terms and conditions apply to their use:

Photocopying
Single photocopies of single articles may be made for personal use as allowed by national copyright laws. Permission of the Publisher and payment of a fee is required for all other photocopying, including multiple or systematic copying, copying for advertising or promotional purposes, resale, and all forms of document delivery. Special rates are available for educational institutions that wish to make photocopies for non-profit educational classroom use. For information on how to seek permission visit www.elsevier.com/permissions or call: (+44) 1865 843830 (UK)/(+1) 215 239 3804 (USA).

Derivative Works
Subscribers may reproduce tables of contents or prepare lists of articles including abstracts for internal circulation within their institutions. Permission of the Publisher is required for resale or distribution outside the institution. Permission of the Publisher is required for all other derivative works, including compilations and translations (please consult www.elsevier.com/permissions).

Electronic Storage or Usage
Permission of the Publisher is required to store or use electronically any material contained in this periodical, including any article or part of an article (please consult www.elsevier.com/permissions). Except as outlined above, no part of this publication may be reproduced, stored in a retrieval system or transmitted in any form or by any means, electronic, mechanical, photocopying, recording or otherwise, without prior written permission of the Publisher.

Notice
No responsibility is assumed by the Publisher for any injury and/or damage to persons or property as a matter of products liability, negligence or otherwise, or from any use or operation of any methods, products, instructions or ideas contained in the material herein. Because of rapid advances in the medical sciences, in particular, independent verification of diagnoses and drug dosages should be made.

Although all advertising material is expected to conform to ethical (medical) standards, inclusion in this publication does not constitute a guarantee or endorsement of the quality or value of such product or of the claims made of it by its manufacturer.

Dental Clinics of North America (ISSN 0011-8532) is published quarterly by Elsevier Inc., 360 Park Avenue South, New York, NY 10010-1710. Months of issue are January, April, July, and October. Business and Editorial Offices: 1600 John F. Kennedy Boulevard, Suite 1800, Philadelphia, PA 19103-2899. Periodicals postage paid at New York, NY and additional mailing offices. Subscription prices are $280.00 per year (domestic individuals), $537.00 per year (domestic institutions), $100.00 per year (domestic students/residents), $340.00 per year (Canadian individuals), $695.00 per year (Canadian institutions), $410.00 per year (international individuals), $695.00 per year (international institutions), and $200.00 per year (international and Canadian students/residents). International air speed delivery is included in all *Clinics* subscription prices. All prices are subject to change without notice. **POSTMASTER:** Send address changes to *Dental Clinics of North America*, Elsevier Health Sciences Division, Subscription Customer Service, 3251 Riverport Lane, Maryland Heights, MO 63043. **Customer Service (orders, claims, online, change of address): Elsevier Health Sciences Division, Subscription Customer Service, 3251 Riverport Lane, Maryland Heights, MO 63043. Tel: 1-800-654-2452 (U.S. and Canada). Fax: 314-447-8029. E-mail: journalscustomer service-usa@elsevier.com (for print support); journalsonlinesupport-usa@elsevier.com (for online support).**

Reprints. For copies of 100 or more, of articles in this publication, please contact the Commercial Reprints Department, Elsevier Inc., 360 Park Avenue South, New York, NY 10010-1710. Tel.: 212-633-3874; Fax: 212-633-3820; E-mail: reprints@elsevier.com.

The Dental Clinics of North America is covered in *MEDLINE/PubMed (Index Medicus), Current Contents/Clinical Medicine, ISI/BIOMED* and *Clinahl.*

Contributors

EDITOR

HARRY DYM, DDS
Chief, Oral and Maxillofacial Surgery; Chairman, Department of Dentistry/Oral and Maxillofacial Surgery, Director of Oral and Maxillofacial Residency Training Program, The Brooklyn Hospital Center, Brooklyn, New York

AUTHORS

SHELLY ABRAMOWICZ, DMD, MPH
Assistant Professor of Surgery and Pediatrics, Division of Oral and Maxillofacial Surgery, Department of Surgery, Children's Healthcare of Atlanta, Emory University School of Medicine, Atlanta, Georgia

GOLALEH BARZANI, DMD
Oral and Maxillofacial Surgery Resident, The Brooklyn Hospital Center, Brooklyn, New York

DUSTIN BOWLER, DDS
Chief Resident, Division of Oral and Maxillofacial Surgery Residency Training Program, The Brooklyn Hospital Center, Brooklyn, New York

RICARDO A. BOYCE, DDS, FICD
Full-time Attending; Director of the General Practice Residency, Department of Dentistry/Oral and Maxillofacial Surgery, The Brooklyn Hospital Center, Brooklyn, New York

LAWRENCE R. BROWN, DDS
Private Practice, Dadeland Oral Surgery Associates; Hospital Affiliate, Associate Privileges, Baptist Hospital of Miami, Miami, Florida

EARL CLARKSON, DDS
Department of Oral & Maxillofacial Surgery, Woodhull Medical Center, Brooklyn, New York

HARRY DYM, DDS
Chief, Oral and Maxillofacial Surgery; Chairman, Department of Dentistry/Oral and Maxillofacial Surgery, Director of Oral and Maxillofacial Residency Training Program, The Brooklyn Hospital Center, Brooklyn, New York

JONATHAN ELMORE, DDS
The Brooklyn Hospital Center, Brooklyn, New York

LESLIE HALPERN, MD, DDS, PhD, MPH
Associate Professor/Program Director, Residency Director, Oral and Maxillofacial Surgery, Meharry Medical College, Nashville, Tennessee

CURTIS J. HOLMES, DDS
Resident, Department of Dentistry and Oral and Maxillofacial Surgery, The Brooklyn Hospital Center, Brooklyn, New York

MEHRAN HOSSAINI-ZADEH, DMD
Professor of Oral and Maxillofacial Surgery, Temple University Kornberg School of Dentistry, Philadelphia, Pennsylvania

MICHAEL P. JOHNSON, DMD
Private Practice, Guilford, Connecticut; Program Director, Oral and Maxillofacial Surgery, Yale-New Haven Hospital, New Haven, Connecticut

TARUN KIRPALANI, DMD
Part-time Attending, Department of Dentistry/Oral and Maxillofacial Surgery, The Brooklyn Hospital Center, Brooklyn, New York

CONSTANTINOS LASKARIDES, DMD, DDS, PharmD, FICD
Associate Professor, Assistant Director, Advanced Residency Program, Oral and Maxillofacial Surgery, Attending Surgeon, Tufts Medical Center, Tufts University, Boston, Massachusetts

JOSHUA M. LEVY, DMD
Resident, Division of Oral and Maxillofacial Surgery, Department of Surgery, Emory University School of Medicine, Atlanta, Georgia

JARED MILLER, DDS
Department of Oral & Maxillofacial Surgery, Woodhull Medical Center, Brooklyn, New York

NAVEEN MOHAN, DDS
Resident, Department of Dentistry/Oral and Maxillofacial Surgery, The Brooklyn Hospital Center, Brooklyn, New York

ORRETT E. OGLE, DDS
Lecturer, Mona Dental Program, Faculty of Medical Sciences, University of the West Indies, Kingston, Jamaica; Former Chief, Oral and Maxillofacial Surgery, Woodhull Medical Center, Brooklyn, New York

ROBERT PELLECCHIA, DDS
Director, Department of Dentistry and Oral Maxillofacial Surgery, Geisinger Medical Center, Danville, Pennsylvania

MIHAI RADULESCU, DMD
Chief Resident, Oral Maxillofacial Surgery, Woodhull Medical Center, Brooklyn, New York

ARVIND BABU RAJENDRA SANTOSH, MDS
Oral and Maxillofacial Pathologist; Lecturer and Research Coordinator, Mona Dental Program, Faculty of Medical Sciences, University of the West Indies, Kingston, Jamaica

FRANCESCO R. SEBASTIANI, DMD
Resident, Oral and Maxillofacial Surgery, The Brooklyn Hospital Center, Brooklyn, New York

JANET H. SOUTHERLAND, DDS, MPH, PhD
Professor, Department of Oral and Maxillofacial Surgery, Meharry Medical College School of Dentistry, Nashville, Tennessee

AVICHAI STERN, DDS
The Brooklyn Hospital Center, Brooklyn, New York

MICHAEL D. TURNER, DDS, MD, FACS
Associate Director, Mount Sinai Beth Israel/Jacobi/Einstein Oral and Maxillofacial Surgery, Institute of Head and Neck and Thyroid Cancer, New York, New York

ROBERT J. WEINSTOCK, DDS
Private Practice, Guilford, Connecticut; Clinical Instructor, Oral and Maxillofacial Surgery, Yale-New Haven Hospital, New Haven, Connecticut

PORCHIA WILLIS, DDS
Chief Resident, PGY 4, Oral and Maxillofacial Surgery, Meharry Medical College, Nashville, Tennessee

JOSHUA WOLF, DDS
Assistant Attending, Oral and Maxillofacial Surgery, The Brooklyn Hospital Center, Brooklyn, New York

JOSEPH ZEIDAN, DMD
Second Year Resident, Division of Oral and Maxillofacial Surgery Residency Training Program, The Brooklyn Hospital Center, Brooklyn, New York

Contents

> Any dental office can face a variety of medical emergencies; therefore, the health care professional and the staff should always be prepared to deal with these emergencies in their office. Preparedness of the dental office staff and their prompt recognition of these emergencies will be the most important factor in dealing with the emergencies in any dental office. Health care professionals should follow the recommendations in this article to maintain a guideline for their staff and office and conduct regular emergency drills to examine the equipment and preparedness of their staff.

> This article highlights the commonly used medications used in dentistry and oral surgery. General dentists and specialists must be knowledgeable about the pharmacology of the drugs currently available along with their risks and benefits. Enteral sedation is a useful adjunct for the treatment of anxious adult and pediatric patients. When enteral sedation is used within the standards of care, the interests of the public and the dental profession are served through a cost-effective, effective service that can be widely available. Oral sedation enables dentists to provide dental care to millions of individuals who otherwise would have unmet dental needs.

> Several sedation options are used to minimize pain, anxiety, and discomfort during oral surgery procedures. Minimizing or eliminating pain and anxiety for dental care is the primary goal for conscious sedation. Intravenous conscious sedation is a drug-induced depression of consciousness during which patients respond purposefully to verbal commands. No interventions are required to maintain a patent airway, and spontaneous ventilation is adequate as well as cardiovascular function. Patients must retain their protective airway reflexes, and respond to and understand verbal communication. The drugs and techniques used must therefore carry a broad margin of safety.

> This article is an update on pain management in the dental care setting for adult and pediatric patients. The 3 main categories of analgesic medications

are examined: (1) opioids, (2) nonsteroidal antiinflammatory drugs (NSAIDs), and (3) nonopioid, non-NSAID medications. Pharmacology, side effects, patient selection, and treatment strategies and principles are examined. The information provided is aimed to facilitate the clinical perspective and update the oral health care clinician on providing safe and effective analgesia to adult and pediatric patients.

Pharmacologic agents play an integral role in the overall management of temporomandibular joint disorder. The general dentist should be familiar with the different classes of drugs currently in use for dealing with this often complex medical/dental problem.

Pain is a universal experience with profound effects on the physiology, psychology, and sociology of the population. Orofacial pain (OFP) conditions are especially prevalent and can be severely debilitating to a patient's health-related quality of life. Evidence-based clinical trials suggest that pharmacologic therapy may significantly improve patient outcomes either alone or when used as part of a comprehensive treatment plan for OFP. The aim of this article is to provide therapeutic options from a pharmacologic perspective to treat a broad spectrum of OFP. Clinical-based systemic and topical applied pharmaceutical approaches are presented to treat the most common OFP syndromes.

The oral ulcerations caused by aphtous lesions, herpetic lesions, candidiasis, ulcerative lichen planus, mucous membrane pemphigoid, and pemphigus vulgaris are managed in a step-up approach that can involve topical, intarlesional, and systemic pharmacologic management. This article reviews the common treatment agents, modalities, and dosages. The emphasis is on local pharmacologic therapies, yet systemic conditions that often present with such oral lesions are briefly reviewed, along with the appropriate management.

The proportion of people over age 60 is growing faster than any other group. Many patients take several medications to manage multiple chronic medical conditions. Poor oral health is common and dental visits by patients over the age of 65 are increasing. The dentist must recognize that these medications may interact with dental treatment. This article reviews the top 10 prescribed drugs as listed in the IMS Institute national prescription audit in January 2015 and reviews the interactions between these medications and dental treatment. The medications reviewed include levothyroxine, acetaminophen/hydrocodone, lisinopril, metoprolol, atorvastatin, amlodipine, metformin, omeprazole, simvastatin, and albuterol.

Michael D. Turner

Saliva is one of the most versatile, multifunctional substances produced by the body and has a critical role in the preservation of the oropharyngeal health. It comprises a serous and mucinous component and is secreted by the major salivary glands. The mucins in the saliva serve to protect and lubricate the hard and soft tissues of the mouth, protecting them from chemical and mechanical damage. Hyposalivation can be managed by various salivary substitutes, peripheral sialagogues, and central sialagogues.

Ricardo A. Boyce, Tarun Kirpalani, and Naveen Mohan

As described in this article, there are many advances in topical and local anesthesia. Topical and local anesthetics have played a great role in dentistry in alleviating the fears of patients, eliminating pain, and providing pain control. Many invasive procedures would not be performed without the use and advances of topical/local anesthetics. The modern-day dentist has the responsibility of knowing the variety of products on the market and should have at least 3 references to access before, during, and after treatment. This practice ensures proper care with topical and local anesthetics for the masses of patients entering dental offices worldwide.

Mehran Hossaini-zadeh

Despite numerous guidelines, joint interprofessional collaboration, and years of data collection, the use of antibiotic prophylaxis before dental procedures remains controversial. There continues to be disagreement on indications, justification, and outcome of the use of various antibiotic prophylaxis regiments. This is complicated by the lack of data demonstrating any positive or negative impact on the care of patients. The dental community has distanced itself from a leadership role in this conversation, based on multiple concerns including fear of litigation, lack of clear pathophysiology, and unclear cause-effect relationship.

Orrett E. Ogle and Arvind Babu Rajendra Santosh

Most pathologic lesions of the jaws or of oral mucosa are treated successfully by surgical interventions. For treatment of the central giant cell lesion, aneurysmal bone cysts, histiocytosis of the mandible, hemangioma, odontogenic keratocyst, Paget disease, oral submucous fibrosis, and oral lichen planus, medical management consisting of intralesional injections, sclerosing agents, and systemic bisphosphonates is as successful as surgical procedures with fewer complications. Pharmacology of agents used and protocols are presented.

DENTAL CLINICS OF NORTH AMERICA

THE CLINICS ARE AVAILABLE ONLINE!
Access your subscription at:
www.theclinics.com

DENTAL CLINICS OF NORTH AMERICA

FORTHCOMING ISSUES

July 2016
Special Care Dentistry
Burton S. Wasserman, Editor

October 2016
Impact of Oral Health on Interprofessional Collaborative Practice
Linda M. Kaste and Leslie R. Halpern, Editors

January 2017
Endodontics
Mo K. Kang, Editor

RECENT ISSUES

January 2016
Oral Radiology: Interpretation and Diagnostic Strategies
Mel Mupparapu, Editor

October 2015
Unanswered Questions in Periodontology
Frank A. Scannapieco, Editor

July 2015
Modern Concepts in Aesthetic Dentistry and Multidisciplined Reconstructive Rounds
John R. Calamia, Richard D. Trushkowsky, Steven B. David, and Alex S. Wolff, Editors

ISSUE OF RELATED INTEREST

Oral and Maxillofacial Surgery Clinics of North America
August 2015 (Vol. 27, No. 3)
Dentoalveolar Surgery
Michael A. Kleiman, Editor
Available at: www.oralmaxsurgery.theclinics.com

THE CLINICS ARE AVAILABLE ONLINE!
Access your subscription at:
www.theclinics.com

Preface

Clinical Pharmacology for Dentists

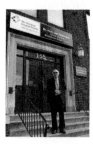

Harry Dym, DDS
Editor

The scope and practice of dentistry in the United States have evolved significantly from its origins as an independent health profession (alongside medicine) in the mid-1800s. The clinical scope of the profession as currently practiced today by thousands of dedicated clinicians encompasses multiple diverse areas that go way beyond the traditional or conventional "drill and fill" most often associated in the past with the dental profession by the general public.

Our profession has rapidly and energetically advanced and significantly expanded our scope of services. Our current clinical roles have evolved to a primary physician model with our area of expertise limited to the maxillofacial region. In fact, the current American Dental Association (ADA) definition of dentistry listed below clarifies this expanded scope of dental care in the United States.

GENERAL DENTISTRY
Definition of Dentistry:

Dentistry is defined as the evaluation, diagnosis, prevention and/or treatment (nonsurgical, surgical or related procedures) of diseases, disorders and/or conditions of the oral cavity, maxillofacial area and/or the adjacent and associated structures and their impact on the human body; provided by a dentist, within the scope of his/her education, training and experience, in accordance with the ethics of the profession and applicable law.

—(As adopted by the 1997 ADA House of Delegates)

Clearly, this definition of dentistry is quite robust and all-encompassing and establishes dentistry as a primary care specialty whose area of interest involves the

Dent Clin N Am 60 (2016) xiii–xv
http://dx.doi.org/10.1016/j.cden.2016.01.001
0011-8532/16/$ – see front matter © 2016 Published by Elsevier Inc.

dental.theclinics.com

maxillofacial area and its interface with the overall health and well-being of the patients we treat.

The modern well-trained and educated general dentist is now licensed to diagnose and treat a multitude of conditions way beyond caries and periodontal disease. Dentists are now actively involved in the diagnosis and treatment of patients with special needs in areas such as sleep apnea, chronic facial pain, oral medicine, clefted patients, traumatic injuries to the mouth and facial region, and the dental management of medically compromised patients.

It is in keeping this expanded and widened scope of care that this issue was conceived and developed. General dentists obviously must be well versed in the pharmacology of the drugs they are most likely to prescribe, but equally so, they must be aware of the common medications their patients are taking and their interactions with the drugs they both administer and prescribe, along with their effects on the oral cavity.

I am extremely pleased with the quality of the work submitted by my esteemed contributors and colleagues, and I am certain that this issue will become an often referenced text by our dental community.

I am once again privileged to have been associated with the *Dental Clinics of North America*—a wonderful series that contributes significantly to the academic and educational advancement of our profession. I am also pleased to have the opportunity to once again work with my capable editor and friend, John Vassallo, who continues to do such an admirable job with these texts, as well as Ms Kristen Helm, Developmental Editor at Elsevier.

I am also deeply indebted to certain individuals with whom I have had the distinct privilege and opportunity to have worked with for decades; who have acted as role models, friends, and confidants; and without whose friendship, my life and career would certainly have been diminished:

- Dr Peter M. Sherman, Chairman of Dentistry/Oral and Maxillofacial Surgery at Woodhull Medical Center, Brooklyn, NY
- Dr Orrett Ogle, Immediate Past Chief of Oral and Maxillofacial Surgery, Woodhull Medical Center, Brooklyn, NY
- Dr Earl Clarkson, Current Director and Chief of Oral and Maxillofacial Surgery, Woodhull Medical Center, Brooklyn, NY

I have had the distinct privilege to have spent my entire professional career at The Brooklyn Hospital Center, where I currently work with a dedicated and committed staff of individuals. I am also forever grateful to the ongoing support to myself and my department of Dentistry/Oral and Maxillofacial Surgery at The Brooklyn Hospital Center, Brooklyn NY by the following individuals:

- Dr Carlos P. Naudon, Chairman Board of Trustees, The Brooklyn Hospital Center
- Mr Gary Terrinoni, CEO and President, The Brooklyn Hospital Center
- Dr Gary Stephens, Chief Medical Officer, The Brooklyn Hospital Center
- Mr John Gupta, Chief Operating Office, The Brooklyn Hospital Center

Much thanks must be extended to my dedicated Executive Assistant/Oral and Maxillofacial Surgery Residency Coordinator, Ms Melissa Molina, and to my capable administrator, Mrs Sheila Kaufman, for their dedicated service.

Finally, this issue is dedicated to my wife, Freida, and my children and grandchildren, who are forever uppermost in my mind and heart and have always supported my professional endeavors.

Harry Dym, DDS
Dentistry/Oral and Maxillofacial Surgery
The Brooklyn Hospital Center
121 Dekalb Avenue, Box 187
Brooklyn, NY 11201, USA

E-mail address:
hdymdds@yahoo.com

Emergency Drugs for the Dental Office

Harry Dym, DDS, Golaleh Barzani, DMD*, Naveen Mohan, DDS

KEYWORDS

- Emergency drugs • Management of airway emergencies • Dental office emergencies

KEY POINTS

- The health care professional and the staff should always be prepared to use emergency drugs to deal with emergency situations in their dental office.
- Preparedness of the dental office staff and their prompt recognition of emergencies will be the most important factor in managing the emergencies in any dental office.
- Health care professionals should follow the recommendations in this article to maintain a guideline for their staff and office and conduct regular emergency drills to examine the equipment and preparedness of their staff.

INTRODUCTION

Medical emergencies in the dental office are an unavoidable part of the profession. Even though precautions to prevent such events are undertaken, these events are inevitable and the dental practitioner must be prepared. Malamed[1] reported in his book that 96.6% of respondents of a survey among practicing dentists had a medical emergency occur in the office.

Emergencies can range from relatively benign conditions to life-threatening situations. Syncope and hyperventilation are two of the most common complications seen in the dental office. One must keep in mind that even these seemingly mild issues can escalate and cause significant morbidity. Although uncommon, major emergencies, including cardiac, pulmonary, and neurologic events, can occur. The dentist must be able to manage such situations until emergency medical responders arrive to the clinic.

Lastly, urgent or emergent situations can occur at any point during the patients' visit to the dental office. The patients' anxiety about the procedure can cause an event in the waiting room or even intraoperatively. Medications administered can also cause adverse reactions intraoperatively or even postoperatively.

Department of Oral and Maxillofacial Surgery, The Brooklyn Hospital Center, 121 Delslb Avenue, Brooklyn, NY 11201, USA
* Corresponding author.
E-mail address: gbarzani@gmail.com

Dent Clin N Am 60 (2016) 287–294
http://dx.doi.org/10.1016/j.cden.2015.11.001
0011-8532/16/$ – see front matter © 2016 Elsevier Inc. All rights reserved.

This article aims to provide the dental practitioner with an overview of emergency adjuncts and medications. It is advisable for dental practitioners to also have formal training to manage emergencies, including basic life support and advance cardiac life support.

Emergency Equipment

Most essential emergency equipment in the dental office includes basic devices used for management of airway emergencies (**Box 1**). Dental office staff should be prepared at all times to provide 100% oxygen through a portable source, such as an E cylinder or an installed oxygen portal on the wall with use of a face mask, nasal cannula, or use of nonrebreather mask. Oral airway equipment, such as nasopharyngeal and oropharyngeal airway devices, can also be very useful in managing airway obstructions in case of airway emergencies. Dental professionals and office staff should routinely run emergency drills in their dental office (**Box 2**). It is the responsibility of the dental professional to assure that all the emergency equipment and oxygen tanks are full and operational at all times. Running emergency drills in the dental office will assure that the staff is prepared to deal with emergencies and the equipment are functioning properly.[2]

Other tools used in the dental office for management of emergencies are those used to assess patients' vital signs. A pulse oximeter, sphygmomanometer, and stethoscope should be readily available in every dental office. If the dental office is equipped with a monitor, the heart rate, blood pressure, and oxygen saturation can be assessed simultaneously. Practitioners should keep in mind that both adult- and child-sized cuffs should be available for use with the sphygmomanometer.

In addition to the aforementioned equipment, it is recommended that dental practitioners are trained and proficient in starting an intravenous (IV) line. Necessary equipment includes IV lines, IV catheters of varying gauges, alcohol gauze, and tourniquets. IV fluids of 1000 mL bags with normal saline 0.9%, dextrose 50%, or lactated ringers should be part of the emergency armamentarium.

Box 1
Basic emergency equipment for the dental office

Portable or installed oxygen portals with nasal cannula

Bag-valve-mask device

Nonrebreather mask with reservoir

Automated external defibrillator

Oropharyngeal and nasopharyngeal airways

Stethoscope and sphygmomanometer

Yankauer suction tips

Magill forceps

Stethoscope

Sphygmomanometer with small, medium, and large cuff sizes

Wall clock with second hand

Adapted from Rosenberg M. Preparing for medical emergencies: the essential drugs and equipment for the dental office. J Am Dent Assoc 2010;141(Suppl 1):16S; with permission.

> **Box 2**
> **Emergency preparedness checklist**
>
> - Everyone in the dental office should have specific assigned duties.
> - Contingency plans are in place in case a staff member is absent.
> - Everyone has received appropriate training in the management of medical emergencies.
> - Everyone is trained in basic life support.
> - The dental office should be equipped with emergency equipment and supplies that are appropriate for that practice.
> - Unannounced emergency drills should be conducted every few months.
> - Emergency telephone numbers should be placed near each phone.
> - Oxygen tanks and oxygen delivery systems should be checked regularly.
> - All emergency medications are checked monthly and replaced if expired or to be expired.
> - All emergency supplies are restocked immediately after use.
> - One staff member is assigned to review this checklist regularly.
>
> *Adapted from* Rosenberg M. Preparing for medical emergencies: the essential drugs and equipment for the dental office. J Am Dent Assoc 2010;141(Suppl 1):15S; with permission.

The American Heart Association now requires every health care professional office to be equipped with an automated external defibrillator (AED). It is the responsibility of the general dentist in charge to assure that his or her staff is trained to operate an AED. This training involves taking basic life support courses and having a current certificate.[3]

EMERGENCY MEDICATIONS

Dental practitioners should maintain an emergency kit with key basic drugs for emergencies in the clinic (**Fig. 1**). This article provides a general guideline for the emergency drugs used in a dental office. These drugs can be administered via various routes, such as subcutaneous, intramuscular, sublingual, IV, or intraosseous routes. It is recommended that the dental practitioners have a designated person assigned to regularly inspect the emergency equipment and the emergency kit to assure all oxygen tanks are full and operational and no emergency medications have expired. The following medication list can serve as a guideline for emergency kits for dental practitioners.

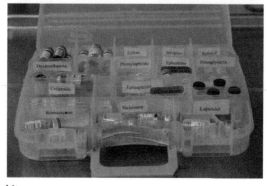

Fig. 1. Emergency kit.

Oxygen

Hypoxemia is a common occurrence in many medical emergencies, highlighting the importance and the need for delivery of supplemental oxygen. Multiple routes are available for delivery of oxygen, and the authors recommend that all offices should have a bag-valve-mask device (Ambu-bag, Ambu, Ballerup, Denmark) and a full-face mask to allow for positive-pressure ventilation (**Fig. 2**).[2,3]

Respiratory Stimulants: Aromatic Ammonia

Syncope is a commonly encountered medical emergency in the dental office. Return to consciousness is typically achieved by placing patients in the Trendelenburg position, administering supplemental oxygen, and using aromatic ammonia. Aromatic ammonia, when cracked or crushed and held 4 to 6 in under the nose, allows the release of a noxious odor that stimulates the respiratory and vasomotor centers of the medulla.[2,3]

Antiplatelets: Aspirin

If patients are experiencing chest pain and there is a suspicion of myocardial infarction or ischemia, aspirin should be given to chew. Rapid and sustained anticoagulative effects are achieved by having patients chew for 30 seconds and then swallow a non–enteric-coated aspirin (325 mg). Caution, however, should be used in administering aspirin to patients with severe bleeding disorders and allergies to aspirin.[2,3]

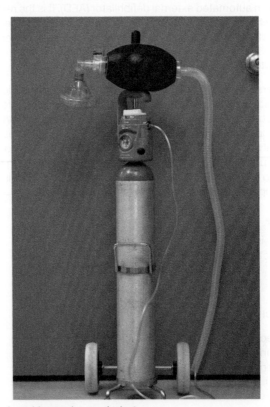

Fig. 2. Oxygen tank and bag-valve-mask device.

β_2-agonists

A bronchodilator, such as albuterol, is used in the treatment of patients with acute wheezing and bronchospasm secondary to asthma. These agents can be used 2 or 3 times every 1 or 2 minutes up to 3 times as needed. Albuterol is available in a metered-dose inhaler and is the most selective of the β_2-agonists, which cause bronchial smooth muscle relaxation. Fewer side effects are reported with albuterol than other bronchodilators.[2,3]

Antihypoglycemic Agents: Glucose

Offices should carry oral hypoglycemic agents to increase blood glucose levels in conscious patients with hypoglycemia. Simple sources, such as fruit juice, cola, or candy, are sufficient for conscious patients; however, oral formulations of glucose should never be administered to unconscious patients because of the risk of aspiration. If patients are unable to swallow and the dentist can obtain IV access, dextrose 50% in water can be administered with IV.[2,3]

Nitroglycerine

Nitroglycerine, a vasodilator, is recommended for the relief of acute chest pain in patients who have a past history of angina or undiagnosed angina with symptoms of myocardial infarction. The most common formulations found in the dental office setting are the 0.4-mg metered aerosol and sublingual tablets. Recommended dose for nitroglycerine tablets is 0.4 mg administered sublingually or in the form of translingual spray every 5 minutes up to 3 doses. The aerosol form does not require special storage and has a longer shelf-life than the tablet form, which requires storage in light-resistant containers and loses potency after 12 weeks. Common side effects of nitroglycerin are headaches, dizziness, and flushing. Nitroglycerine should not be administered to patients taking medication for erectile dysfunction.[2,3]

Epinephrine

Epinephrine, a sympathomimetic drug, acts on α-adrenergic and β-adrenergic receptors. Epinephrine can be administered as auto-injections or preload syringes or ampules: 1:1000 solution subcutaneously, intramuscularly or sublingually; adult dose of 0.3 mg, children 0.15 mg.[3] The primary effects of epinephrine include bronchodilation, vasoconstriction, increased heart rate and contractility, increased cerebral blood flow, and stabilization of mast cells (involved in severe allergic reactions). These effects make epinephrine useful during severe bronchospasm, cardiac arrest, and anaphylaxis.[2,3]

Diphenhydramine

Diphenhydramine is histamine blocker used to reverse the effects of mild or delayed-onset allergic reactions. It is available in oral and parental forms. A dose of 50 mg of diphenhydramine can be administered intramuscularly or 25 to 50 mg orally every 3 to 4 hours.[3]

EMERGENCY MEDICATIONS FOR INTRAVENOUS SEDATION

Dentists and specialists providing IV sedation should also maintain supplemental injectable drugs, including but not limited to analgesics, anticholinergics, anticonvulsants, antihypertensives, corticosteroids, vasopressors, and reversal agents, with the other emergency medications present in the office. The onset of action is faster when drugs are injected via IV. The following medications are typically used when in-office IV sedation is being performed and IV access has already been established. Many of these medications can also be used in an emergency situation involving nonsedated patients.

Anticholinergics

Muscarinic receptors are the target of anticholinergic medications. When activated, these receptors cause parasympathetic effects on specific organs. The 3 primary anticholinergic medications are atropine, glycopyrrolate, and scopolamine. These medications are useful in the management of hypotension. Atropine has the fastest onset time and is used to treat bradycardia in emergency situations. It blocks vagal stimulation to the heart allowing for unopposed sympathetic stimulation. The typical dose to treat bradycardia is 0.5 mg IV. Additional drug can be titrated to effect with a maximum dose of 0.04 mg/kg. Dosing of less than 0.4 mg has been shown to cause bradycardia.[4]

Ephedrine

Aside from parasympathetic suppression, another method of managing hypotension is adrenergic agonism. Ephedrine displays both α_1 and β_1 adrenergic agonism. In turn, the drug causes increased peripheral vascular resistance, positive cardiac chronotropic, and positive cardiac inotropy.[5,6] It is useful in the treatment of moderate to severe hypotension, particularly in situations when patients are bradycardic. Typical dosing is 5-mg bolus every 10 minutes and titrated to desired effect. Onset time can be up to 10 minutes.[6]

Phenylephrine

Phenylephrine is another useful adrenergic agonist used in the management of hypotension. Unlike ephedrine, phenylephrine is a selective α_1 agonist. Usage results in peripheral vasoconstriction causing increased blood pressure. This medication is useful when patients have tachycardia or a normal heart in the presence of hypotension. It has a fast onset and short duration of action of 5 to 10 minutes.[5] A total of 100 μg should be administered every 10 to 15 minutes for the hypotension. Reflex bradycardia typically accompanies administration. The clinician should be mindful of the heart rate when treating hypotension with this medication.

Naloxone

Fentanyl is almost universally used in IV sedations in the dental office. Respiratory depression and oversedation can occur when fentanyl is overdosed. Naloxone is an opioid antagonist that will reverse all of the effects of opioids, including analgesia, respiratory depression, and chest wall rigidity.[7] Dosing is 0.4 mg to 2 mg IV and can be titrated in increments of 0.1 mg to effect.[4] Caution must be exercised, as the duration of action of naloxone is 30 to 45 minutes. If residual opioids are still present, it is possible for their effects to manifest again.

Flumazenil

Along opiates, benzodiazepines are used in most IV sedations, specifically midazolam. Effects of this class of medication include anterograde amnesia, sedation, and anxiolysis. In association with other medications, respiratory and central nervous system can occur requiring reversal agents.[8] Usual dose is 0.1 mg to 0.2 mg incrementally titrated to 1.0 mg.[4] Like naloxone, the effects the benzodiazepine medication can be present after flumazenil has been metabolized. Caution should be exercised when flumazenil is used in patients with epilepsy.

Labetalol

Labetalol is used in the management of hypertension. This medication blocks α_1 and β_1 adrenergic receptors. In turn, it decreases peripheral vascular resistance and sympathetic stimulation to the heart. In larger doses, labetalol can block β_2 adrenergic receptors and lead to increased airway resistance. Dosage recommendations are 20 mg initially followed by an additional 20 mg at 10-minute intervals.[9,10] Precaution must be used in patients with asthma, bradycardia, and congestive heart failure as the agent can exacerbate these conditions.

MEDICATION STORAGE AND MONITORING

The emergency kit, medications, and oxygen should be placed in an area that is readily accessible and familiar to personnel in the event of an emergency.

The following are suggestions to ensure patient safety and effective monitoring of medications:

- Hold frequent (semiannual or quarterly) emergency drills in which every staff member's role is detailed.
- Store all emergency drugs and equipment in an easily accessible area.
- Perform an annual review to check for drug expiration dates and the level of the oxygen tanks.
- Develop cheat sheets for what procedure to follow based on the nature of the emergency.
- Have the telephone numbers of emergency personnel or the local volunteer ambulance service readily available.
- Patient emergencies can occur in the office waiting area, so have airway equipment that is mobile and easily transferable rather than fixed to a room.

SUMMARY

Any dental office can be faced with variety of medical emergencies; therefore, the health care professional and the staff should always be prepared to deal with these emergencies in their office. Preparedness of the dental office staff and their prompt recognition of these emergencies will be the most important factor in dealing with the emergencies in any dental office. Health care professionals should follow the recommendations in this article to maintain a guideline for their staff and office and conduct regular emergency drills to examine the equipment and preparedness of their staff.

REFERENCES

1. Malamed S. Introduction. In: Malamed S, editor. Medical emergencies in the dental office. 7th edition. St Louis (MO): Elsevier Mosby; 2015. p. 1–13.
2. Rosenberg M. Preparing for medical emergencies: the essential drugs and equipment for the dental office. J Am Dent Assoc 2010;141(Suppl 1):14S–9S.
3. Dym H. Preparing the dental office for medical emergencies. Dent Clin North Am 2008;52:605–8.
4. Haas DA. Management of medical emergencies in the dental office. Anesth Prog 2006;53:20–4.
5. Feiner J. Autonomic nervous system. In: Miller RD, Pardo MC, editors. Basics of anesthesia. 6th edition. Philadelphia: Elsevier Saunders; 2011. p. 66–77.

6. Adlesic EC. Cardiovascular anesthetic complications and treatment in oral surgery. Oral Maxillofacial Clin N Am 2013;25:487–506.

7. Garcia P, Whalin MK, Sebel PS. Intravenous anesthetics. In: Hemmings HC, Egan TD, editors. Pharmacology and physiology for anesthesia. Philadelphia: Elsevier Saunders; 2013. p. 137–58.

8. Fukam MC, Ganzberg SI. Pharmacology of outpatient anesthesia medications. In: Miloro M, Ghali GE, Larsen PE, et al, editors. Peterson's principles of oral and maxillofacial surgery. 3rd edition. Shelton (CT): People's Medical Publishing House – USA; 2012. p. 43–62.

9. Jeske AH. L. In: Jeske AH, Flaitz CM, Shlafer M, et al, editors. Mosby's dental drug reference. 11th edition. St Louis (MO): Elsevier Mosby; 2014. p. 718–86.

10. Saef SN, Bennett JD. Basic principles and resuscitation. In: Bennett JD, Rosenberg MB, editors. Medical emergencies in dentistry. Saunders; 2002. p. 3–59.

Oral Sedation in the Dental Office

Francesco R. Sebastiani, DMD[a], Harry Dym, DDS[b],*, Joshua Wolf, DDS[a]

KEYWORDS

• Anxiolysis • Conscious sedation • Clinical technique • Safety • Regulation

KEY POINTS

• There is a strong need and demand for adult and pediatric enteral sedation services in dentistry.
• Knowledge of the potential risks and benefits of oral sedatives is absolutely necessary to allow the clinician to use an effective anesthesia technique safely in the office setting.
• This article highlights the pharmacology of the medications commonly used for oral conscious sedation in dentistry as well as clinical guidelines for administration.
• Patient safety is the paramount consideration. Oral administration to achieve conscious sedation requires state regulation to ensure safety.

Dental anxiety has been shown to be one of the biggest barriers for patients in seeking needed care. An estimated 100 million people in the United States (approximately 30%) are in need of dental care but neglect the dental visit. A survey conducted in the United States found that 18% of adults would visit the dentist more frequently if they were given a drug to make them less nervous.[1] With the strong need to treat fearful and anxious adult patients, effective sedation and pain control have become integral components of dental care.

General dental practitioners have used in-office oral sedation for more than 160 years during routine dental practice. The oral route has remained the safest, most established, and most commonly used route of drug administration. Advantages of the oral route of drug administration in adults versus other routes of drug administration include:

1. Lower incidence of adverse reactions
2. Decreased severity of adverse reactions
3. High degree of patient acceptance and compliance
4. Convenience of administration

[a] Oral and Maxillofacial Surgery, The Brooklyn Hospital Center, 121 Dekalb Avenue, Brooklyn, NY 11201, USA; [b] Oral and Maxillofacial Surgery, Department of Dentistry, The Brooklyn Hospital Center, 121 Dekalb Avenue, Box 187, Brooklyn, NY 11201, USA
* Corresponding author.
E-mail address: hdymdds@yahoo.com

Dent Clin N Am 60 (2016) 295–307
http://dx.doi.org/10.1016/j.cden.2015.11.002
0011-8532/16/$ – see front matter © 2016 Elsevier Inc. All rights reserved.

5. Low cost
6. Additional equipment or personnel not needed

Oral medications are well suited for anxiolysis (minimal sedation) and conscious sedation (moderate sedation) in dentistry. Anxiolysis is a drug-induced state in which patients respond appropriately to verbal commands. Although cognitive function and coordination may be impaired, ventilatory and cardiovascular functions are unaffected.[2] Anxiolysis is the lightest level of sedation (**Fig. 1**).

Oral medication to achieve anxiolysis in adult patients seems to have a wide margin of safety. When the intent is minimal sedation for adults, the appropriate initial dosing of a single enteral drug is no more than the maximum recommended dose (MRD) of a drug that can be prescribed for unmonitored home use.[2] The MRD is the maximum US Food and Drug Administration (FDA)–recommended dose of a drug as printed in FDA-approved labeling for unmonitored home use. Incremental and supplemental dosing both apply to the administration of minimal sedation. Incremental dosing is the administration of multiple doses of a drug until a desired effect is reached, but not to exceed the MRD. During minimal sedation, supplemental dosing is a single additional dose of the initial dose of the initial drug that may be necessary for prolonged procedures. The supplemental dose should not exceed one-half of the initial total dose and should not be administered until the dentist has determined that the clinical half-life of the initial dosing has passed. The total aggregate dose must not exceed 1.5 times the MRD on the day of treatment for minimal sedation.[2] Regulatory agencies in all 50 United States and Canada allow anxiolysis without an additional permit beyond completion of an accredited predoctoral dental training program.

The American Dental Association (ADA) first developed clinical guidelines, including educational requirements, for the use of sedation in dentistry in 1996 and most recently released an update in 2012. In the 2012 ADA clinical guidelines, it is stated that, "For all levels of sedation and anesthesia, dentists, who are currently providing sedation and anesthesia in compliance with their state rules and/or regulations prior to adoption of this document, are not subject to these educational requirements. However, all dentists providing sedation and general anesthesia in their offices or the offices of other dentists should comply with the Clinical Guidelines in this document."[3] The 2012 ADA Clinical Guidelines for the Use of Sedation and General Anesthesia by Dentists state that to administer minimal sedation (anxiolysis) the dentist must have successfully completed:

1. Training to the level of competency in minimal sedation consistent with that prescribed in the ADA Guidelines for Teaching Pain Control and Sedation to Dentists and Dental Students, or a comprehensive training program in moderate sedation that satisfies the requirements described in the Moderate Sedation section of the ADA Guidelines for Teaching Pain Control and Sedation to Dentists and Dental Students at the time training was commenced; or

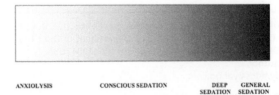

ANXIOLYSIS   CONSCIOUS SEDATION   DEEP   GENERAL
                                                SEDATION   SEDATION

Fig. 1. The spectrum of sedation. (*From* Goodchild JH, Feck AS, Silverman MD. Anxiolysis in general dental practice. Dent Today 2003;22(3):106–11; with permission.)

2. An advanced education program accredited by the ADA Commission on Dental Accreditation that affords comprehensive and appropriate training necessary to administer and manage minimal sedation commensurate with these guidelines; and
3. A current certification in Basic Life Support (BLS) for Healthcare Providers

Administration of minimal sedation by another qualified dentist or independently practicing qualified anesthesia health care provider requires operating dentists and their clinical staff to maintain current certification in Basic Life Support for Healthcare Providers.[2]

Conscious sedation is defined as, "a minimally depressed level of consciousness that retains the patient's ability to independently and continuously maintain an airway and respond appropriately to physical stimulation or verbal command and that is produced by a pharmacological or non-pharmacological method or a combination thereof."[3] All patients pass through anxiolysis before entering conscious sedation. The same drugs that are prescribed for anxiolysis produce oral conscious sedation usually at a dosage greater than 1.5 times the FDA-approved maximum recommended dosage or in combination with other central nervous system (CNS)–altering medications.

According to the 2012 ADA Clinical Guidelines for the Use of Sedation and General Anesthesia by Dentists to administer moderate (conscious) sedation dentists must have successfully completed:

1. A comprehensive training program in moderate sedation that satisfies the requirements described in the Moderate Sedation section of the ADA Guidelines for Teaching Pain Control and Sedation to Dentists and Dental Students at the time training was commenced; or
2. An advanced education program accredited by the ADA Commission on Dental Accreditation that affords comprehensive and appropriate training necessary to administer and manage moderate sedation commensurate with these guidelines; and
3. (i) A current certification in Basic Life Support for Healthcare Providers and (ii) either current certification in advanced cardiac life support (ACLS) or completion of an appropriate dental sedation/anesthesia emergency management course on the same recertification cycle that is required for ACLS

Administration of moderate sedation by another qualified dentist or independently practicing qualified anesthesia health care provider requires the operating dentist and his/her clinical staff to maintain current certification in Basic Life Support for Healthcare Providers.[3]

Per state regulation, oral conscious sedation (moderate sedation) may be safely and effectively administered in the dental office. New York state requirements for a Dental Enteral Conscious Sedation Certificate include 20 clinically oriented experiences in the use of enteral conscious sedation techniques; 18 hours of training, including but not limited to instruction in nitrous oxide and emergency medicine; BLS; and 6 hours of continuing education.[4] In addition, a minimum of 2 individuals must be present in the operatory; such individuals must include the dentist and 1 additional qualified individual. In New York and specified other states, the dentist shall not administer conscious sedation (enteral or parenteral) to more than 1 patient at a time. Six hours of training every 3 years is required for the dentist to renew an oral sedation permit in New York. American dentists can find state-specific regulations at the following link to the chart of state statutory requirements for conscious sedation permits provided by the ADA: http://www.ada.org/~/media/ADA/Advocacy/Files/anesthesia_sedation_permit.ashx.

Benzodiazepines are the preferred drugs for the management of dental fear and preoperative anxiety. Benzodiazepines are anxiolytic, have sedative properties, and produce anterograde amnesia. These drugs are indicated for the management of mild to moderate anxiety. Benzodiazepines act by facilitating the physiologic inhibitory effects of gamma-aminobutyric acid (GABA), the major inhibitory neurotransmitter in the brain.[5] Benzodiazepines have a high therapeutic index (ratio of the toxic dose of a drug to its therapeutic dose), and therefore possess a high margin of safety, which is the primary advantage compared with other classes of sedative-hypnotics, especially the barbiturates, which have a much lower therapeutic index. Benzodiazepines have proved to be fairly innocuous in intentional or accidental overdose when taken without additional drugs.[6]

Benzodiazepines are effective as single agents, thus drug cocktails are not necessary. Benzodiazepines vary by onset time, duration, metabolism, and in degree of sedation. Triazolam, diazepam, lorazepam, and alprazolam are the most effective and commonly administered benzodiazepines for anxiolysis and conscious sedation in dentistry.[6]

Triazolam (Halcion) was first introduced in the 1980s. It is the most prescribed psychoactive drug and the most popular drug prescribed by dentists to alleviate pretreatment patient anxiety in the United States. Triazolam has been described as a nearly ideal anxiolytic for oral sedation in dentistry because of its short half-life of 1.5 to 5.5 hours and absence of active metabolites.[6] A high level of sleep and amnesic effect is produced by triazolam, with little residual drowsiness or hangover effect. Triazolam has about a 45% bioavailability and an onset of action of approximately 1 hour. If administered sublingually, the rate of onset is improved to about 30 minutes and bioavailability is increased. The reported duration of triazolam is an average 1 to 2 hours.[5]

Triazolam is available in 0.125-mg and 0.25-mg tablets. The average dose is 0.25 mg and the FDA MRD is 0.5 mg. As pregnancy category X, triazolam is contraindicated in pregnant patients.[5] Caution should be taken when using it in the elderly or debilitated because excessive sedation is possible. The initial recommended dose in elderly patients is 0.125 mg. Overdose may occur at 4 times the MRD of 0.5 mg, which is 2 mg or 8 tablets (0.25 mg) (**Table 1**).

Table 1 Triazolam (Halcion)	
Dose (mg)	0.25–0.5 Average: 0.25 MRD: 0.5
Onset	1 h 30 min; sublingual
Duration (h)	1–2
Contraindications	Pregnancy
Precautions	Excessive sedation possible in elderly
Availability	Tablets: 0.125, 0.25 mg
Active Metabolites	None
Pregnancy Category	X
Classification	Sedative/hypnotic

Diazepam (Valium) was synthesized in 1959 and marketed in 1963. Diazepam was the leader among prescription drugs by the 1970s, and remained so until recently. After oral administration, diazepam has an onset of about 1 hour, achieving 90% of maximal clinical effect. Peak onset of plasma levels occurs within 2 hours. From the presence of active metabolites and prolonged plasma half-life of 20 to 70 hours, a long-lasting effect may occur with prolonged oral administration.[5] Because of the presence of active metabolites, patients may experience a hangover effect. Diazepam is well tolerated in elderly patients. The recommended dose of diazepam for anxiolytic premedication is 5 to 10 mg 1 hour before treatment. It is available in 2-mg, 5-mg, and 10-mg tablets and 10 mg/5 mL syrup (**Table 2**).

Lorazepam was marketed in 1977 under the trade name Ativan. The drawback to the use of lorazepam is the longer onset time of 1 to 2 hours. Thus, administration may be best suited for patients at home before the dental visit. Lorazepam has a profound amnestic and effective antianxiety affect. Its usage is well tolerated in elderly individuals. Lorazepam is contraindicated in patients with narrow-angle glaucoma and with a known allergy to benzodiazepines. Caution must be taken to not oversedate the patient and in patients with a depressive disorder or psychosis. Reported side effects include sedation (15.9%), dizziness (6.9%), weakness (4.2%), and ataxia (3.4%).[5] For preoperative anxiety control, a dose of 2 to 4 mg may be given or prescribed 1 to 2 hours before the dental appointment (**Table 3**).

Alprazolam (Xanax) is another benzodiazepine in the antianxiety drug class. It is most commonly used for patients with panic-type anxiety. Alprazolam's properties include an onset time of 1 hour and duration of 1 to 2 hours. It is contraindicated in patients with acute narrow-angle glaucoma and benzodiazepine allergy. Caution about intensified sedation is needed if coadministered with cytochrome P (CYP) 3A4 inhibitors.[5] Alprazolam is available in 0.25-mg, 0.5-mg, and 1-mg tablets (**Table 4**).

Oxazepam was synthesized in 1961 and marketed in 1965 under the trade name Serax. Oxazepam is desirable for use in patients with short-term anxiety. It has a rapid onset, short elimination half-life of 5.7 to 10.9 hours, and no active metabolites.[5] Oxazepam is not affected by the CYP system, thus is less prone to undesirable drug interactions. It has a low incidence of drowsiness and is a metabolite of valium. Oxazepam is available in 10-mg, 15-mg, and 30-mg capsules and 15-mg tablets (**Table 5**).

Nonbenzodiazepine anxiolytics-hypnotics are chemically unrelated to other sedative-hypnotics but have a pharmacologic effect similar to benzodiazepines. These drugs are GABA receptor alpha-1 subunit agonists producing sedation and

Table 2 Diazepam (Valium)	
Dose (mg)	2–20
Onset (h)	1
Duration (h)	1–3
Contraindications	Allergy, acute narrow-angle glaucoma
Precautions	Sedation intensified with CYP3A4 and CYP2C19 inhibitors
Availability	Tablets: 2, 5, 10 mg Syrup: 10 mg/5 mL
Active Metabolites	Yes
Pregnancy Category	D
Classification	Antianxiety

Abbreviation: CYP, cytochrome P.

Table 3 Lorazepam (Ativan)	
Dose (mg)	2–4
Onset (h)	1–2
Duration (h)	2–4
Contraindications	Allergy, acute narrow-angle glaucoma
Precautions	Oversedation, depressive disorders, psychosis
Availability	Tablets: 0.5, 1, 2 mg
Active Metabolites	None
Pregnancy Category	D
Classification	Antianxiety Sedative/hypnotic

amnesia. The amnestic effect is not as profound as that produced by benzodiazepines. Nonbenzodiazepine anxiolytics-hypnotics produce less memory and cognitive impairment than benzodiazepines. They are biotransformed by several CYP enzymes in addition to CYP3A4, thus CYP3A4 inhibitors and inducers have a lesser effect.[5] Zolpidem, zaleplon, and ezopiclone are effective nonbenzodiazepine anxiolytics-hypnotics used in dentistry.

Zolpidem (Ambien) is a nonbenzodiazepine sedative-hypnotic approved for use in the United States in 1993. It is a strong sedative with mild anxiolytic, myorelaxant, and anticonvulsant properties. Zolpidem is the drug of choice for pregnant patients.[6] It has been proved to be effective in inducing and maintaining sleep in adults. Zolpidem is rapidly absorbed from the gastrointestinal tract, with an onset of action of approximately 1 hour and peak effect in 1.6 hours.

There is an increased risk of further depressed respiratory drive if zolpidem is used in patients with compromised respiratory function. There has been reported a slightly greater than 3% risk of dizziness, headache, allergy, back pain, drowsiness, lethargy, nausea, dyspepsia, diarrhea, myalgia, arthralgia, and dry mouth with zolpidem use.[5] Dose in adults is 5 to 10 mg by mouth; an initial dose of 5 mg orally is recommended in elderly and debilitated patients because of increased sensitivity (**Table 6**).

Zaleplon (Sonata) is an additional nonbenzodiazepine, imidazopyridine class sedative-hypnotic. Zaleplon is similar to zolpidem both pharmacologically and pharmacokinetically. Zaleplon should be used with a high degree of caution in imidazopyridine class hypersensitivity, impaired hepatic function, and elderly and pregnant

Table 4 Alprazolam (Xanax)	
Dose (mg)	0.25–1
Onset (h)	1
Duration (h)	1–2
Contraindications	Allergy, acute narrow-angle glaucoma
Precautions	Sedation intensified with CYP3A4 inhibitors
Availability	Tablets: 0.25, 0.5, 1 mg
Active Metabolites	None
Pregnancy Category	D
Classification	Antianxiety

Table 5 Oxazepam (Serax)	
Dose (mg)	10–30
Onset (h)	1
Duration (h)	2–4
Contraindications	Allergy
Precautions	Elderly, debilitated patients
Availability	Capsules: 10, 15, 30 mg Tablets: 15 mg
Active Metabolites	None
Pregnancy Category	D
Classification	Antianxiety

patients. Common adverse reactions include drowsiness, amnesia, paresthesias, abnormal vision, dizziness, headache, hangover effect, rebound insomnia, and confusion.[5] Adult dose is 5 to 10 mg by mouth; it is available in 5-mg and 10-mg capsules.

Anxiolysis and enteral conscious sedation both require evaluation of patients, monitoring, documentation, facilities, equipment, and personnel requirements as described in ADA guidelines. The following are the 2012 ADA clinical guidelines for minimal sedation, with additions specifically stated for moderate sedation.

PATIENT EVALUATION

Patients considered for minimal sedation must be suitably evaluated before the start of any sedative procedure. In healthy or medically stable individuals (ASA I, II) this may consist of a review of their current medical history and medication use.

However, patients with significant medical considerations (ASA III, IV) may require consultation with their primary care physician or consulting medical specialist.

PREOPERATIVE PREPARATION

- The patient, parent, guardian, or care giver must be advised regarding the procedure associated with the delivery of any sedative agents and informed consent for the proposed sedation must be obtained.

Table 6 Zolpidem (Ambien)	
Dose (mg)	5–10
Onset (h)	1
Duration (h)	2–3
Contraindications	Allergy
Precautions	Reduce dose in elderly
Availability	Tablets: 5, 10 mg
Active Metabolites	None
Pregnancy Category	B
Classification	Sedative/hypnotic

- Determination of adequate oxygen supply and equipment necessary to deliver oxygen under positive pressure must be completed (Ambu bag, Oxygen).
- Baseline vital signs must be obtained unless the patient's behavior prohibits such determination.
- A focused physical evaluation must be performed as deemed appropriate.
- Preoperative dietary restrictions must be considered based on the sedative technique prescribed.
- Preoperative verbal and written instructions must be given to the patient, parent, escort, guardian, or care giver.

PERSONNEL AND EQUIPMENT REQUIREMENTS

Personnel:

- At least 1 additional person trained in Basic Life Support for Healthcare Providers must be present in addition to the dentist.

Equipment:

- A positive pressure oxygen delivery system suitable for the patient being treated must be immediately available (Ambu bag, Oxygen).
- When inhalation equipment is used, it must have a fail-safe system that is appropriately checked and calibrated. The equipment must also have either (1) a functioning device that prohibits the delivery of less than 30% oxygen or (2) an appropriately calibrated and functioning in-line oxygen analyzer with audible alarm.
- An appropriate scavenging system must be available if gases other than oxygen or air are used.
- For moderate sedation, the equipment necessary to establish intravenous (IV) access must be available.

MONITORING AND DOCUMENTATION
Monitoring for Minimal Sedation

A dentist or, at the dentist's direction, an appropriately trained individual must remain in the operatory during active dental treatment to monitor the patient continuously until the patient meets the criteria for discharge to the recovery area. The appropriately trained individual must be familiar with monitoring techniques and equipment.

Monitoring for Moderate Sedation

A qualified dentist administering moderate sedation must remain in the operatory room to monitor the patient continuously until the patient meets the criteria for recovery. When active treatment concludes and the patient recovers to a minimally sedated level a qualified auxiliary staff may be directed by the dentist to remain with and continue to monitor the patient as explained in the guidelines until the patient is discharged from the facility. The dentist must not leave the facility until the patient meets the criteria for discharge and is discharged from the facility.

Monitoring must include:

- Consciousness:
  Level of consciousness (eg, responsiveness to verbal command) must be continually assessed.
- Oxygenation:
  Color of mucosa, skin, or blood must be evaluated continually.

Oxygen saturation by pulse oximetry may be clinically useful and should be considered for minimal sedation.

For moderate sedation, oxygen saturation must be evaluated by pulse oximetry continuously.

- Ventilation for minimal sedation:

  The dentist and/or appropriately trained individual must observe chest excursions continually.

  The dentist and/or appropriately trained individual must verify respirations continually.

- Ventilation for moderate sedation:

  The dentist must observe chest excursions continually.

  The dentist must monitor ventilation. This monitoring can be accomplished by auscultation of breath sounds, monitoring end-tidal CO_2, or by verbal communication with the patient.

- Circulation:

  Blood pressure and heart rate should be evaluated preoperatively, postoperatively, and intraoperatively as necessary.

Documentation

An appropriate time-oriented anesthetic record must be maintained, including the names of all drugs administered, including local anesthetics, dosages, and monitored physiologic parameters.

RECOVERY AND DISCHARGE

- Oxygen and suction equipment must be immediately available if a separate recovery area is used.
- The qualified dentist or appropriately trained clinical staff must monitor the patient during recovery until the patient is ready for discharge by the dentist.
- The qualified dentist must determine and document that the level of consciousness, oxygenation, ventilation, and circulation are satisfactory before discharge.
- Postoperative verbal and written instructions must be given to the patient, parent, escort, guardian, or care giver.
- If a pharmacologic reversal agent is administered before discharge criteria have been met, the patient must be monitored for a longer period than usual before discharge, because resedation may occur once the effects of the reversal agent have waned.

EMERGENCY MANAGEMENT

- If a patient enters a deeper level of sedation than the dentist is qualified to provide, the dentist must stop the dental procedure until the patient returns to the intended level of sedation.
- The qualified dentist is responsible for the sedative management; adequacy of the facility and staff; diagnosis and treatment of emergencies related to the administration of minimal and moderate sedation; and providing the equipment, drugs, and protocol for patient rescue.[3]

Oral antianxiety drugs are administered by the dentist in a rationale technique. If indicated, the dentist may prescribe a medication for the patient to take the night before the appointment at bedtime. On the day of the appointment, if the patient is deemed responsible, the prescribed drug may be taken by the patient at home, ideally 1 hour before (for most drugs) the appointment time, in which case a responsible adult must escort the patient to the dental office. To ensure proper dosage and time of administration, the dentist may administer the dose in the dental office approximately 1 hour before the start of the dental appointment. After administration, the patient should remain under constant supervision, ideally in the treatment room. After 45 minutes, the dentist should evaluate the comfort level of the patient and the efficacy of the oral drug, and make the clinical decision on when to proceed with treatment.

If the current level of sedation produced by the oral medication is less than desired, the dentist may introduce nitrous oxide-oxygen (N_2O-O_2). N_2O-O_2 may be used in combination with a single enteral drug in minimal sedation. N_2O-O_2 when used in combination with sedative agents may produce minimal, moderate, or deep sedation, or general anesthesia.[2] The flow of N_2O-O_2 must be carefully titrated to the desired level of sedation throughout the procedure. Vital signs are monitored and recorded every 5 minutes on the anesthesia-sedation record. On termination of N_2O-O_2 use, the patient should breathe 100% oxygen for a minimum of 5 minutes and recovery should be assessed. Postoperative vital signs are documented on the anesthesia-sedation record. If deemed ready for discharge, postoperative instructions should be read, and a written copy given, to both the patient and the patient's escort, who must be a responsible adult. Later in the afternoon or evening the dentist or nurse should call the patient to review postoperative instructions and answer any questions.

Adhering to state regulation of enteral administration of sedatives to achieve conscious sedation, dentists may implement multidose enteral sedation. The Dental Organization for Conscious Sedation (DOCS) has developed a multidose enteral sedation protocol and educated more than 5000 dentists over the past several years. Preoperative and postoperative patient instructions are shown in **Box 1**.

The DOCS protocol is initiated with an oral dose of 0.25 mg of triazolam 1 hour before the appointment by the patient at home. The dose is reduced to 0.125 mg in

---

Box 1
Preoperative and postoperative patient instructions

Preoperative

1. Take regular medications unless specified by physician or dentist
2. Do not eat or drink for 8 hours before the dental appointment
3. Patient must be driven to the office by a responsible companion
4. No smoking or drinking alcohol for 8 hours before the dental appointment
5. Sedative medications must be taken according to dentists' instructions

Postoperative

1. Take all regular or prescribed medications as outlined by physician or dentist
2. No alcohol for 12 hours postsurgery
3. No driving for 12 hours postsurgery
4. Do not operate machinery for 12 hours postsurgery
5. Must have a responsible companion drive patient home and observe recovery
6. Phone number where dentist can be reached must be provided

From Goodchild JH, Feck AS, Silverman MD. Anxiolysis in general dental practice. Dent Today 2003;22(3):106–11; with permission.

elderly patients or patients who are overly sensitive to benzodiazepines. The dentist should assess the patient on arrival at the office. Assessment of the need for further medication is conducted with the dentist sitting at eye level with the patient and asking the patient to rate the level of sedation using a 10-point scale (1 = relaxed, 10 = excited).[1] The patient's quality and speed of speech as well as the patient's ability to make eye contact should be evaluated. The patient should be asked by the dentist whether more sedation is desired. No additional medication should be administered when acceptable sedation is achieved. **Table 7** shows the DOCS criteria for administering additional oral medication.

The patient should be monitored for heart rate and oxygen saturation continuously and blood pressure at 5-minute intervals. Reassessment of the patient's level of sedation should be conducted after 30 to 45 minutes, and additional sublingual triazolam administered if necessary. The goal of incremental dosing is to achieve the lowest dose for a comfortable patient experience during treatment. Per the DOCS protocol, before administering the local anesthetic, 20% to 30% nitrous oxide should be introduced.[1] The nitrous oxide should then be discontinued and the dental procedure started. Patient monitoring should occur every 5 minutes, including verbal responsiveness. For treatment longer than 2 hours in which the dentist and patient agree that the level of sedation is inadequate, additional triazolam can be administered to the patient.

In case of an overdose emergency, use of a pharmacologic antagonist (reversal drug) must never be substituted for maintenance of the airway and ventilation with 100% oxygen. Flumazenil (Romazicon) is the benzodiazepine reversal agent, and it competes with benzodiazepines for the receptor site (competitive inhibition). Flumazenil is used to reverse CNS and respiratory depressant effects and decrease recovery time. It possesses a short half-life resulting in short duration. Do not be hesitant to use flumazenil if you are having trouble getting patients to respond to verbal commands or the constant physiologic monitoring indicates a trend toward nonmanageable oxygen desaturation.[7] Readministration may be necessary because resedation can occur, especially if the benzodiazepine has a long-acting effect. It is prudent to keep and monitor the patient for resedation at least an hour after flumazenil reversal use.

Flumazenil administered by IV, sublingual, intramuscular, and rectal routes reversed midazolam-induced respiratory depression in a dog model.[8] The IV route was significantly faster than the other routes (120 seconds vs 262 seconds with the sublingual route). There was no significance between the non-IV routes. Flumazenil 0.2 mg by submucosal injection into the maxillary posterior vestibule produced an incomplete and transient attenuation of moderate/deep sedation produced by incremental sublingual doses of triazolam.[9] It takes approximately a 1 mg submucosal administration of

Table 7 DOCS criteria for administering additional oral medication	
Patient Response	Recommended Sublingual Dose (mg)
Clear response, high scale rating, good eye contact and posture	Triazolam 0.5
Clear, but slightly delayed response and moderate eye contact	Triazolam 0.25
Slightly slurred and delayed response, inconsistent eye contact	Triazolam 0.125
Slurred and delayed response, quiet and confused, no eye contact	No additional medication

Overdose may develop at 4X MRD of Triazolam.

flumazenil to be as effective as a 0.2-mg IV administration. This amount equates to about 5 carpules of local anesthetic (**Table 8**).

Oral sedatives can also have an important role in treating children. For most patients, acceptable behavior can be achieved by traditional nonpharmacologic management techniques; however, for a small percentage of patients, oral sedatives can help behavior management and anxiety issues. The primary use of pharmacologic sedation in children is similar to that in adults. It also includes minimizing the negative psychological response to treatment by reducing anxiety and minimizing the long-term negative psychological feelings about dentistry.

Many drugs are available for children for the relief of anxiety through oral administration and must be given in amounts depending on the patient's weight and the comfort level of the practitioner. Many of these drugs have also been given in combinations. Some of the most common drugs are drugs given to adult patients, including midazolam, tramadol, meperidine, and zolpidem. Hydroxyzine is one of the antihistaminic drugs used for its sedative effect alone before a dental procedure.[10] All of the oral sedatives can also be combined with nitrous oxide for increased effect.

In a Cochrane Review, the range of dosages of oral midazolam cited in the literature was from 0.2 mg/kg to 1 mg/kg, whereas the range of chloral hydrate was from 40 mg/kg to 70 mg/kg.

The study concluded that dosages, mode of administration, and time of administration varied widely in the literature regarding sedation in dental patients and the best evidence, although weak, was for oral midazolam as an effective sedative agent for children undergoing dental treatment in doses between 0.25 mg/kg and 0.75 mg/kg.[11]

When dealing with sedatives and children, practitioners should understand the differences in airway anatomy and physiology between children and adult patients in emergencies (which is beyond the scope of this article) and be prepared with the appropriate-sized equipment.

Dental practitioners using oral sedation in children must be vigilant to the possibility of hypoxemia because of the reduced oxygen reserve in children versus adults. Pulse oximetry must be used and frequent ongoing monitoring performed. Similar to adult patients, children require all the essential items and requirements as noted earlier regarding preoperative evaluation, intraoperative monitoring, and postprocedure discharge evaluation. However, dental offices engaged in the enteral sedation of children must be equipped with the appropriate child-sized resuscitation equipment, including oral and nasal airways, laryngeal mask airways, endotracheal tubes, laryngoscopes, and full-face mask ambu bags.

Table 8 Flumazenil (Romazicon)	
Dose (mg)	0.2 IV (over 15 s) or Sublingual
Additional Dose (mg)	0.2 IV or IM
Maximum Dose	1.0 (5 doses)
Sublingual Location	0.2mg (0.1mg/cc) initial dose 2-3 mm under mucosa just off midline under tongue into venous plexus, 2nd dose in 2-3 min (if needed)
Adverse Effects	Agitation, confusion, dizziness, nausea
Precautions	May precipitate withdrawal syndrome (chronic benzodiazepine use). May produce seizures and cardiac dysrhythmias with tricyclic antidepressants
Availability	0.1 mg/mL IV solution (10 mL maximum)

Abbreviation: IM, intramuscular.

Although many enteral drugs are available for the sedation of children, the senior author (HD) agrees with the many studies found in the literature that oral midazolam at a dose of 0.5 mg/kg is ideal and will provide safe and effective sedation for most children requiring minor procedures, with few to no side effects.[12]

When oral conscious sedation is used within the standards of care, the interests of the public and the dental profession are served through a cost-effective service that can be widely available. Oral sedation will continue to enable dentist to provide dental care to millions of individuals who otherwise would have unmet dental needs.

SUMMARY

Enteral sedation is a useful adjunct for the dental treatment of both anxious adults and pediatric patients. General dentists and specialists must be knowledgeable in the pharmacology of the medications currently available along with their potential risks and benefits.

REFERENCES

1. Dionne RA, Yagiela JA, Coté CJ, et al. Balancing efficacy and safety in the use of oral sedation in dental outpatients. J Am Dent Assoc 2006;137(4):502–13.
2. American Dental Association. Guidelines for teaching pain control and sedation to dentists and dental students. ADA House of Delegates. Chicago: American Dental Association; 2007.
3. American Dental Association. Guidelines for the use of conscious sedation, deep sedation and general anesthesia for dentists. Chicago: American Dental Association; 2012.
4. American Dental Association and Department of State Government Affairs. Conscious sedation permit requirement. Available at: http://www.ada.org/~/media/ADA/Advocacy/Files/anesthesia_sedation_permit.ashx. Accessed September 2, 2009.
5. Malamed SF. Sedation: a guide to patient management [Print]. 5th edition. St Louis (MO): Mosby; 2009.
6. Giovannitti JA, Trapp LD. Adult sedation: oral, rectal, IM, IV. Anesth Prog 1991; 38(4–5):154–71.
7. Goodchild JH, Feck AS, Silverman MD. Anxiolysis in general dental practice. Dent Today 2003;22(3):106–11.
8. Heniff MS, Moore GP, Trout A, et al. Comparison of routes of flumazenil administration to reverse midazolam-induced respiratory depression in a canine model. Acad Emerg Med 1997;4:1115–8.
9. Hosaka K, Jackson D, Pickrell JE, et al. Flumazenil reversal of sublingual triazolam. A randomized controlled clinical trial. JADA 2009;140:559–66.
10. Chowdhury J, Vargas KG. Comparison of chloral hydrate, meperidine, and hydroxyzine to midazolam regimens for oral sedation of pediatric dental patients. Pediatr Dent 2005;27(3):191–7.
11. Lourenço-Matharu L, Ashley PF, Furness S. Sedation of children undergoing dental treatment. Cochrane Database Syst Rev 2012;(3):CD003877.
12. Davies FC, Waters M. Oral midazolam for conscious sedation of children during minor procedures. J ACCID Emerg Med 1998;(4):244–8.

Conscious Intravenous Sedation in Dentistry
A Review of Current Therapy

Janet H. Southerland, DDS, MPH, PhD[a],*, Lawrence R. Brown, DDS[b,c]

KEYWORDS

- IV conscious sedation • Moderate sedation • Sedation guidelines
- Pharmacotherapeutics • Airway assessment • Monitoring • Dental pain
- Dental anxiety

KEY POINTS

- The use of intravenous (IV) conscious sedation in dentistry has gained significant popularity over the last decades to help manage pain and anxiety in the dental office setting.
- The goals of successful sedation should include a physical and psychological evaluation. The plan should be realistic and should (1) determine the patient's physical status and length of the procedure, (2) determine the patient's psychological status, (3) determine whether sedation is indicated, (4) determine whether treatment modifications are needed, (5) determine which drug regimen is appropriate, and (6) determine whether contraindications exist for conscious sedation or the drugs to be used.
- IV conscious sedation is also referred to as parenteral or moderate sedation.
- Moderate sedation is defined as a drug-induced depression of consciousness during which patients respond purposefully to verbal commands, either alone or accompanied by light tactile stimulation. No interventions are required to maintain a patent airway, and spontaneous ventilation is adequate as well as cardiovascular function.
- For practitioners providing moderate sedation in their offices, it is imperative that they are knowledgeable about guidelines and are adequately trained to safely administer moderate sedation. Further, practitioners and their staff providing sedation need requisite training in basic life support, advanced cardiac resuscitation, and/or pediatric advanced cardiac resuscitation techniques.

INTRODUCTION

Thanks to the efforts of Dr Horace Wells and his student, Dr William T.G. Morton, sedation has become an integral part of the practice of dentistry. Dr Wells is credited with the introduction of nitrous oxide, or laughing gas, as a way to control pain and anxiety

[a] Department of Oral and Maxillofacial Surgery, Meharry Medical College School of Dentistry, 1005 Dr. DB Todd Jr. Boulevard, Nashville, TN 37208, USA; [b] Dadeland Oral Surgery Associates, 8950 S.W. 74th Court, Suite 1610, Miami Florida 33156; [c] Baptist Hospital Of Miami, 8900 North Kendall Drive, Miami Florida 33176
* Corresponding author.
E-mail address: jsoutherland@mmc.edu

Dent Clin N Am 60 (2016) 309–346
http://dx.doi.org/10.1016/j.cden.2015.11.009
0011-8532/16/$ – see front matter © 2016 Elsevier Inc. All rights reserved.

during dental procedures. To demonstrate the effectiveness of nitrous oxide during dental surgery, on December 11, 1844, Dr Wells successfully used nitrous oxide on himself while having a colleague extract one of his wisdom teeth. The following year he performed a similar experiment at Harvard using a real patient and the patient cried out during the procedure, resulting in Wells being ridiculed by those attending the lecture.[1] Although Wells was not as successful as he had hoped, a former student 2 years later, Dr William T.G. Morton, successfully administered sulfuric ether to a patient in front of a group of physicians and students at Harvard University to remove a tumor.[2] The combined efforts of these two pioneers introduced the spectrum of sedation that is, used to effectively minimize pain, anxiety, and discomfort during oral surgery procedures. Minimizing or eliminating pain and anxiety for dental care is the primary goal for conscious sedation.

This article provides dental practitioners, surgeons, and recent graduates with a review of the literature and the most up-to-date guidelines and methods used in the practice of intravenous (IV) conscious sedation. Goals of successful sedation should include a physical and psychological evaluation. The plan should be realistic and should:

1. Determine the patient's physical status and the length of the procedure
2. Determine the patient's psychological status
3. Determine whether sedation is indicated
4. Determine whether treatment modifications are needed
5. Determine which drug regimen is appropriate
6. Determine whether contraindications exist for conscious sedation or the drugs to be used

New guidelines for training and monitoring have emerged. The American Society of Anesthesiologists (ASA) currently mandates that "during moderate or deep sedation, the adequacy of ventilation shall be evaluated by continual observation of qualitative clinical signs and monitoring for the presence of exhaled carbon dioxide unless precluded or invalidated by the nature of the patient, procedure, or equipment."[3] This guideline is one of the most recent that is discussed in this article.

MODERATE/CONSCIOUS SEDATION

IV conscious sedation, also referred to as parenteral or moderate sedation, is defined as a drug-induced depression of consciousness during which patients respond purposefully to verbal commands, either alone or accompanied by light tactile stimulation. No interventions are required to maintain a patent airway, and spontaneous ventilation is adequate, as well as cardiovascular function.[4] In addition, patients must retain their protective airway reflexes, and be able to respond to and understand verbal communication. The drugs and techniques used must therefore carry a margin of safety broad enough to make loss of consciousness and airway control unlikely.[5]

Conscious sedation is intended to allow the patient to maintain protective reflexes, but sedation represents a continuum and at times an individual patient may experience a deeper sedation than was anticipated. It is extremely important that the practitioner has the requisite knowledge, training, and skill to manage all levels of sedation adequately, identify unintended outcomes, and manage an emergency until either assistance arrives or the patient is successfully recovered to baseline status.[6] Therefore, understanding the levels of anesthesia is helpful in guiding provider in selection of the proper sedation technique and drugs. The levels of anesthesia are listed in **Table 1**.

Table 1
Definitions for different levels of sedation and anesthesia

Minimal or anxiolysis	A drug-induced state during which patients respond normally to verbal commands. Although cognitive function and physical coordination may be impaired, airway reflexes, ventilation, and cardiovascular functions are unaffected
Moderate or conscious sedation	A drug-induced depression of consciousness during which patients respond purposefully** to verbal commands, either alone or accompanied by light tactile stimulation. No interventions are required to maintain a patent airway, and spontaneous ventilation is adequate. Cardiovascular function is usually maintained
Deep/analgesia	A drug-induced depression of consciousness during which patients cannot be easily aroused but respond purposefully following repeated or painful stimulation. The ability to independently maintain ventilation function may be impaired. Patients may require assistance in maintaining a patent airway, and spontaneous ventilation may be inadequate. Cardiovascular function is usually maintained
General	A drug-induced loss of consciousness during which patients cannot be aroused, even by painful stimulation. The ability to independently maintain ventilatory function is often impaired. Patients often require assistance in maintaining a patent airway, and positive pressure ventilation may be required because of depressed spontaneous ventilation or drug-induced depression of neuromuscular function. Cardiovascular function may be impaired

Adapted from American Society of Anesthesiologists. Continuum of depth of sedation: definition of general anesthesia and levels of sedation/analgesia (approved by the ASA House of Delegates on October 13, 1999, and last amended on October 15, 2014).

The use of IV conscious sedation in dentistry has gained significant popularity over the last decades. Along with this popularity has come continued concerns with deaths associated with administration of conscious sedation as well as the need for adequate training/guidelines for practitioners and their staff to improve patient safety in the dental office setting. Although morbidity and mortality outcomes still exist, the extent of adverse outcomes is not clearly documented in the literature. A study published by the *Journal of the American Dental Association* in 2001 comparing 4 IV sedation drug regimens in 997 patients concluded that the drugs and doses evaluated were of therapeutic benefit in the outpatient setting and there was minimal incidence of potentially serious adverse effects. This study helped to reinforce the safety of the use of conscious sedation using different drug combinations with careful titration and adequate provider training.[7] In contrast, a more recent study published in the *Journal of Public Safety* by Karamnov and colleagues,[8] in a retrospective review conducted on 143,000 moderate sedation cases performed outside the operating room, showed that adverse events were associated with patient characteristics and procedure types. Patient harm was associated with age, body mass index (BMI), comorbidities, female sex, and gastroenterology procedures.[8] Having a good working knowledge of pharmacodynamics, titration of medications to the adequate level of sedation, and strict guidelines, along with use of monitoring devices, has had a significant impact on patient safety and improved outcomes in conscious sedation (discussed later).

Even with improved practice guidelines and knowledge, adverse outcomes have not been eliminated. Guidelines established by the ASA in 2001 and updated in 2002 provided the foundation for provision of sedation in most practice settings.[4,9]

In addition to the ASA, the American Association of Oral and Maxillofacial Surgeons, the American Dental Association (ADA), and the American Academy of Pediatric Dentistry (AAPD) have all developed sedation guidelines relating to administering sedation during dental and surgical procedures as well as the requisite education and skills.[10–12]

The ASA task force for the establishment of guidelines for monitoring patient sedation by nonanesthesiologists in 1996 replaced conscious sedation with the more precise term sedation-analgesia, but the term conscious sedation continues to be widely used, along with the term moderate sedation.[9] The ADA has also produced several documents to guide the use of sedation for dental practitioners that include Guidelines for the Use of Sedation and General Anesthesia by Dentists, Guidelines for Teaching Pain Control and Sedation to Dentists and Dental Students, and ADA Policy Statement: The Use of Sedation and General Anesthesia by Dentists. Similar to the ASA, the ADA provides a definition for moderate sedation in the dental office setting.[4]

Recently underway, the ADA is in the process of updating the guidelines for sedation. The ADA Council on Dental Education and Licensure has called for comments and input from its communities of interest regarding the anesthesia guidelines, with an imposed deadline of June 29, 2015. Some of the proposals recommend changes in definitions, educational requirements, terminology, and clinical and educational guidelines. For example, under section I, Definitions, the definition given earlier is recommended to be modified as follows "moderate sedation - a drug-induced depression of consciousness during which patients respond purposefully to verbal commands, ..." The following definition applies to the administration of moderate or greater sedation: "titration - administration of incremental doses of a drug until a desired effect is reached. Knowledge of each drug's time of onset, peak response and duration of action is essential to avoid over sedation. Although the concept of titration of a drug to effect is critical for patient safety, when the intent is moderate sedation one must know whether the previous dose has taken full effect before administering an additional drug increment." In addition, a recommended change under section III, Education Requirements, states that to administer moderate sedation, the dentist must "demonstrate competency"; this reference to competency has been newly added. The guidelines for conscious sedation administration and training differ only slightly between most governing bodies. Credentialing is required by most dental boards nationally and some internationally and it is imperative that practitioners providing this service are knowledgeable about guidelines and adequately trained to safely administer moderate sedation. Further, practitioners and their staff providing sedation need requisite training in basic life support, advanced cardiac resuscitation (ACLS), and/or pediatric advanced cardiac resuscitation techniques.[13]

PREOPERATIVE ASSESSMENT

Having a satisfactory outcome from IV sedation and anesthesia greatly depends on the experience of the provider, patient selection, and the sedation plan (preoperative and postoperative). Having an approach to sedation that is consistent is valuable for obtaining predictable outcomes during and after the procedure. It is critical that the approach to sedation involves a preoperative evaluation of the patient that includes a comprehensive medical and dental history and physical examination. Additional information should include an anesthesia history and any record of adverse reactions to sedation or anesthesia. The patient should be queried on past medical history involving any major medical problems and systems disease and family history of disease. The patient should also provide a list of past surgeries, food and drug allergies, and a list of current medications. A report of current or past history of drug use or abuse should also be obtained, including history of smoking and alcohol use.

Medical History, Dental and Physical Examination

A complete and comprehensive medical and dental examination, including family history, should be taken and should cover all systems. Any positive responses should be thoroughly discussed and documented. The history is divided into major sections: the chief complaint, history of present illness, past medical history, review of systems, family history, and social history. Past medical history review elaborates on medical dental and psychological illnesses, hospitalizations, experiences with anesthesia, past surgeries, medication, and allergies. Review of systems involves gathering information covering general health, head, ears, eyes, nose, and throat, and signs and symptoms of diseases involving the cardiovascular, respiratory, gastrointestinal, genitourinary, integumentary, nervous, psychiatric, endocrine, hematologic, and musculoskeletal systems, and medical treatments (drugs and other physiologically active compounds). Patients with conditions of most concern should be evaluated more closely when considering IV sedation. The aging of the population and advancements in technology and medical discovery have resulted in an increase in the number of individuals living with chronic diseases. Significant among them are about 610,000 Americans who die from heart disease each year, which represents 1 in every 4 deaths and, depending on the extent of disease, presents significant challenges for delivery of conscious sedation.[14] Conditions of most concern in this group are ischemic disease resulting in angina, myocardial infarction, heart failure, valvular disease, and cardiac arrhythmias. Liver disease, renal function, and respiratory disorders are also important to evaluate as they relate to administering conscious sedation because of concerns of drug administration/overdose and metabolism, as well as airway compromise. In addition to the medical history, any adverse reaction to anesthesia should be discussed with the patient. Most individuals who have had problems with anesthesia are able to recall most details concerning the incident. For individuals who have not been exposed to sedation or anesthesia, family history may be helpful in identifying those at risk for complications with sedation. Information concerning past hospitalizations and surgeries is also helpful in determining the presence of disease and the degree of severity before developing a sedation plan.

Medications

The medications list is also an essential component of the medical history. It provides valuable insight into the patient's medical status and possible drug interactions. The inquiry should include medications that are prescribed as well as those that are over-the-counter, alternative, or homeopathic medications. The need to discontinue medications before IV sedation is generally not indicated. However, there are certain medications that may require the practitioner to alter the sedation plan by supplementation or altering drug dosages. Chronic glucocorticoid use, insulin use, anticoagulant therapy, and the use of sympathomimetics may increase risks if not managed properly before the sedation appointment. Allergies to any medications or foods should be evaluated as well. Reported allergies should be investigated and the clinician should determine whether the reaction is related to delayed hypersensitivity or is an immunoglobulin E–mediated response.[15,16]

If the allergy cannot be clearly delineated, the patient may need to be referred for allergy testing.

Physical Evaluation

The physical examination requires collection of baseline information such as vital signs (blood pressure, pulse and oxygen saturation). Also of importance are patient characteristics such as age, weight, height, and BMI. Once a complete history is obtained for the patient's physical status, the patient is assigned a classification based on the ASA classification system developed in 1941 and revised in 1984. This scale has been used widely and a recent study concluded that the scale has inherent subjectivity, with moderate inter-rater reliability in clinical practice, and also shows validity as a marker of a patient's preoperative health status.[17]

The classification system is still widely used and has been shown to be effective in evaluating physical status for sedation and general anesthesia. The classification system is shown in **Table 2**.

Table 2	
ASA classification system for administration of anesthesia	
ASA I	Healthy (ie, nonsmoking, no or little alcohol use)
ASA II	Mild systemic disease (ie, current smoker, well-controlled disease, pregnancy, obesity)
ASA III	Severe systemic disease (ie, 1 or more moderate to severe diseases)
ASA IV	Severe systemic disease that is a constant threat to life (ie, unstable disease myocardial infarction, cardiovascular accident)
ASA V	Patient who is not expected to survive without surgical intervention
ASA VI	Organ donor, patient is brain dead
	*The addition of E denotes emergency surgery (an emergency is defined as existing when delay in treatment of the patient would lead to a significant increase in the threat to life or body part)

Adapted from American Society of Anesthesiologists (ASA). ASA physical status classification system. Available at: http://www.asahq.org/resources/clinical-information/asa-physical-status-classification-system.

Patients who are classified as ASA I or II may receive a physical that is focused on sedation, whereas those at III and IV or with more unstable disease may require a more comprehensive evaluation. Based on ASA recommendations, review of the medical history and medications should take place for healthy or medically stable individuals (ASA I or II) within 30 days. Also, individuals with significant medical considerations (ASA III or IV) may require consultation with their primary care physicians or consulting medical specialists, including an immediate preoperative review before administration of sedation.[4] Along with the physical examination and classification of physical status, the airway needs to be examined and scored to ensure that a patent airway is available before the sedation appointment. This step is essential to the preoperative evaluation. The Mallampati or Modified Mallampati airway system of classification is most commonly used and is the standard of care (**Fig. 1, Table 3**).[18,19] This indirect approach originally consisted of 3 categories, and a fourth category was added by Samsoon and Young[20] in 1987 creating the modified scale. An additional modification has been proposed that would expand the scale with class 0, which is defined as the ability to see any part of the epiglottis on mouth opening and tongue protrusion.[20] Other systems used to classify airway difficulty include the Cormack-Lehane classification system, the Simplified Airway Risk Index, and thyromental distance.

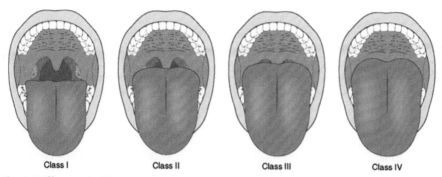

Class I   Class II   Class III   Class IV

Fig. 1. Different classifications. (*From* Sweitzer BJ. Preoperative evaluation and medication. In: Miller RD, Pardo MC. Basics of anesthesia. 6th edition. Philadelphia: Saunders, 2011; with permission.)

Table 3 Mallampati classification system	
Class I	Complete visualization of the uvula, tonsillar pillars, and soft palate
Class II	Partial visibility of the uvula and complete soft palate
Class III	Only the soft palate is visible
Class IV	Only the hard palate is visible

From Mallampati SR. Clinical sign to predict difficult tracheal intubation (hypothesis). Can Anaesth Soc J 1983;30:316–7.

Increases in score generally result in increases in risks in management of the airway. Any airway disorders should be documented, as well as severity. Individuals with obstructive sleep apnea or reactive airway disorders such as severe asthma or chronic obstructive pulmonary that are not stable may not be candidates for moderate sedation in the office setting.

Airway class III or VI classifications can be more difficult to manage under deeper levels, are at greater risk for obstruction, and are more difficult to intubate. Preoperative instructions should cover preoperative fasting to avoid airway compromise and possible aspiration. The guidelines provided by the ASA should be closely adhered to in providing conscious sedation to avoid potential complications (**Table 4**).[21]

PHARMACOTHERAPEUTICS

All doses of medication given should be verified with the manufacturer's package insert. In addition, all drugs to be administered should be properly labeled before the sedation procedure. Doses outlined the article for medications should not be relied on as accurate or definitive. Dosing should be based on the individual patient.

Table 4	
Nil-by-mouth guidelines for adult and pediatric patients	
Clear liquids	2 h
Breast milk	4 h
Infant formula	6 h
Nonhuman milk	6 h
Light meal	6 h
Fatty	8 h

Data from American Society of Anesthesiologists. Practice guidelines for preoperative fasting and the use of pharmacologic agents to reduce the risk of pulmonary aspiration: application to healthy patients undergoing elective procedures. Anesthesiology 2011;114:495.

Inhalation Agents

Nitrous oxide

Nitrous oxide is an inhaled anesthetic. Its potency is defined by the minimum alveolar concentration (MAC) that produces immobility to a skin incision in 50% of the patients who are subjected to such stimuli.[22] The MAC for nitrous oxide at 1 atm in adults is 104%.[23] It has a blood gas partition coefficient of 0.47. When nitrous oxide and a potent inhalation anesthetic are given concurrently, the wash-in of the anesthetic administered in a small concentration may be increased if the uptake of the second anesthetic is large.[24] However, more recent evidence suggests that this second gas effect may not have any clinical significance and, if it does exist, it is minimal.[25,26] Another well-known phenomenon associated with nitrous oxide is the concept of diffusion hypoxia. When the surgical procedure is completed and the inhalation gases are turned off this may be seen during the first 10 minutes of recovery. There is a rapid outflow of nitrous oxide, and this was originally called diffusion anoxia by Fink.[27] The 2 mechanisms thought to be responsible for the hypoxia are a direct displacement of oxygen and a diluting of carbon dioxide in the alveolar compartment by the outflow of nitrous oxide, thereby decreasing the respiratory drive and ventilation.[28]

Many anesthesiologists administer 100% O_2 during the first 5 to 10 minutes of recovery. Nitrous oxide is contraindicated in patients with pneumothorax or in procedures in which air embolus is a risk, as well as in middle ear surgical procedures.[29] Nitrous oxide is 34 times more soluble than nitrogen in blood. As mentioned earlier, it has a blood gas partition coefficient of 0.47 at 37°C. It defuses into cavities that contain nitrogen more rapidly than nitrogen escapes, thereby increasing the volume of the cavity. Nitrous oxide can enter any gas-filled cavity, such as obstructed bowel,[30] pneumothorax and endotracheal tube cuffs,[31] and bubbles in veins,[32] and it should be avoided in laparoscopic surgery. The National Institute of Occupational Safety and Health set a limit of chronic exposure to nitrous oxide as 25 ppm because of its effects on organ systems and teratogenicity.[33] Nitrous oxide has a rapid onset of less than 5 minutes and when it is discontinued the patient's return to baseline status is rapid. When nitrous oxide is combined with midazolam or fentanyl, alone or in combination, a deeper level of sedation can be reached with lower dosages of the benzodiazepine or narcotic required. Fifty percent nitrous with oxygen can produce minimal sedation and 70% nitrous combined with oxygen can produce moderate sedation (**Fig. 2**).

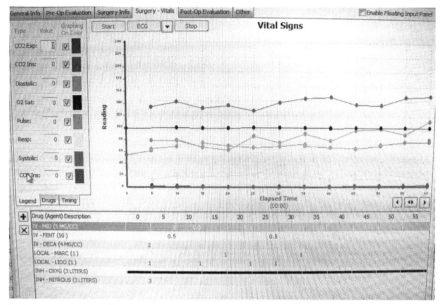

Fig. 2. Current technology allowing real-time recording of patients' vital signs and IV medications/inhalation agents by electronic medical records. The nitrous oxide is only used for the first 5 minutes of the procedure, improving the ease of catheter placement.

Sedative-Hypnotic Agents

Sedative-hypnotics are drugs that depress or slow down the body's functions. Their effects range from calming down anxious people to promoting sleep. At high doses, the drugs can cause unconsciousness and death. Barbiturates and benzodiazepines are the two major categories of sedative-hypnotics.

Benzodiazepines

Diazepam (Valium) and midazolam (Versed) are widely used in dentistry for moderate sedation. Midazolam is the first synthesized water-soluble benzodiazepine.[34] They both are lipid soluble at physiologic pH, with midazolam being more lipid soluble in vivo.[35] Each milliliter of diazepam (5 mg) contains 0.4 mL of propylene glycol, 0.1 mL of alcohol, 0.015 mL of benzyl alcohol, and sodium benzoate/benzoic acid in water for injection (pH 6.2–6.9). Midazolam is formulated with 1 mg or 5 mg/mL of midazolam plus 0.89% sodium chloride and 0.019% disodium edetate, with 1% benzyl alcohol as a preservative. The pH is adjusted to 3 with hydrochloric acid and sodium hydroxide. As noted earlier, midazolam's lipid solubility is pH dependent and, because of its pH- dependent solubility, it is water soluble when formulated in its buffered acidic medium at pH 3.5.[36] Because it is highly lipophilic, it has a fast onset in the central nervous system (CNS) and a large volume of distribution.[37] The benzodiazepines are metabolized in the liver. Midazolam is considered a short-acting benzodiazepine and diazepam a longer lasting benzodiazepine based on their metabolism and clearance. The patient's age and weight, and function of the patient's hepatic and renal systems all affect the duration of action and effect of the drug.

The benzodiazepines all have amnesic, hypnotic, sedative, anxiolytic, anticonvulsant, as well as centrally produced muscle relaxant properties.[36] Midazolam is 3 to 6 times as potent as diazepam.[38] The benzodiazepines occupy the gamma-aminobutyric acid (GABA) receptor. GABA is the major inhibitory neurotransmitter in the brain.[39] By occupying the GABA receptor the benzodiazepines exert their effect and the percentage of receptors occupied determines the effect that is seen. A benzodiazepine receptor with less than 20% occupancy may have the ability to produce a decrease in anxiety; 30% to 50% of occupied receptor sites may show sedation and greater than 60% of occupied sites produce unconsciousness.[40] Midazolam binds to the $GABA_A$ receptor and then there is a chloride ion influx and hyperpolarization and the cell becomes resistant to neuronal excitation.[41] Benzodiazepines decrease cerebral blood flow and increase the seizure threshold of local anesthetics in mice exposed to lethal doses of anesthetics.[42]

Benzodiazepines decrease respiratory rate and, when combined with opioids, there is a greater effect on respiratory depression. Midazolam can cause a minimal lowering of arterial blood pressure. The combination of nitrous oxide and midazolam has minimal hemodynamic effects compared with the combination of opioids and benzodiazepines, which can have a significant effect by lowering blood pressure.[43] Patients presenting to the dental office may be nervous or anxious about the visit or procedure, especially if it involves a surgical procedure or any procedure in which injections are required. Aside from inhalation with nitrous oxide, midazolam could be considered preoperatively in the oral form for pediatric patients or intravenously depending on the patient's willingness to accept an IV line to decrease anxiety and produce amnesia. By implementing nitrous oxide into the sedation technique, clinicians can achieve a cutaneous feeling of numbness of the extremities, which provides a more pleasant experience when placing the catheter for the IV line. A new IV fluid bag appropriate for the patient (for injection only) is chosen and always attached to a sterile disposable tubing line that runs from the fluid bag to the already placed disposable angiocatheter. All tubing, catheters, and syringes are disposed of after the procedure. (Note: All doses of medication should be verified with the manufactured package insert. The doses noted in this section for medication should NOT be relied upon as accurate nor definitive). Midazolam intravenously has a rapid onset because of its lipid solubility, and its peak effect is in about 2 to 4 minutes. The adult dose is 0.5 mg to 1.0 mg IV administered over 2 minutes and titrated until the desired level of sedation is obtained. The pediatric dose range is 0.025 mg/kg IV to 0.5 mg/kg IV with an onset of about 1 to 3 minutes and duration of action of 45 to 60 minutes intravenously.[44] Using midazolam in children may produce hyperexcitability and further anxiousness to the point of combativeness.[45] The level of consciousness may not correlate with the amnesia effect of the benzodiazepines. Patients may be awake or seem alert during the procedure but have no recall of it when questioned postoperatively.[46] Midazolam is contraindicated in patients with acute narrow-angle glaucoma or a hypersensitivity to the drug. Benzodiazepines can cause respiratory depression and upper airway obstruction.[47–49] In children, respiratory depression may be significant, especially in patients with enlarged tonsils. The combination of opioid and benzodiazepines in children has, as expected, an additive effect so the total effect is greater than the effect of each individual drug.[50,51] Midazolam produces anterograde amnesia. Children who had dental extractions with midazolam better tolerated additional dental treatment than those treated without midazolam.[52]

Barbiturates
Barbiturates have the basic structure of barbituric acid.[53] These drugs act as CNS depressants, and can therefore produce a wide spectrum of effects, from mild sedation to total anesthesia. Barbiturates are a family of compounds that have sedative and hypnotic activities and act as nonselective CNS depressants.[54] The GABA receptor is one of barbiturates' main sites of action, and therefore it is thought to play a pivotal role in the development of tolerance to and dependence on barbiturates.[55] The most common use for barbiturates currently is as anesthesia for surgery. Current indications for the

barbiturates include short-term treatment of insomnia and as a preanesthetic agent. Amobarbital (Amytal) and butabarbital (Soneryl, Butisol) are currently available short-acting barbiturates for parenteral administration, being used largely as preanesthetic agents.[56] Other short-acting agents in use include secobarbital, which is available as a 100-mg capsule generically and under the brand name Seconal; it is also classified as a schedule II substance because there is the potential for physical and psychological dependence and abuse.[57] Very-short-acting drugs in use include pentobarbital (Nembutal), methohexital (Brevital), and thiopental (Pentothal).[58-60] Further medium-acting agents, such as butalbital (Fiorinal, Fioricet), Talbutal (Lotusate) and long-acting mephobarbital (Mebaral) and methylphenobarbital (Prominal), are available.[61,62]

Barbiturates induce several hepatic cytochrome P (CYP) enzymes (most notably CYP2C9, CYP2C19, and CYP3A4), leading to exaggerated effects from many pro-drugs and decreased effects from drugs that are metabolized by these enzymes to inactive metabolites. This property can result in fatal overdoses from drugs such as codeine, tramadol, and carisoprodol, which become considerably more potent after being metabolized by CYP enzymes.[63] Although all known members of the class possess relevant enzyme induction capabilities, the degree of inhibition overall, as well as the impact on each specific enzyme, span a broad range, with secobarbital being the most potent enzyme inducer and butalbital and talbutal being among the weakest enzyme inducers in the class.

In addition to their sedative-hypnotic properties, this class also has anxiolytic and anti-convulsant properties. Barbiturates also have analgesic effects; however, these effects are weak, preventing barbiturates from being used in surgery in the absence of other analgesics. They have addiction potential, both physical and psychological. Barbiturates have now largely been replaced by benzodiazepines in routine medical use, mainly because benzodiazepines are significantly less dangerous in overdose because there is no specific reversal agent for barbiturate overdose.[64,65] The longest-acting barbiturates have half-lives of a day or more, and subsequently result in bioaccumulation of the drug in the system. The therapeutic use of long-acting barbiturates wears off significantly faster than the drug can be eliminated, allowing the drug to reach toxic concentrations in the blood following repeated administration (even when taken at the therapeutic/prescribed dose) despite the user feeling little or no effect from the plasma-bound concentrations of the drug.[66] Individuals who consume alcohol or who are given sedatives after the drug effects have worn off, but before it has cleared the system, could experience an exaggerated effect from the sedatives, which can be incapacitating or even fatal.

There are special risks to consider for older adults, women who are pregnant, and babies. When a person ages, the body becomes less able to rid itself of barbiturates. As a result, people more than 65 years of age are at higher risk of experiencing the harmful effects of barbiturates, including drug dependence and accidental overdose.[67] A rare adverse reaction to barbiturates is Stevens-Johnson syndrome, which primarily affects the mucous membranes.[68,69]

Barbiturates in overdose with other CNS depressants (eg, alcohol, opiates, benzodiazepines) are even more dangerous because of additive CNS and respiratory depressant effects.[70] In the case of benzodiazepines, not only do they have additive effects but barbiturates also increase the affinity of the benzodiazepine binding site, leading to exaggerated benzodiazepine effects.[71,72] Frequent side effects include drowsiness, sedation, hypotension, nausea, headache, and skin rash.

Propofol (Diprivan)
Although this article is about moderate sedation, propofol should also be mentioned. Propofol use often causes patients to be in a state of deep sedation or general

anesthesia, with the inability of the patient to maintain an airway continuously and independently. Therefore propofol may be considered an agent that often produces a level of deep sedation/general anesthesia and therefore should not be used in a facility where only moderate sedation is approved. Regardless, all facilities providing sedation, whether moderate or deep, should be prepared to manage the complications that may arise, including, but not limited to, airway compromise and apnea. Propofol is a sedative-hypnotic that is used for the induction and maintenance of anesthesia.[73] Diprivan is composed of 1% propofol, 10% soybean oil, 1.25% egg yolk phosphatide, 2.25% glycerol, ethylenediaminetetraacetic acid, and sodium hydroxide to maintain a pH of 7.0 to 8.5.[33] It is highly lipophilic with a rapid distribution to vessel-enhanced organs and therefore has a rapid induction. It has rapid redistribution and hepatic and extrahepatic clearance, which is why it has a short duration of action and requires frequent repeated doses or a continuous infusion to maintain the desired level of anesthesia.[74–76] Propofol is a sedative-hypnotic and its effects on the CNS is thought to be the result of increasing the GABA-induced chloride current through binding to the beta subunit of the $GABA_A$ receptor.[36]

Propofol inhibits acetylcholine release by its action on $GABA_A$ receptors in the hippocampus and prefrontal cortex.[77] This acetylcholine release inhibition is thought to be responsible for the sedative effect of propofol.[78] Propofol also has an inhibitory effect on the N-methyl-D-aspartate (NMDA) receptor via the sodium channel, which may also contribute to the action of the drug on the CNS.[79] Propofol has antiemetic properties and produces a sense of well-being.[80] Propofol decreases intraocular pressure,[81,82] as well as intracranial pressure. Propofol can cause a decrease in respiratory rate and apnea. Propofol causes bronchodilation in patients with chronic obstructive pulmonary disease.[83] There is a decrease in arterial blood pressure seen with propofol. It has both a depressant and vasodilation effect on the heart that may be dose and plasma concentration related.[84]

Propofol used for sedation is best administered by an infusion pump but incremental dosing also can be done. An infusion rate for sedation in which local anesthesia is used in healthy adults is 30 to 60 µg/kg/min.[85,86] In pediatric patients the dosage required can range from a bolus of 1 to 2 mg/kg with an infusion rate of 50 to 250 µg/kg/min.[44,87] With propofol there may be pain on injection, hypotension, and apnea on induction. The use of an opioid along with propofol increases the incidence of apnea,[88,89] as well as decreasing the arterial blood pressure.[90] In pediatric patients the arterial blood pressure was decreased more, and the total dosage was greater, when an infusion was used compared with intermittent boluses.[91] In pediatric patients, IV lidocaine should be considered to relieve the pain associated with injection. Bradycardia can be seen in both adults and children with propofol.[92] Propofol has a negative effect on airway patency and respiration in children.[33] The airway narrows in children during infusion but remains patent.[93] All open vials of propofol must be discarded within 6 hours because of the potential growth of Escherichia coli, Staphylococcus aureus, Pseudomonas aeruginosa, and Candida albicans.[94–96] Egg allergy in adults and children is not considered a contraindication to propofol use; however, it is recommended to avoid propofol in children with documented anaphylaxis to eggs.[97]

Narcotics Analgesics

Opioids
Morphine is the prototype opioid for all other opioids. Previously, it was an integral part of the sedation regimen for prolonged procedures, but morphine has no application in modern IV sedation procedures. Its main usefulness is in acute pain management. The onset of morphine is slow: 5 to 10 minutes following IV administration and up to

20 minutes following intramuscular injection. It produces analgesia, euphoria, and sedation lasting from 2 to 4 hours. Its use is limited by side effects such as histamine release, postural hypotension, and nausea and vomiting.[98]

Meperidine (Demerol) is the prototype of the phenylpiperidine series of opioids, which includes fentanyl, sufentanil, alfentanil, and remifentanil. Meperidine is an opioid narcotic that binds to opioid receptors in the CNS. The dose for adults is generally 25 to 50 mg in incremental doses to a maximum dose of 150 mg; for elderly patients (65 years and older) the dose is 25 mg in incremental doses to a maximum dose of 75 mg. The elderly are more susceptible to CNS depression.[99] In addition, they are more susceptible to seizures from accumulation of normeperidine, a metabolite of meperidine, as a result of reduced renal function. For years meperidine was the mainstay of IV sedation regimens for procedures of all durations. It has a more rapid onset than morphine, within 3 to 5 minutes following IV administration, making it easier to titrate than morphine. The peak effect is 1 hour, and duration of action is 2 to 4 hours.[100] Meperidine is 10 times less potent than morphine, producing sedation and analgesia lasting 45 to 90 minutes.[101] Meperidine was first investigated as an atropinelike agent and is unique among opioids in that it may produce tachycardia and drying of secretions.[102] It also releases histamine, and may produce orthostatic hypotension with rapid position change. Severe asthma is a relative contraindication. Other side effects include dysphoria, especially in the absence of pain, and nausea and vomiting. Meperidine is associated with increased neuronal activity that may result in CNS excitation.[103] Its metabolite, normeperidine, is twice as potent as meperidine in producing CNS excitation and convulsions. Meperidine is contraindicated in patients taking monoamine oxidase inhibitors because concentrations of normeperidine are increased with these drugs.[104] Although meperidine is still used on a limited basis for dental sedation, its main use is currently in the management of postanesthetic shivering. Opioids in general reduce thermoregulation thresholds similarly to potent inhalational agents.

Fentanyl, sufentanil, alfentanil, and remifentanil are synthesized opioid compounds that are phenylpiperidine derivatives.[104] The brain and spinal cord contains the mu receptors, which are responsible for modulating the effects of opioids.[105] Opioids produce analgesia, decrease respiratory drive, and increase sedation at the mu receptor. Neuronal excitation is decreased by the action of the opioids on the receptors, which depends on the suppression of the Ca^{2+} channel and activation of the K^+ channel.[104]

Opioids decrease cerebral blood flow with nitrous oxide. Giovannitti[106] in 2013 provided a table comparing common drugs in this class in terms of potency, peak effect, duration, and half-life (**Table 5**).[107] There are reports of no significant effect on intracranial pressure in patients with head trauma and opioids have been used safely in such patients.[106] Other reports have shown a slight increase in intracranial pressure

Table 5 Comparative effects of commonly used opioids in oral surgery						
	Meperidine	Morphine	Fentanyl	Sufentanil	Alfentanil	Remifentanil
Comparative potency	0.1	1	75–125	500–1000	10–25	250
Peak Effect (min)	5–7	20–30	3–5	3–5	1.5–2	1.5–2
Duration (h)	2–3	3–4	0.5–1	0.5–1	0.2–0.3	0.1–0.2
Half-life (h)	3–4	2–4	1.5–6	2.5–3	1–2	0.15–0.3

From Giovannitti JA Jr. Pharmacology of intravenous sedative/anesthetic medications used in oral surgery. Oral Maxillofac Surg Clin North Am 2013;25(3):439–51; with permission.

in head injured patients with morphine and fentanyl. The increase in intracranial pressure is thought to be multifactorial.[108] Muscle tone and muscle rigidity can be increased with opioids. The rigidity can lead to severe respiratory problems. In an awake patient this may be shown by hoarseness. It also can be shown just as, or immediately after, a patient losses consciousness. The muscle rigidity is not caused by a direct action on the muscle fiber, but is thought to be CNS regulated; especially the nucleus pontes raphae.[109] The closure of vocal cords is thought to be the reason for difficulty in the ventilation of patients after opioid administration.[104]

Pretreatment with midazolam has been shown to decrease episodes of muscle rigidity as well as treat the rigidity episode. The office should have a neuromuscular blocker available in case of an episode of severe rigidity. Rigidity can occur hours after the last dose of opioid has been administered.[107] Opioids decrease the respiratory drive to increases in CO_2. The mu receptor–stimulating opioids cause a direct depression of the respiratory center in the brainstem.[110] Elderly patients are more sensitive to the opioid-induced respiratory depression and analgesic effect of the opioids.[111] Opioids are associated with an increased incidence of postoperative nausea and vomiting and an antiemetic such as ondansetron (serotonin antagonist) should be considered.[112] Fentanyl is highly lipophilic and therefore widely distributed to body tissues. The lungs show a first pass effect and take up to 75% of the IV fentanyl, which is rapidly released.[113] Fentanyl is metabolized in the liver by N-dealkylation and hydroxylation and the primary metabolite, norfentanyl, can be found in the urine for up to 48 hours after IV fentanyl.[104] A dose of 100 μg (0.1 mg) (2 mL) is equal to 10 mg of morphine in its analgesic effect. The onset of action is immediate and the duration of action is 30 to 60 minutes after a 2-mL dose. IV anesthesia with fentanyl injections should be initially titrated. Low-dose fentanyl 1 to 3 μg/kg IV can produce analgesia for minor painful surgical procedures. Maintenance can be achieved using nitrous oxide 50% to 60% with or without a benzodiazepine. Boluses of 25 to 50 μg every 15 to 30 minutes can be used, or an infusion pump may be used.

Fentanyl is 100 times more potent than morphine and is a pure opioid; it produces no amnesia. It has a rapid onset of less than 1 minute and a peak effect in about 2 to 3 minutes, with a duration of action of about 20 to 40 minutes. In pediatrics the IV dose is 0.5 to 1.0 μg/kg, which is titrated every 5 minutes to the desired effect, not to exceed 5 μg/kg.[114] Similar to adults, there is chest wall rigidity and vocal cord closure that may be associated with its use or rapid administration usually in high doses.[115] Chest wall rigidity is usually not seen with low doses of fentanyl. Patients should be observed in the recovery, because the effects on respiratory depression can be longer than the analgesic effect of fentanyl. Remifentanil is a rapid-acting opioid. It has a rapid onset and short duration of action. A high incidence of apnea and chest wall rigidity is associated with it, and its use by nonanesthesiologists is not recommended in pediatrics.[116,117]

Dissociative Agents

This classification includes agents that cause interruption of cerebral association pathways between the limbic system and cortical system. It produces a catalepsylike state, in which the individual feels dissociated from the environment, and it also induces marked analgesia.[118]

Phencyclidines (ketamine)

Ketamine produces amnesia and analgesia. It exerts its dissociative effect on the limbic/thalamic system. Ketamine is an antagonist of the NMDA receptors and an agonist of the opioid receptors.[118] Ketamine can cause increased heart rate, cardiac output, and blood pressure. Ketamine causes bronchial smooth muscle relaxation. It improves pulmonary status in patients with reactive airway disease and bronchospasm.[119] Ketamine also produces an associated increased salivation that can cause upper airway obstruction leading to a laryngospasm. It is not recommended for use in patients with coronary artery disease. Ketamine usually allows spontaneous respirations.[120] It does have associated psychological effects. Ketamine has 2 isomers: S-(+) and R-(−). The S-(+) is the more potent isomer with fewer side effects.[36] Ketamine is metabolized by the liver and its metabolite norketamine has about 30% less activity than ketamine.[121] Ketamine produces an anesthetized state called dissociative anesthesia; patients are in a cataleptic state in which the eyes are open but they do not respond to pain.[115] Because of its high lipid solubility, it crosses the blood-brain barrier rapidly and has a rapid onset of 30 seconds. Patients usually show pupil dilatation, nystagmus, and increased salivation. In pediatric patients the starting doses[122] are 1 to 2 mg/kg intramuscularly and 0.25 to 1.0 mg/kg intravenously, and 4 to 6 mg/kg orally.[123–125] Onset after IV administration is about 1 minute, with a duration of action of 10 to 15 minutes. After intramuscular injection, the onset is about 5 minutes and duration of action is 30 to 120 minutes.[115]

The combination of ketamine with a benzodiazepine prolongs the effect of ketamine.[126] There is no known antagonist of ketamine. Ketamine increases cerebral blood flow and intracranial pressure. Patients with increased intracranial pressure, such as with head trauma, should not be administered ketamine because it can further increase intracranial pressure and cause apnea.[127] It is also contraindicated in patients with open eye injury, psychiatric disorders, as well as ischemic heart disease.[128] Ketamine is also associated with nonpurposeful extremity movements. One of its negative aspects is the emergence phenomena seen with its use. There are illusions, fear, hyperexcitability,[129] and what is described as an out-of-body experience.[130] The incidence of the emergence phenomena is lower in children than in adults and is multifactorial. Midazolam and other benzodiazepines have been shown to decrease the incidence of the emergence phenomena.[131]

As noted earlier, ketamine has not been shown to have a major effect on respiratory depression unless used in high doses.[132] It is an excellent drug for patients with airway disease and bronchospasm because of its smooth muscle relaxation. It has been used to treat patients with resistant status asthmaticus.[133] Although it is an excellent drug for asthmatic patients, it is associated with increased salivation that can lead to laryngospasm and silent aspiration.[134] Ketamine is often used for pediatric sedation in the outpatient setting for dental treatment[126] and is reported to have fewer emergent effects in children than in adults.[135] Ketamine is usually combined with an antisialogogue such as glycopyrrolate, 0.01 mg/kg, or atropine, 0.02 mg/kg, to decrease secretions that may lead to laryngospasm.[136]

Etomidate (Amidate)

Etomidate is often used as part of a rapid sequence induction and a modulator at the GABA receptors. GABA is a chemical messenger that inhibits the activity of brain cells. Boosting GABA levels both calms the brain and increases dopamine levels in the nucleus accumbens.[137–139] It has a half-life of 75 minutes, is highly protein bound in blood plasma, and is metabolized by hepatic and plasma esterases to inactive products. Excretion is 85% in urine and 15% in the bile. It is used as an anesthetic agent because it has a rapid onset of action and a safe cardiovascular risk profile, and therefore is less likely to cause a more significant reduction in blood pressure than other induction agents.[140,141] Other useful qualities of etomidate are that dosing is easy, suppression of ventilation is minimal, histamine liberation is inhibited, and it can be used safely in patients with myocardial and cerebral ischemia.[138]

Major adverse outcomes involve corticosteroid synthesis suppression in the adrenal cortex by inhibiting 11-beta-hydroxylase, an enzyme that is important in adrenal steroid production (it leads to primary adrenal suppression).[142,143] Komatsu and colleagues[143] in 2013 conducted a retrospective study of almost 32,000 patients and found that etomidate, when used for the induction of anesthesia, was associated with a 2.5-fold increase in the risk of dying compared with those given propofol. Patients given etomidate also had significantly greater odds of having cardiovascular morbidity and significantly longer hospital stay. These results, especially given the large size of study, strongly suggest that, at the least, clinicians should use etomidate judiciously.[144] In addition, the use of etomidate with opioids and/or benzodiazepines may potentiate etomidate-related adrenal insufficiency.[145]

Reversal Agents and Fluids

Flumazenil

Flumazenil (Romazicon) is a competitive antagonist at the $GABA_A$ receptor and can reverse the effects of benzodiazepines. With the rapid clearance of flumazenil the possibility of resedation exists. When flumazenil is used to reverse the action of midazolam the possibility of resedation is less than when it is used to reverse other benzodiazepines because of midazolam's rapid clearance compared with other benzodiazepines.[145] Flumazenil reverses the respiratory depression, amnesia, and sedative effect of the benzodiazepine.[40] Its action is rapid, with a peak effect occurring at 1 to 3 minutes.[40] The dosage if benzodiazepine overdose is suspected is 0.1 to 0.2 mg IV to a total of 3 mg in incremental doses every 1 to 2 minutes.[36]

In adults, a dose of 17 μg/kg has been shown to antagonize the effects of benzodiazepines, and in children a dose of 24 μg/kg has shown to have the same effect.[146] After reversal or antagonism with flumazenil patients should be observed in the recovery room because of the possibility of resedation. Seizures have been reported when larger doses of flumazenil are used.[147]

Naloxone

Naloxone (Narcan) is an opioid antagonist that can reverse the respiratory depression, urinary retention, rigidity, and nausea and vomiting associated with opioids. Its use is associated with an increased heart rate, increased blood pressure, and cases of pulmonary edema.[148,149] Dosages range from 0.4 to 0.8 mg in adults. It has a rapid onset of action of about 1 to 2 minutes and in doses of 0.5 to 1.0 μg/kg every 2 to 3 minutes, restores spontaneous respiration.[150]

Because of the short half-life of naloxone (30–60 minutes) renarcotization can be seen.[104] Note that, by titration, the respiratory depression of the opioids can be reversed with little effect on the analgesia. For treating muscle rigidity associated with the opioids, both naloxone and succinylcholine may be used, with the disadvantage of naloxone reversing the analgesia opioid effect. For pediatric patients less than the age of 5 years a dose of 100 μg/kg is recommended, and for children more than 5 years old (weighing >20 kg) a dose of 2 mg of naloxone is recommended by the American Academy of Pediatrics.[151]

Intravenous Fluids

For the purposes of office-based IV anesthesia, general practitioners use IV fluids mainly to dilute the administered anesthetic medications given to the patient. Crystalloids are used in the office setting to provide water and electrolytes as well as to expand intravascular fluid.[152] The fluid deficit for an adult who has been fasting for 8 hours can be estimated to be 2 mL/kg for each hour before surgery. Therefore a

70-kg patient who has been nil by mouth for 8 hours has a deficit of 1120 mL. Most office dental procedures last 1 to 2 hours, and within the first hour of the procedure one-half of the deficit is replaced (560 mL), and within the second hour of the procedure one-half of the initial amount given over the first hour (280 mL) is replaced. The 4-2-1 rule for pediatric patients is often used to calculate the daily maintenance fluid requirements of 4 mL/kg/h for the first 10 kg of weight, 2 mL/kg/h for the second 10 kg of weight, and 1 mL/kg/h for each additional kilogram.[153] Intraoperatively for pediatric patients 20 to 40 mL/kg of lactated Ringer solution may be given to replace the fluid deficit.[153]

Crystalloids when used alone without colloids for replacement of blood volume are at a 3:1 ratio, which is 3 mL of crystalloid for every 1 mL of blood loss. Most office-based dental procedures do not require colloids for replacement therapy. Presently in the United States IV fluids are on an allocation and extremely difficult to obtain. When they are used for office-based dental anesthesia a minimum of a 1-L bag is required.

Normal saline (0.9% weight/volume) intravenous infusion blood pressure

Each 100 mL of 0.9% NaCl contains sodium chloride United States Pharmacopeia (USP) 0.9 g; water for injection. The concentration of electrolytes is sodium 154 mEq/L and chloride 154 mEq/L. It has an osmolarity of 308 mOsm/L and a pH of about 5.5. Sodium chloride for injection is sterile, isotonic, nonpyrogenic, and has no antimicrobial or bacteriostatic agents. The infusion provides fluids and electrolytes. Sodium is the major extracellular cation, whereas chloride is the major extracellular anion. Normal saline IV fluid is used for extracellular fluid replacement. Relative contraindications include patients with renal failure, congestive heart failure, and pulmonary edema. It is recommended to check the IV bag for precipitate if additional medications are added, such as antibiotic or steroids.

Dextrose 0.5% and 0.9% sodium chloride injection United States pharmacopeia

The management and sedation of diabetic patients are beyond the scope of this article; however, a fluid containing dextrose should be considered in such patients. Each 100 mL contains hydrous dextrose 5 g; sodium chloride 0.9 g; water for injection USP. It has a pH of approximately 4.4 and an osmolarity of 560 mOsm/L. It is a hypertonic solution and contains 154 mEq/L of sodium and 154 mEq/L of chloride. The dextrose provides a source of calories, and functions as free water because it is rapidly metabolized.[152] Dextrose-containing solutions must be used with caution in patients with diabetes mellitus and clinicians must consider the patient's potassium status because hypokalemia is a risk. Dextrose-containing solutions should also be considered for patients with a history of fainting associated with long periods of fasting.

MONITORING
Arterial Blood Pressure

The standard for monitoring arterial blood pressure is a minimum of every 5 minutes for patients who are receiving anesthesia.[154] For the purposes of in-office dental procedures in which moderate sedation is used, noninvasive blood pressure monitoring is accomplished using a cuff device. Offices providing moderate sedation should be equipped with a monitor that is automated to provide noninvasive blood pressure monitoring at set intervals, oxygen saturation (pulse oximetry), carbon dioxide monitoring with respiration (capnography), and electrocardiogram readings (minimum 3-lead electrocardiogram [ECG]).

Noninvasive blood pressure units provide automated readings of the systolic, diastolic, and mean arterial blood pressure at set times without operator assistance. The pressure at which the peak amplitudes of arterial pulsations are detected corresponds with the mean arterial pressure.[155,156] The systolic and diastolic pressures are determined by formulas that evaluate the rate of change of the pressure pulsations.[157] Systolic blood pressure is the pressure at which pulsations are increasing and are at 25% to 50% of maximum, and diastolic is when the pulse amplitude has decreased from the peak value by 80%.[158] In summary, noninvasive blood pressure is based on oscillometry, which in 1931 was introduced by von Recklinghausen.[159] The systolic blood pressure is measured at the beginning of an increase in cuff pressure oscillations, and the mean arterial pressure correlates with the point of maximal oscillations. The diastolic blood pressure is measured at the point the oscillations start to diminish (weaken).[157] The complications associated with an automated noninvasive blood pressure monitor include stasis, pain, nerve compression,[160] and thrombophlebitis. Care must be taken not to place a blood pressure cuff on the arm of a patient who has an arteriovenous shunt.

Pulse Oximetry

Office-based anesthesia with any type of sedation requires pulse oximeter monitoring for a baseline reading as well as intraoperative and postoperative monitoring of arterial oxygen saturation. There are 4 types of hemoglobin (Hb) noted: oxyhemoglobin (HbO_2), reduced Hb, methemoglobin (metHb), and carboxyhemoglobin.[161] Because metHb and carboxyhemoglobin do not contribute to oxygen transport and are usually present under certain conditions, it is the functional saturation (the ratio of HbO_2 to HbO_2 plus reduced Hb) that is reflected.[161] When carboxyhemoglobin and metHb are zero, O_2Hb percentage and arterial saturation of oxygen (SaO_2) are the same.[161] Carboxyhemoglobin reflects an overestimation of oxygen saturation because the photodetector senses it as HbO_2[162] and methemogobinemia results in desaturation but the oximeter reading reflects a greater oxygen saturation than is present.[163] The oximeter calculates arterial oxygen saturation of Hb by spectrophotoelectric oximeter analysis.[164] This technique measures the amount of light that is transmitted through a pulsatile soft tissue bed between a 2-wavelength light source of 660 nm (red light) and 930 nm (near-infrared light) and a detector.[165] The SaO_2 is estimated by the transmission of 2 wavelengths of light (660 nm and 930 nm) through a pulsatile tissue bed where it is absorbed by tissue, capillary, venous, and arterial blood (**Fig. 3**).[166]

In one pediatric study in which pulse oximetry was used, with data available to the anesthesia team during the procedure, versus a pulse oximeter used intraoperatively but no data or alarms available, there were twice as many desaturation events in the blinded group; the desaturation was detected by the monitor before the anesthesiologist; major desaturations were not associated with changes in blood pressure, heart rate, or respiratory rate; and desaturation episodes occurred in both groups regardless of the

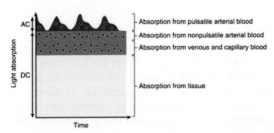

Fig. 3. The SaO_2 is estimated by the transmission of 2 wavelengths of light (660 nm [red light] and 930 nm [infrared light]) through a pulsatile tissue bed where it is absorbed by tissue, capillary, venous, and arterial blood. (*From* Chitilian HV, Kaczka DW, Vidal M. Respiratory monitoring. In: Miller RD, ed. Miller's anesthesia. 8th edition. Philadelphia: Saunders, 2014; with permission.)

anesthesia team's experience.[167,168] Of key importance that the monitor reflection of a decreasing saturation lags behind the true desaturation of the patient.

There are many factors that can lead to false oxygen saturation readings, including MetHb, carboxyhemoglobin, dyes, nail polish, external light, movement, electrosurgery, room or digit temperature, jaundice, and sensor fit. Two important elements to which the clinician must attend are, first, the correlation between oxygen saturation and ventilation, and, second, the Hbo_2 saturation curve. Pulse oximetry is not a reliable or accurate monitor for ventilation because the Spo_2 is not significantly affected by Pco_2 (Bohr effect), and the pulse oximeter can fail to warn of hypoventilation.[169] Also, when the Hbo_2 saturation curve is evaluated, an Hbo_2 saturation between 90% and 100% is associated with a Po_2 between 60 and 100 mm Hg. When office-based IV sedation is monitored by pulse oximetry the goal is to maintain the Sao_2 at greater than 90%. With an O_2 saturation greater than 90% and a reasonable cardiac output, it can be assumed that there is adequate O_2 tissue perfusion. Less than a Po_2 of 60 mm Hg (arterial O_2 content) there is a rapid and steep decline in the Hbo_2 saturation (**Fig. 4**).[166]

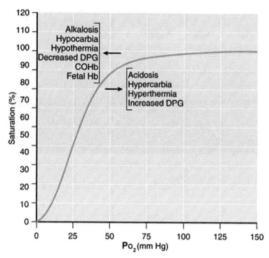

Fig. 4. In evaluating the Hbo_2 saturation curve, an Hbo_2 saturation between 90% and 100% is associated with a Po_2 between 60 and 100 mm Hg. When office-based IV sedation is monitored by pulse oximetry the goal is to maintain the Sao_2 at greater than 90%. With an O_2 saturation greater than 90% and a reasonable cardiac output it can be assumed that there is adequate O_2 tissue perfusion. At a Po_2 of less than 60 mm Hg (arterial O_2 content) there is a rapid and steep decline in the Hbo_2 saturation. (*From* Chitilian HV, Kaczka DW, Vidal M. Respiratory monitoring. In: Miller RD, ed. Miller's anesthesia. 8th edition. Philadelphia: Saunders, 2014; with permission.)

Capnography

Capnography is the measurement of carbon dioxide (CO_2) in expired gas. Expired CO_2 is a reliable indication that the sedated patient in the dental office is ventilating spontaneously or, if intubated, that the endotracheal tube is in the trachea and adequate ventilation is being performed. Most capnographs use infrared absorption.[170] In the office setting a small side-stream sample port is used that is usually incorporated into the nasal hood or nasal cannula and a tubing is run from the port to a moisture separator attached to the monitor. This measurement is an estimate of the arterial Pco_2. Sampling CO_2 from a face mask is not reliable to determine $Paco_2$ because the values of the end-tidal partial pressure of CO_2 (Petco$_2$) measured are much lower; however, this technique is acceptable to measure the rate of respiration.[171] Because this is an open system with multiple connections, tube lengths, dead space, and contaminations by environmental air, there are many possible errors that can lead to false readings. However, usually a waveform can be obtained to assess the patient's ventilation measuring Petco$_2$. False readings are also possible if nitrous oxide–oxygen is used along with a scavenger that is on low wall suction; this too leads to lower Petco$_2$. The waveform represents the inspired and expired gas flow (Petco$_2$) (**Figs. 5** and **6**).

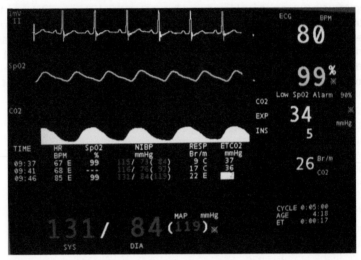

Fig. 5. Capnography is the measurement of CO_2 in expired gas. The waveform represents the inspired and expired gas flow (Petco$_2$).

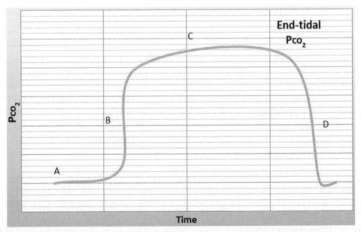

Fig. 6. With inspiration and at the beginning of expiration, there is no CO_2 as dead space is being exhaled. As expiration continues (A), there is an increase in CO_2 represented by an upward deflection of the waveform to a plateau (B). The plateau usually has a slight rise to it over time (C), with most expired air being exhaled during the first half of the exhalation time. The peak level is reached at the final phase of exhalation and is called the Petco$_2$. The downward deflection of the capnogram (D) represents the beginning of inspiration.

The expired gas must travel from the port in the facemask through the tubing and condensation unit to the sensor cell in the monitor. This process requires time and represents dead space. The waveform can be seen in **Fig. 6**.

With inspiration and at the beginning of expiration, there is no CO_2 because dead space is being exhaled (see **Fig. 6**A). As expiration continues, there is an increase in CO_2 represented by an upward deflection of the waveform to a plateau (see **Fig. 6**B). The plateau usually has a slight rise to it over time (see **Fig. 6**C), most of the expired air being exhaled during the first half of exhalation time. The peak level is reached at the final phase of exhalation and is called the $Petco_2$.[171] The downward deflection of the capnogram (see **Fig. 6**D) represents the beginning of inspiration. With inspiration, the CO_2 concentration decreases toward the value as inspired CO_2 and depends on flow rates, breathing circuit, and whether any dead space with remaining CO_2 is present.[171] End-expiratory CO_2 partial pressure ranges between 35 and 45 mm Hg. If there are increases of values of CO_2 greater than 45 mm Hg, it is known as hypercapnia and may be related to malignant hyperthermia, fever, decreased ventilation, respiratory distress, or chest wall rigidity (fentanyl). If the $Petco_2$ is less than 35 mm Hg it may represent hyperventilation or dilution by additional gas flows, pulmonary emboli, or circuit disconnection. Capnography is also the standard to ensure endotracheal intubation into the trachea.[172,173] It is crucial in the detection of malignant hyperthermia as well as in its treatment.[174] Bronchospasm causes an increase in the slope of the plateau on the capnograph with expiration and, with appropriate treatment, the plateau returns to the normal shape.[164]

Electrocardiogram

The basic ECG complex is reviewed here and some examples are given of rhythm strips that may be seen in the dental office. The ECG is a measurement of the electrical voltages produced in the heart. The recognition and treatment of irregularities in the heartbeat or arrhythmias should be reviewed in the ACLS protocol. ECG monitoring is required when the sedation level is deep or when the patient is under general anesthesia. For moderate sedation, ECG monitoring is required if there is a cardiovascular disease history or when a dysrhythmia is anticipated or detected. It is recommended that an ECG monitor be used for any in-office sedation procedure. The ECG is a measurement of the electrical voltages produced in the heart. These voltages are measured from the production of potentials by the atrial and ventricular muscle fibers. The first wave noted is the P wave, which represents atrial stimulation and depolarization. It usually precedes a QRS and is an upward deflection. It represents atrial systole. The PR interval is the time that the impulse travels from the sinoatrial node until the start of ventricular depolarization.[175] The QRS complex represents ventricular depolarization after stimulation.[175] The ST segment and T and U waves represent ventricular repolarization. ECG paper has measurements that are horizontal and vertical. Each small box is 1 mm^2. The ECG paper travels at 25 mm/s, therefore each small box running in a horizontal direction between the darker running vertical lines measures 0.04 seconds. The vertical measurements are 1 mm, which represents each small box and coincides with the amplitude of each waveform. A 1-mV signal produces a 10-mm deflection (1 mV = 10 mm).[176] In summary, the amplitude is measured in voltage and the width in time; usually the amplitude is recorded in millimeters not millivolts.

The PR interval is measured from the P wave to the beginning of the QRS complex. It is the time taken for the stimulus to spread through the atria and pass through the atrioventricular junction (0.12–0.20 seconds).[176] The QRS complex measures ventricular depolarization and measures 0.1 seconds. The ST segment represents ventricular repolarization and is measured from the end of the QRS to the beginning of the T wave. The ST segment may be elevated or depressed, such as is seen with a myocardial infarct.[176] Ventricular repolarization is reflected by a T wave that is positive; however, T waves of different morphology may represent a myocardial infarct or potassium level abnormalities.[176] The QT interval is usually 0.44 seconds. It represents the return of the ventricles to the resting state. Certain pathologic conditions and medications can prolong the QT interval, such as a myocardial infarct or cardiac ischemia, quinidine, and procainamide. QT elongation can increase the patient's susceptibility to lethal arrhythmias.[176] The QT interval may be shortened by medications such as digitalis and serum abnormalities such as hypercalcemia. The U wave represents the last phase of ventricular repolarization.[176]

For dental professionals who do office-based moderate sedation, a cardiac monitor is required. The office-setting ECG is usually completed using a 3-lead rhythm strip with positive V1 placed on the right side between the fourth and fifth intercostal spaces.[176] The second and third are placed on the right and left shoulder with the right acting as a negative electrode and the left serving as a ground.

Arrhythmias

The recognition and treatment of arrhythmias is beyond the scope of this article; however, a brief review is included. Arrhythmias are divided into tachyarrhythmia greater than 100 beats/min, bradyarrhythmias less than 100 beats/min, and conduction blocks.[177] Patients with preexisting cardiac disease have a higher incidence of arrhythmias during anesthesia than those without disease.[178] Dental surgery may be associated with stimulation of the sympathetic and parasympathetic nervous systems and therefore arrhythmias may be seen.[179] The arrhythmias should be identified and treated if the patient is symptomatic or it can lead to more severe dysrhythmias.

1. Sinus bradycardia: the heart rate is less than 60 beats/min. If less than 40 beats/min and hypotension (unstable), the clinician should consider treatment with atropine 0.5 mg to 1.0 mg every 3 to 5 minutes to a maximum total of 3.0 mg. If no response, the clinician may consider an external pacemaker. Sinus bradycardia may be associated with sick sinus syndrome in which sinus node dysfunction leads to bradycardias, heart blocks, alternating bradyarrhythmias, and tachyarrhythmia.[180]

2. Sinus tachycardia: the heart rate is greater than 100 beats/min and can go up to 200 beats/min. Causes of sinus tachycardia include pain, poor local anesthesia, hypovolemia, hypercarbia, hypoxia, drugs such as epinephrine, fever, and loss of blood.[181] The cause of a tachycardia should be addressed by various treatment modalities, such as improving the local anesthetic, deepening the level of anesthesia, administering 100% oxygen, and considering volume replacement. Significant blood loss or dehydration is not expected with an in-office dental procedure. In a patient with preexisting ischemic heart disease who develops tachycardia with ST changes during anesthesia, esmolol could be considered to prevent the ischemia from worsening.[177] Based on 2010 ACLS guidelines for stable ventricular tachycardia, clinicians can try vagal maneuvers, and, if no resolution, adenosine 6 mg IV push over 1 to 3 seconds can be administered. If there is no improvement, clinicians can repeat a adenosine 12 mg IV push over 1 to 3 seconds.

3. Premature ventricular beats (premature ventricular contractions): ventricular premature beats arise in the ventricles and are depolarizations that result in a widening QRS complex. They are common during anesthesia and make up 15% of arrhythmias. They are seen much more regularly in anesthetized patients with preexisting

cardiac disease.[177] The number of premature ventricular beats ranges from 1 to multiple. Two consecutive premature ventricular is a couplet and 3 in a row is considered ventricular tachycardia. Ventricular premature beats can lead to ventricular tachycardia or ventricular fibrillation. In a dental office setting during anesthesia the clinician should consider the cause of the premature ventricular contractions; pain, hypoxia, existing heart disease, acute myocardial infarct, hypokalemia, and the local anesthesia are possibilities. Again, treatment is directed to identify the underlying cause, such as pain or hypoxemia, and to follow ACLS protocol and consider IV lidocaine.

4. Pulseless ventricular tachycardia/ventricular fibrillation: these rhythms must be recognized and treated following the ACLS protocol because they can be lethal. The cause may be an acute myocardial infarction, hypoxia, or medication reaction. The patient becomes unresponsive and unconscious with no detectable pulse or blood pressure. An early warning sign may be chest pain, or shortness of breath. cardiopulmonary resuscitation (CPR) must be initiated and an automated external defibrillator (AED) attached. The AED determines whether the rhythm can be shocked and its use should not be delayed (**Fig. 7**). IV access should be established, intubation attempted, and medications such as epinephrine and amiodarone available for use. Recommendations include a review of CPR and ACLS, as well as certification in both by an approved American Heart Association course provider.

5. Angina (rule out acute myocardial infarction): in the dental office setting most patients with angina complain of shortness of breath and chest pain. It may be difficult to distinguish between angina and an acute myocardial infarction without a 12-lead ECG. However, the use of oxygen 4 L/min, aspirin (325 mg by mouth to chew), and nitroglycerin sublingual (0.4 mg 0.006 grains) every 5 minutes for 3 doses as long as the systolic blood pressure is greater than 90 mm Hg, and then morphine sulfate 2 mg IV should be given only if the third dose of nitroglycerin

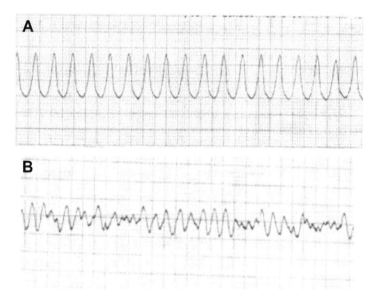

Fig. 7. (*A*) Ventricular tachycardia. (*B*) Ventricular fibrillation.

does not relieve the chest pain. The dental procedure should be terminated and a 3-lead ECG can be used to try to determine any rhythm strip abnormalities. Depending on the location of the myocardial infarct, various ECG changes may be noticed, such as peaked or depressed T waves, abnormal Q waves, and loss of normal R wave progression.[182]

CONSIDERATION FOR INTRAVENOUS CONSCIOUS/MODERATE SEDATION IN PEDIATRIC PATIENTS

One of the many reasons for sedation in pediatric patients is to obtain a more cooperative patient with less movement so that extensive dental treatment can be accomplished. In addition, similar to adult patients, sedation is also used to reduce anxiety and pain. Pediatric patients are defined by the AAPD as being from birth to age 21 years. Inhalation as well as IV sedation techniques are also used in pediatric patients not only for significant behavioral concerns but for those who have special needs or have extensive treatment concerns. As with adult moderate sedation, sedation of children can also result in significant risk. The requirements for sedation for pediatric patients mirror those outlined for adults. When planning moderate sedation for pediatric patients it is important to understand that they may require meticulous scrutiny above and beyond what is required for adult patients in the preoperative, operative, and postoperative stages. However, in recent years, increasing liability insurance costs and risks associated with office-based moderate sedation have caused more pediatric dentists to favor oral sedation.[183,184] A study supported by the National Center for Biotechnology Information assessed 95 cases involving the relationship between adverse outcomes and medications used in pediatric patients. Associations evaluated included individual and classes of drugs, routes of administration, drug combinations and interactions, medication errors and overdoses, patterns of drug use, practitioners, and venues of sedation. Adverse sedation events were frequently associated with drug overdoses and drug interactions, particularly when 3 or more drugs were used. Adverse outcomes were associated with all routes of drug administration and all classes of medication, and dental specialists had the greatest frequency of negative outcomes associated with the use of 3 or more sedating medications. In addition, nitrous oxide in combination with any other class of sedating medication was frequently associated with adverse outcomes.[185]

An analysis of data from 1990 to 2000 from the Pediatric Perioperative Cardiac Arrest Registry (POCA) showed that 36% of closed claims reports of pediatric anesthesia were from dental/ear-nose-throat/maxillofacial procedures. Also, cardiovascular and respiratory events were responsible for most intraoperative cardiac arrests. In addition, equipment-related and medication-related causes were common. The POCA analysis reported that an incorrect dose was involved in half of the medication-related events.[186] Compared with the POCA study, another study by Cote and colleagues[184] in an incident analysis of contributing factors to adverse outcomes in pediatric sedation found that most cardiac arrests seemed to be related to an initial respiratory arrest, consistent with previously reported complications associated with pediatric moderate sedation in the non–operating room setting. The predominance of respiratory arrests, number of sedations, and age distribution of patients suggested that depth of sedation might be a critical common pathway in the cases examined.[187] Recently, the focus has been on the physiologic monitoring of sedated children because lack of proper monitoring has led to significant morbidity and mortality.[188] The goal is improving the safety of conscious sedation through improved physiologic monitoring and adequate provider training. Advanced training in recognition and management of pediatric emergencies is critical in providing safe sedation and anesthetic care. The AAPD recommends a systematic approach that includes no administration of sedating medication without the safety net of medical supervision, careful presedation evaluation for underlying medical or surgical conditions that would place the child at increased risk from sedating medications, appropriate fasting for elective procedures and a balance between depth of sedation and risk for those who are unable to fast because of the urgent nature of the procedure, a focused airway examination for large tonsils or anatomic airway abnormalities that might increase the potential for airway obstruction, a clear understanding of the pharmacokinetic and pharmacodynamic effects of the medications used for sedation as well as an appreciation for drug interactions, appropriate training and skills in airway management to allow rescue of the patient, age-appropriate and size-appropriate equipment for airway management and venous access, appropriate medications and reversal agents, sufficient numbers of people to perform the procedure and monitor the patient, appropriate physiologic monitoring during and after the procedure, a properly equipped and staffed recovery area, recovery to the presedation level of consciousness before discharge from medical supervision, and appropriate discharge instructions.[189]

Preoperative

The medical and dental histories should include past medical history, particularly history of upper respiratory infection or history of reactive airway diseases, anesthesia record, recent illness, other systems diseases, medications, allergies or any adverse reactions, family history, past dental history, diet, and an ASA classification. Pediatric patients should be accompanied to and from their treatment appointments by a parent, legal guardian, or other responsible person in order to provide informed consent and postoperative care. It may be necessary to have 2 or more adults accompany a child who requires transport in a car safety seat.[190]

Unlike the adult physical examination, in which the same routine can often be followed at every encounter, the pediatric examination must be modified for each patient. Interacting with children of different ages and temperaments in different settings can be challenging. The physical examination should include the patient's age, weight, height, baseline vital signs, airway examination, head, eyes, ears, nose, and throat (HEENT), pulmonary function, and cardiovascular function. Guidelines for sedation recommend that patients in ASA classes I and II are generally considered appropriate candidates for minimal, moderate, or deep sedation. Children in ASA classes III and IV, children with special needs, and those with anatomic airway abnormalities or large tonsils present challenges that require additional consideration.[191] The use of the Mallampati classification for assessment is also needed to properly evaluate the airway.

Children of all ages should be nil by mouth for clear liquids 2 hours before undergoing sedation. Recommendations for duration of nil by mouth for solid food and nonclear liquids vary by age, as follows: less than 6 months, 4 to 6 hours; 6 to 36 months, 6 hours; greater than 36 months, 6 to 8 hours. Also, it is important in the systems review that adequate cardiovascular, renal, and liver function are included for effective and safe moderate sedation in this patient population. In addition, note that, in the cardiovascular system evaluation, children often have an audible murmur at some point between infancy and adolescence. Most murmurs occur in normal hearts and are benign. Murmurs that have a structural cause may indicate a need for preoperative antibiotic prophylaxis, and consultation with a cardiologist may be indicated before the sedation procedure.[192]

Equipment, Supplies, and Monitoring

Suction and airway equipment should always be nearby and ready to use if necessary. The components required are an appropriately sized positive pressure oxygen delivery system, and various suction devices. Other equipment and supplies should include assorted IV catheters, tourniquets, alcohol wipes, tape, syringes, IV tubing, pediatric and adult drip, pediatric burette, extension tubing, IV fluids, pediatric IV board, IV needles, intraosseous bone marrow needle, and sterile gauze pads. Some of the equipment suggested to manage the airway that should be available for patient recovery and/or rescue are face masks (infant, child, small adult, medium adult, large adult), breathing bag and valve set, oropharyngeal airways (infant, child, small adult, medium adult, large adult), nasopharyngeal airways (small, medium, large), laryngoscope, blades and handles (with extra batteries and light bulbs), and nasogastric tubes.[193]

Competent and well-trained practitioners and their staff should observe their patients continuously. The monitoring should include all parameters described previously for moderate sedation. The name, route, site, time of administration, and dosage of all drugs administered should be recorded meticulously. The inspired concentrations of inhalation sedation agents and oxygen and the duration of administration should also be documented. Appropriate monitoring of patients should involve continuous oxygen saturation and heart rate monitoring, record of vital signs and blood pressure every 5 minutes for conscious sedation as well as a record of drug dose and time administered, a record of the state of consciousness and response to stimulation, and end-tidal CO_2.

Medications

A variety of sedative medications have been used in moderate sedation procedures for children. The most common classes of drugs are opioids (fentanyl), benzodiazepines (midazolam), barbiturates (methohexital), as well as miscellaneous agents such as nitrous oxide, ketamine, propofol, and dexmedetomidine. Dosing should be based on the weight of the child. For those children who are overweight or obese, calculating the BMI may be helpful in avoiding adverse outcomes. Children who are overweight and have a high BMI may be at greater risk when administering sedation. A study by Kang and colleagues[193] in 2012 evaluated the impact of childhood obesity on adverse events observed during sedation for dental procedures. BMI data were available for 103 children, and patients who had 1 or more adverse events had higher mean weight and BMI. Although the findings were not statistically significant, the investigators concluded that children who are overweight or obese may experience more adverse events during sedation for dental procedures.[194] Another student found that pediatric patients with high BMIs were at greater risk for nausea or emesis during ketamine sedation and recommended antiemetic prophylaxis for this group of patients before performing ketamine sedation.[195]

Local Anesthetic Agents

Also of importance in children is local anesthetics. All local anesthetic agents are cardiac depressants and may cause CNS excitation or depression, and special attention should be paid to dosage in small children.[196,197] Many of the anesthetics also contain epinephrine, which can adversely affect cardiovascular and CNS function if given intravascularly or in higher than recommended doses. To ensure that patients do not receive an excessive dose, the maximum allowable safe dosage in milligrams per kilogram should be calculated before administration. There may be enhanced sedative effects when the highest recommended doses of local anesthetic drugs are used in combination with other sedatives narcotics. During administration of local anesthetic drugs, aspiration should be done frequently to minimize the likelihood that anesthetic is delivered into a vessel. Also, the lowest doses should be used when injecting into vascular tissues.[198]

Whether the medication is for sedation or local anesthesia, the dose should be calculated by weight and it is important to keep in mind that the response to a single drug or combination of drugs can vary significantly from one child to the next. In addition, there is an increasing concern with obesity among pediatric populations, and evaluation of the patient's BMI may also play a role in dose calculation.[199,200] Consideration in dosing should be based on starting with the lowest recommended dose (or even half that) and then titrating as needed. Practitioners and sedation teams should always be prepared to support and/or rescue a patient who has moved to a deeper level of sedation. Reversal agents should be immediately available and the correct doses prepared. The agents that should be on hand are naloxone and flumazenil. Rescue drugs are based on individual skill and preference and may include albuterol for inhalation, ammonia spirits, atropine, diphenhydramine, diazepam, epinephrine (1:1000, 1:10,000; the recommended epinephrine dose for children is 0.01 mg/kg, up to 0.3 mg or 0.01 mL/kg), flumazenil, glucose (25% or 50%), lidocaine, lorazepam, methylprednisolone, naloxone, oxygen, epinephrine, rocuronium or succinylcholine, and sodium bicarbonate.

Postprocedure Care

Guidelines recommended for postprocedure care are that cardiovascular function and airway patency are satisfactory and stable, the patient is easily arousable and protective reflexes are intact, the patient can talk (if age appropriate), and that the patient can sit up unaided (if age appropriate). For a very young or handicapped children incapable of the usual responses, the presedation level of responsiveness or a level as close as possible to the normal level for that child should be achieved and the state of hydration should be adequate.[193] A patient back to the baseline state should be normotensive. A child who is not tachycardic is likely to be well resuscitated; a child with tachycardia or hypotension may be hypovolemic. It is also important to evaluate the influence of anxiety and pain, which can increase the heart rate and blood pressure as well. Also, sedation is stimulus dependent, it may be likely based on the medications given that a child could become more sedated after than during the procedure, which can lead to hypoventilation and hypoxia. Some agents are associated with specific aftercare needs. For example, ketamine may cause ataxia for 12 to 24 hours, and the child's activities should be restricted during this period to prevent further injury.[201,202]

SUMMARY

Moderate sedation continues to be an integral part of providing high-quality dental care. The goal is to minimize physical pain, discomfort, and negative psychological responses by providing sedation, amnesia, and analgesia during painful, uncomfortable, or extensive dental procedures. Also, in administering moderate sedation, no interventions should be required to maintain a patent airway, spontaneous ventilation should be adequate, and cardiovascular function should be maintained. Guidelines for providing moderate sedation that is safe and effective are available for administering medications, equipment use, monitoring, as well as the necessary training for providers and support staff. The understanding that moderate sedation is also part of a continuum and that deeper levels of sedation are possible because of several factors should be noted and be a part of the plan and preparation for the sedation procedure. In general, depth of sedation is evaluated by observation of the patient, monitoring, and standardized sedation assessment scales. Recent interest in electroencephalogram-based depth of anesthesia (DoA) monitoring devices as an additional method to monitor level of consciousness during sedation may prove that this is a useful tool for dental providers. Types of monitors available include Bispectral, E-Entropy and Narcotrend-Compact M monitors. The basis for this process involves an algorithmic analysis of a patient's electroencephalogram.[203] A proposed systematic review published by Cochrane is underway to determine whether this additional DoA monitoring during procedural sedation and analgesia in the hospital and other settings improves patient safety by reducing the risk of hypoxemia. The investigators hypothesized that earlier identification of deeper than intended levels of sedation using these monitors would lead to more effective titration of sedative and analgesic medications and will result in reduction in the risk of sedation-related adverse events caused by oversedation.[203] The outcome of the analysis of the studies may be important in helping to establish DoA monitoring as another valuable part of the conscious sedation armamentarium.

REFERENCES

1. Wells H. A history of the discovery of the application of nitrous oxide gas, ether, and other vapors, to surgical operations. Hartford (CT): J Gaylord Wells; 1847.
2. Stearns FP. Cambridge sketches. Philadelphia; London: JB Lippincott; 1905. p. 9–355.
3. Weaver J. The latest ASA mandate: CO_2 monitoring for moderate and deep sedation. Anesth Prog 2011;58(3):111–2.
4. American Society of Anesthesiologists. Continuum of depth of sedation: definition of general anesthesia and levels of sedation/analgesia (approved by the ASA House of Delegates on October 13, 1999, and last amended on October 15, 2014).
5. Collado V, Faulks D, Nicolas E, et al. Conscious sedation procedures using intravenous midazolam for dental care in patients with different cognitive profiles: a prospective study of effectiveness and safety. PLoS One 2013;8(8):e71240.
6. Guidelines for the use of sedation and general anesthesia by dentists. Available at: http://www.ada.org/~/media/ADA/About%20the%20ADA/Files/anesthesia_use_guidelines.ashx. Accessed October 25, 2015.
7. Dionne RA, Yagiela JA, Moore PA, et al. Comparing efficacy and safety of four intravenous sedation regimens in dental outpatients. J Am Dent Assoc 2001; 132(6):740–51.
8. Karamnov S, Sarkisian N, Grammer R, et al. Analysis of adverse events associated with adult moderate procedural sedation outside the operating room. J Patient Saf 2014;10(3):125–32 [Epub ahead of print].
9. American Society of Anesthesiologists Task Force on Sedation and Analgesia by Non-Anesthesiologists. Practice guidelines for sedation and analgesia by non-anesthesiologists. Anesthesiology 2002;96:1004–17.
10. American Association of Oral and Maxillofacial Surgeons (AAOMS). Parameters and pathways: clinical practice guidelines for oral and maxillofacial surgery anesthesia in outpatient facilities. Rosemont (IL): American Association of Oral and Maxillofacial Surgeons; 2001. Available at: www.aaoms.org/index.php.
11. Guidelines for the use of sedation and general anesthesia by dentists. Available at: http://www.ada.org/~/media/ADA/Advocacy/Files/anesthesia_use_guidelines.ashx. Accessed June 01, 2015.

12. American Academy of Pediatric Dentistry (AAPD). Monitoring and management of pediatric patients during and after sedation for diagnostic and therapeutic procedures: an update. Developed through a collaborative effort between the American Academy of Pediatrics and the AAPD. Available at: www.aapd.org/policies. Accessed May 30, 2015.

13. ADA Council on Dental Education: Proposed revisions to ADA Guidelines for the use of sedation and general anesthesia by dentists and the guidelines for teaching pain control and sedation to dentists and dental students. Available at: http://www.ada.org/en/publications/ada-news/2015-archive/may/comments-sought-on-proposed-sedation-anesthesia-guideline-revisions. Accessed May 30, 2015.

14. Centers for Disease Control and Prevention, National Center for Health Statistics. Underlying cause of death 1999-2013 on CDC WONDER Online Database, released 2015. Data are from the Multiple Cause of Death Files, 1999-2013, as compiled from data provided by the 57 vital statistics jurisdictions through the Vital Statistics Cooperative Program. Available at: http://wonder.cdc.gov/ucd-icd10.html. Accessed December 09, 2015.

15. Mertes PM, Demoly P, Stenger R. Disease summaries: allergy to anesthetic agents. World Allergy Organization Journal 2007. Available at: http://www.worldallergy.org/professional/allergic_diseases_center/anaesthetic_agents/.

16. Johansson SG, Bieber T, Dahl R, et al. Revised nomenclature for allergy for global use: report of the Nomenclature Review Committee of the World Allergy Organization, October 2003. J Allergy Clin Immunol 2004;113:832-6.

17. Sankar A, Johnson SR, Beattie WS, et al. Reliability of the American Society of Anesthesiologists physical status scale in clinical practice. Br J Anaesth 2014;113(3):424-32.

18. Mallampati SR. Clinical sign to predict difficult tracheal intubation (hypothesis). Can Anaesth Soc J 1983;30:316-7.

19. Mallampati SR, Gatt SP, Gugino LD, et al. A clinical sign to predict difficult tracheal intubation: a prospective study. Can Anaesth Soc J 1985;32:429-34.

20. Samsoon GL, Young JR. Difficult tracheal intubation: a retrospective study. Anaesthesia 1987;42(5):487-90.

21. American Society of Anesthesiologists. Practice guidelines for preoperative fasting and the use of pharmacologic agents to reduce the risk of pulmonary aspiration: application to healthy patients undergoing elective procedures. Anesthesiology 2011;114:495.

22. Quasha AL, Eger EI II, Tinker JH. Determination and applications of MAC. Anesthesiology 1980;53:315.

23. Coté CJ, Lerman J, Ward RM, et al. Pharmacokinetics and pharmacology of drugs used in children. In: Coté CJ, Lerman J, Anderson BJ, editors. A practice of anesthesia for infants and children. 5th edition. Philadelphia: Elsevier Health Sciences; 2013. p. 111.

24. Eger EI. Anesthetic uptake and action. Baltimore (MD): Williams & Wilkins; 1974.

25. Lin CY, Wang JS. Supramaximal second gas effect—a nonexistent phenomenon. Anesth Analg 1993;77:870-2.

26. Sun X-G, Su F, Shi YQ, et al. The "second gas effect" is not a valid concept. Anesth Analg 1999;88:188-92.

27. Fink BR. Diffusion anoxia. Anesthesiology 1955;16:511-9.

28. Rackow H, Salanitre E, Frumin MJ. Dilution of alveolar gases during nitrous oxide excretion in man. J Appl Physiol 1961;16:723-8.

29. Thomsen KA, Terkildsen K, Arnfred J. Middle ear pressure variations during anesthesia. Arch Otolaryngol 1985;82:609–11.
30. Eger EI, Saidman LJ. Hazards of nitrous oxide anesthesia in bowel obstruction and pneumothorax. Anesthesiology 1965;26:61–6.
31. Munson ES, Stevens DS, Redfern RE. Endotracheal tube obstruction by nitrous oxide. Anesthesiology 1980;52:275–6.
32. Mehta M, Sokoll MD, Gergis SD. Effects of venous air embolism on the cardiovascular system and acid base balance in the presence and absence of nitrous oxide. Acta Anaesthesiol Scand 1984;28:226–31.
33. Coté CJ, Lerman J, Ward RM, et al. Pharmacokinetics and pharmacology of drugs used in children. In: Coté CJ, Lerman J, Todres ID, editors. A practice of anesthesia for infants and children. 4th edition. Philadelphia: Elsevier Health Sciences; 2009. p. 118, 120, 122.
34. Walser A, Benjamin L, Flynn T. Quinazolines and 1, 4-benzodiazepines. 84. Synthesis and reactions of imidazo (1,5)(1.4)-benzodiazepines. J Org Chem 1978;43:939.
35. Greenblatt DJ, Shader RI, Abernethy DR. Drug therapy. Current status of benzodiazepines. N Engl J Med 1983;309:354–8.
36. Reeves JG, Glass PSA, Lubarsky DA, McEvoy MD. Intravenous nonopioid anesthetics. In: Miller's anesthesia: 2-volume set (anesthesia). 6th edition. New York: Elsevier/Churchill Livingstone; 2005. p. 320, 335, 337, 345.
37. Arendt RM, Greenblatt DJ, deJong RH, et al. In vitro correlates of benzodiazepine cerebrospinal fluid uptake, pharmacodynamic action and peripheral distribution. J Pharmacol Exp Ther 1983;227:98–106.
38. Mould DR, DeFeo TM, Reele S, et al. Simultaneous modeling of the pharmacokinetics and pharmacodynamics of midazolam and diazepam. Clin Pharmacol Ther 1995;58:35–43.
39. Stanford AD, Corcoran C, Malaspina D. Schizophrenia. In: Rowland LP, editor. Merritt's neurology. 11th edition. Philadelphia: Lippincott Williams & Wilkins; 2005. p. 1139.
40. Amrein R, Hetzel W, Hartmann D, et al. Clinical pharmacology of flumazenil. Eur J Anaesthesiol Suppl 1988;2:65–80.
41. Mendelson WB. Neuropharmacology of sleep induction by benzodiazepines. Crit Rev Neurobiol 1992;6:221–32.
42. de Jong RH, Bonin JD. Benzodiazepines protect mice from local anesthetic convulsions and deaths. Anesth Analg 1981;60:385–9.
43. Reves J, Croughwell N. Valium-fentanyl interaction. In: Reves J, Hall K, editors. Common problems in cardiac anesthesia. Chicago: Year Book; 1987. p. 356.
44. Cravero JP, Blike GT. Review of pediatric sedation. Anesth Analg 2004;99:1355–64.
45. Golparvar M, Saghaei M, Sajedi P, et al. Paradoxical reaction following intravenous midazolam premedication in pediatric patients—a randomized placebo controlled trial of ketamine for rapid tranquilization. Paediatr Anaesth 2004;14:924–30.
46. George KA, Dundee JW. Relative amnesic actions of diazepam, flunitrazepam and lorazepam in man. Br J Clin Pharmacol 1977;4:45–50.
47. Litman RS, Berkowitz RJ, Ward DS. Levels of consciousness and ventilatory parameters in young children during sedation with oral midazolam and nitrous oxide. Arch Pediatr Adolesc Med 1996;150:671–5.
48. Alexander CM, Gross JB. Sedative doses of midazolam depress hypoxic ventilatory responses in humans. Anesth Analg 1988;67:377–82.
49. Drummond GB. Comparison of sedation with midazolam and ketamine: effects on airway muscle activity. Br J Anaesth 1996;76:663–7.

50. Yaster M, Nichols DG, Deshpande JK, et al. Midazolam-fentanyl intravenous sedation in children: case report of respiratory arrest. Pediatrics 1990;86:463–7.
51. Krauss B, Green SM. Sedation and analgesia for procedures in children. N Engl J Med 2000;342:938–45.
52. Jensen B, Schroder U. Acceptance of dental care following early extractions under rectal sedation with diazepam in preschool children. Acta Odontol Scand 1998;56:229–32.
53. Ernst BJ, Clark GF, Grundmann O. The physicochemical and pharmacokinetic relationships of barbiturates - from the past to the future. Curr Pharm Des 2015;21(25):3681–91.
54. Coupey SM. Barbiturates. Pediatr Rev 1997;18(8):260–4.
55. Heyer EJ, Macdonald RL. Barbiturate reduction of calcium-dependent action potentials: correlation with anesthetic action. Brain Res 1982;236(1):157–71.
56. Goldfrank LR, Flomenbau NE. Sedative-hypnotic agents. In: Goldfrank's toxicologic emergencies. 5th edition. Prentice Hall; 1994. p. 787–804.
57. Katzung BG. Sedative-hypnotics. In: Basic and clinical pharmacology. 6th edition. Appleton & Lange; 1995. p. 333–49.
58. Mason KP, Zurakowski D, Karian VE, et al. Sedatives used in pediatric imaging: comparison of IV pentobarbital with IV pentobarbital with midazolam added. AJR Am J Roentgenol 2001;177:427–30.
59. Zgleszewski SE, Zurakowski D, Fontaine PJ, et al. Is propofol a safe alternative to pentobarbital for sedation during pediatric diagnostic CT? Radiology 2008; 247(2):528–34.
60. Martone CH, Nagelhout J, Wolf SM. Methohexital: a practical review for outpatient dental anesthesia. Anesth Prog 1991;38(6):195–9.
61. Russo H, Bressolle F. Pharmacodynamics and pharmacokinetics of thiopental. Clin Pharmacokinet 1998;35(2):95–134.
62. Mendelson WB. Clinical distinctions between long-acting and short-acting benzodiazepines. J Clin Psychiatry 1992;53(Suppl):4–7.
63. Roberts DM, Buckley NA. Enhanced elimination in acute barbiturate poisoning - a systematic review. Clin Toxicol (Phila) 2011;49(1):2–12.
64. Johns MW. Sleep and hypnotic drugs. Drugs 1975;9(6):448–78.
65. Jufe GS. New hypnotics: perspectives from sleep physiology. Vertex 2007; 18(74):294–9.
66. Mihic J, Harris RA. Barbiturates. Hypnotics and sedatives. In: Brunton LL, Chabner BA, Knollman BC, editors. Goodman & Gilman's the pharmacological basis of therapeutics. 12th edition. New York: McGraw-Hill; 2011. p. 469–74.
67. Ross-Flanigan N, Uretsky S. Barbiturates. Gale encyclopedia of surgery: a guide for patients and caregivers. 2004. Available at: http://www.encyclopedia.com/doc/1G2-3406200057.html. Accessed December 16, 2015.
68. Mockenhaupt M, Messenheimer J, Tennis P, et al. Risk of Stevens-Johnson syndrome and toxic epidermal necrolysis in new users of antiepileptics. Neurology 2005;64(7):1134–8.
69. Mamishi S, Fattahi F, Pourpak Z, et al. Severe cutaneous reactions caused by barbiturates in seven Iranian children. Int J Dermatol 2009;48(11):1254–61.
70. Griffin CE, Kaye AM, Bueno FR, et al. Benzodiazepine pharmacology and central nervous system-mediated effects. Ochsner J 2013;13(2):214–23.
71. Buckley NA, McManus PR. Changes in fatalities due to overdose of anxiolytic and sedative drugs in the UK (1983-1999). Drug Saf 2004;27(2):135–41.
72. Spina E, Perucca E. Clinical significance of pharmacokinetic interactions between antiepileptic and psychotropic drugs. Epilepsia 2002;43(Suppl 2):37–44.

73. Sebel PS, Lowdon JD. Propofol: a new intravenous anesthetic. Anesthesiology 1989;71:260–77.
74. Fulton B, Sorkin EM. Propofol. An overview of its pharmacology and a review of its clinical efficacy in intensive care sedation. Drugs 1995;50:636–57.
75. Bryson HM, Fulton BR, Faulds D. Propofol. An update of its use in anaesthesia and conscious sedation. Drugs 1995;50:513–59.
76. Smith I, White PF, Nathanson M, et al. An update on its clinical use. Anesthesiology 1994;81:1005–43.
77. Kikuchi T, Wang Y, Sato K, et al. In vivo effects of propofol on acetylcholine release from the frontal cortex, hippocampus and striatum studied by intracerebral microdialysis in freely moving rats. Br J Anaesth 1998;80:644–8.
78. Pain L, Jeltsch H, Lehmann O, et al. Central cholinergic depletion induced by 192 IgG-saporin alleviates the sedative effects of propofol in rats. Br J Anaesth 2000;85:869–73.
79. Lingamaneni R, Birch ML, Hemmings HC Jr. Widespread inhibition of sodium channel -dependent glutamate release from isolated nerve terminals by isoflurane and propofol. Anesthesiology 2001;95:1460–6.
80. McDonald NJ, Mannion D, Lee P, et al. Mood evaluation and outpatient anaesthesia. A comparison between propofol and thiopentone. Anaesthesia 1988;43(Suppl):68–9.
81. Mirakhur R, Shepherd W. Intraocular pressure changes with propofol ('Diprivan'): comparison with thiopentone. Postgrad Med J 1985;61(Suppl 3):41–4.
82. Mirakhur RK, Shepherd WF, Darrah WC. Propofol or thiopentone: effects on intraocular pressure associated with induction of anaesthesia and tracheal intubation (facilitated with suxamethonium). Br J Anaesth 1987;59:431–6.
83. Conti G, Dell'Utri D, Vilardi V, et al. Propofol induces bronchodilation in mechanically ventilated chronic obstructive pulmonary disease (COPD) patients. Acta Anaesthesiol Scand 1993;37:105–9.
84. Pagel PS, Warltier DC. Negative inotropic effects of propofol as evaluated by the regional preload recruitable stroke work relationship in chronically instrumented dogs. Anesthesiology 1993;78:100–8.
85. Mackenzie N, Grant IS. Propofol for intravenous sedation. Anaesthesia 1987;42:3–6.
86. Fanard L, Van Steenberge A, Demeire X, et al. Comparison between propofol and midazolam as sedative agents for surgery under regional anaesthesia. Anaesthesia 1988;43(Suppl):87–9.
87. Coté CJ, Stafford MA. The principle of pediatric sedation. Boston: Tufts University School of Medicine; 1998.
88. Turtle MJ, Cullen P, Prys-Roberts C, et al. Dose requirements of propofol by infusion during nitrous oxide anaesthesia in man. II: Patients premedicated with lorazepam. Br J Anaesth 1987;59:283–7.
89. Sanderson JH, Blades JF. Multicentre study of propofol in day case surgery. Anaesthesia 1988;43(Suppl):70–3.
90. Van Aken H, Meinshausen E, Prien T, et al. The influence of fentanyl and tracheal intubation on the hemodynamic effects of anesthesia induction with propofol/N2O in humans. Anesthesiology 1988;68:157–63.
91. Klein SM, Hauser GJ, Anderson BD, et al. Comparison of intermittent versus continuous infusion of propofol for elective oncology procedures in children. Pediatr Crit Care Med 2003;4:78–82.
92. Tramer MR, Moore RA, McQuay HJ. Propofol and bradycardia: causation, frequency and severity. Br J Anaesth 1997;78:642–51.

93. Evans RG, Crawford MW, Noseworthy MD, et al. Effect of increasing depth of propofol anesthesia on upper airway configuration in children. Anesthesiology 2003;99:596–602.

94. Crowther J, Hrazdil J, Jolly DT, et al. Growth of microorganisms in propofol, thiopental, and a 1:1 mixture of propofol and thiopental. Anesth Analg 1996;82: 475–8.

95. Sosis MB, Braverman B, Villaflor E. Propofol, but not thiopental, supports the growth of Candida albicans. Anesth Analg 1995;81:132–4.

96. Wachowski I, Jolly DT, Hrazdil J, et al. The growth of microorganisms in propofol and mixtures of propofol and lidocaine. Anesth Analg 1999;88:209–12.

97. Murphy A, Campbell DE, Baines D, et al. Allergic reactions to propofol in egg-allergic children. Anesth Analg 2011;113:140–4.

98. Hirayama T, Ishii F, Yago K, et al. Evaluation of the effective drugs for the prevention of nausea and vomiting induced by morphine used for postoperative pain: a quantitative systematic review. Yakugaku Zasshi 2001;121:179–85.

99. Lacy CF, Armstrong LL, Goldman MP, et al. Drug information handbook. 11th edition. Hudson (OH): American Pharmaceutical Association; Lexi-Comp; 2003–2004.

100. Horn E, Nesbit SA. Pharmacology and pharmacokinetics of sedatives and analgesics. Gastrointest Endosc Clin N Am 2004;14(2):247–68.

101. Latta KS, Ginsberg B, Barkin RL. Meperidine: a critical review. Am J Ther 2002; 9:53–68.

102. Hershey LA. Meperidine and central neurotoxicity. Ann Intern Med 1983;98: 548–9.

103. Seifert CF, Kennedy S. Meperidine is alive and well in the new millennium: evaluation of meperidine usage patterns and frequency of adverse drug reactions. Pharmacotherapy 2004;24:776–83.

104. Fukuda K. Intravenous opioid anesthetics. In: Miller RD, Cucchiara RF, editors. Miller's anesthesia: 2-volume set (anesthesia). 6th edition. New York: Elsevier/Churchill Livingstone; 2005. p. 380, 383, 390, 402, 421.

105. Mansour A, Fox CA, Akil H, et al. Opioid-receptor mRNA expression in the rat CNS: anatomical and functional implications. Trends Neurosci 1995;18:22–9.

106. Lauer KK, Connolly LA, Schmeling WT. Opioid sedation does not alter intracranial pressure in head injured patients. Can J Anaesth 1997;44:929–33.

107. Goldberg M, Ishak S, Garcia C, et al. Postoperative rigidity following sufentanil administration. Anesthesiology 1985;63:199–201.

108. de Nadal M, Munar F, Poca MA, et al. Cerebral hemodynamic effects of morphine and fentanyl in patients with severe head injury: absence of correlation to cerebral autoregulation. Anesthesiology 2000;92:11–9.

109. Blasco TA, Lee D, Amalric M, et al. The role of the nucleus raphe pontis and the caudate nucleus in alfentanil rigidity in the rat. Brain Res 1986;386:280–6.

110. Tabatabai M, Kitahata LM, Collins JG. Disruption of the rhythmic activity of the medullary inspiratory neurons and phrenic nerve by fentanyl and reversal with nalbuphine. Anesthesiology 1989;70:489–95.

111. Bailey PL, Wilbrink J, Zwanikken P, et al. Anesthetic induction with fentanyl. Anesth Analg 1985;64:48–53.

112. Rung GW, Claybon L, Hord A, et al. Intravenous ondansetron for postsurgical opioid-induced nausea and vomiting. S3A-255 Study Group. Anesth Analg 1997;84:832–8.

113. Roerig DL, Kotrly KJ, Vucins EJ, et al. First pass uptake of fentanyl, meperidine, and morphine in the human lung. Anesthesiology 1987;67:466–72.

114. Kennedy RM, Porter FL, Miller JP, et al. Comparison of fentanyl/midazolam with ketamine/midazolam for pediatric orthopedic emergencies. Pediatrics 1998; 102:956–63.

115. Kaplan RF, Cravero JP, Yaster M, et al. Sedation for diagnostic and therapeutic procedures outside the operating room. In: Coté CJ, Lerman J, Todres ID, editors. A practice of anesthesia for infants and children. 4th edition. Philadelphia: Elsevier Health Sciences; 2009. p. 1045–6.

116. Krauss B, Green SM. Procedural sedation and analgesia in children. Lancet 2006;367:766–80.

117. Parashchanka A, Schelfout S, Coppens M. Role of novel drugs in sedation outside the operating room: dexmedetomidine, ketamine and remifentanil. Curr Opin Anaesthesiol 2014;7(4):442–7.

118. Maxwell LG, Tobias JD, Cravero JP, et al. Adverse effects of sedatives in children. Expert Opin Drug Saf 2003;2:167–94.

119. Hirshman CA, Downes H, Farbood A, et al. Ketamine block of bronchospasm in experimental canine asthma. Br J Anesth 1979;51:713–8.

120. Tobias JD. End-tidal carbon dioxide monitoring during sedation with a combination of midazolam and ketamine for children undergoing painful, invasive procedures. Pediatr Emerg Care 1999;15:173–5.

121. Cheng G. The pharmacology of ketamine. In: Schüttler J, Schwilden H, editors. Ketamine. Berlin: Springer-Verlag; 1969. p. 1.

122. Hannallah RS, Patel RI. Low-dose intramuscular ketamine for anesthesia pre-induction in young children undergoing brief outpatient procedures. Anesthesiology 1989;70:598–600.

123. Gutstein HB, Johnson KL, Heard MB, et al. Oral ketamine preanesthetic medication in children. Anesthesiology 1992;76:28–33.

124. Tobias JD, Phipps S, Smith B, et al. Oral ketamine premedication to alleviate the distress of invasive procedures in pediatric oncology patients. Pediatrics 1992; 90:537–41.

125. Reinemer HC, Wilson CF, Webb MD. A comparison of two oral ketamine-diazepam regimens for sedating anxious pediatric dental patients. Pediatr Dent 1996;18:294–300.

126. Okamoto GU, Duperon DF, Jedrychowski JR. Clinical evaluation of the effects of ketamine sedation on pediatric dental patients. J Clin Pediatr Dent 1992;16: 253–7.

127. Shapiro HM. Intracranial hypertension: therapeutic and anesthetic considerations. Anesthesiology 1971;43:445–71.

128. Reves JG, Lell WA, McCracken LE Jr, et al. Comparison of morphine and ketamine anesthetic techniques for coronary surgery: a randomized study. South Med J 1978;71:33–6.

129. Corssen G, Reves J, Stanley T. Dissociative anesthesia. In: Corssen G, Reves J, Stanley T, editors. Intravenous anesthesia and analgesia. Philadelphia: Lea & Febiger; 1988. p. 99.

130. Garfield JM, Garfield FB, Stone JG, et al. A comparison of psychologic responses to ketamine and thiopental-nitrous oxide-halothane anesthesia. Anesthesiology 1972;36:329–38.

131. White PF, Way WL, Trevor AJ. Ketamine-its pharmacology and therapeutic uses. Anesthesiology 1982;56:119–36.

132. Dillon J. Clinical experience with repeated ketamine administration for procedures requiring anesthesia. In: Kreuscher H, editor. Ketamine. Berlin: Springer-Verlag; 1969.

133. Sarma VJ. Use of ketamine in acute severe asthma. Acta Anaesthesiol Scand 1992;36:106–7.
134. Taylor PA, Towey RM. Depression of laryngeal reflexes during ketamine anaesthesia. BMJ 1971;2:688–9.
135. Sussman DR. A comparative evaluation of ketamine anesthesia in children and adults. Anesthesiology 1974;40:459–64.
136. Gingrich BK. Difficulties encountered in a comparative study of orally administered midazolam and ketamine. Anesthesiology 1994;80:1414–5.
137. Hohl CM, Kelly-Smith CH, Yeu TC, et al. The effect of a bolus dose of etomidate on cortisol levels, mortality, and health services utilization: a systematic review. Ann Emerg Med 2010;56(2):105–13.
138. Vanlersberghe C, Camu F. Etomidate and other non-barbiturates. Handb Exp Pharmacol 2008;182(182):267–82.
139. Zed PJ, Abu-Laban RB, Harrison DW. Intubating conditions and hemodynamic effects of etomidate for rapid sequence intubation in the emergency department: an observational cohort study. Acad Emerg Med 2006;13(4):378–83.
140. Sokolove PE, Price DD, Okada P. The safety of etomidate for emergency rapid sequence intubation of pediatric patients. Pediatr Emerg Care 2000;16(1):18–21.
141. Patel A, Wordell C, Szarlej D. Alternatives to sodium amobarbital in the Wada test. Ann Pharmacother 2011;45(3):395–401.
142. Wagner RL, White PF, Kan PB, et al. Inhibition of adrenal steroidogenesis by the anesthetic etomidate. N Engl J Med 1984;310(22):1415–21.
143. Komatsu R, Yo J, Mascha EJ, et al. Anesthetic induction with etomidate, rather than propofol, is associated with increased 30-day mortality and cardiovascular morbidity after noncardiac surgery. Anesth Analg 2013;117(6):1329–37.
144. Daniell H. Opioid and benzodiazepine contributions to etomidate-associated adrenal insufficiency. Intensive Care Med 2008;34(11):2117–8.
145. Lauven PM, Schwilden H, Stoeckel H, et al. The effects of a benzodiazepine antagonist Ro 15-1788 in the presence of stable concentrations of midazolam. Anesthesiology 1985;63:61–4.
146. Jones RD, Chan K, Roulson CJ, et al. Pharmacokinetics of flumazenil and midazolam. Br J Anaesth 1993;70:286–92.
147. Davis CO, Wax PM. Flumazenil associated seizure in an 11-month-old child. J Emerg Med 1996;14:331–3.
148. Prough DS, Roy R, Bumgarner J, et al. Acute pulmonary edema in healthy teenagers following conservative doses of intravenous naloxone. Anesthesiology 1984;60:485–6.
149. Partridge BL, Ward CF. Pulmonary edema following low dose naloxone administration. Anesthesiology 1986;65:709–10.
150. Bailey PL, Clark NJ, Pace NL, et al. Antagonism of postoperative opioid-induced respiratory depression: nalbuphine versus naloxone. Anesth Analg 1987;66:1109–14.
151. American Academy of Pediatrics Committee on Drugs: naloxone dosage and route of administration for infants and children: addendum to emergency drug doses for infants and children. Pediatrics 1990;86:484–5.
152. Kaye AD, Kucera IJ. Intravascular fluid and electrolyte physiology. In: Miller's anesthesia: 2-volume set (anesthesia). 6th edition. New York: Elsevier/Churchill Livingstone; 2005. p. 1785.
153. McClain CD, McManus ML. Fluid management. In: A practice of anesthesia for infants and children. 5th edition. Philadelphia: Elsevier Health Sciences; 2013. p. 165–9.

154. American Society of Anesthesiologists. Standards for basic anesthetic monitoring, ASA standards, guidelines and statements. Park Ridge (IL): American Society of Anesthesiologist; 1993. p. 5.
155. Posey JA, Geddes LA, Williams H, et al. The meaning of the point of maximum oscillations in cuff pressure in the indirect measurement of blood pressure. Part 1. Cardiovasc Res Ctr Bull 1969;8:15–25.
156. Yelderman M, Ream AK. Indirect measurement of mean blood pressure in the anesthesized patient. Anesthesiology 1979;50:253–6.
157. Mark JB, Slaughter TF. Cardiovascular monitoring. In: Miller's anesthesia: 2-volume set (anesthesia). 6th edition. New York: Elsevier/Churchill Livingstone; 2005. p. 1270. Fig. 32–33.
158. Gorback MS. Considerations in the interpretation of systemic pressure monitoring. In: Lumb PD, Bryan-Brown CW, editors. Complications in critical care medicine. Chicago: Year Book; 1988. p. 296.
159. von Recklinghausen H. Neue Wege zur Blutdruckmessung. Berlin: Springer-Verlag; 1931.
160. Sy WP. Ulnar nerve palsy possibly related to use of automatically cycled blood pressure cuff. Anesth Analg 1981;60:687–8.
161. Szocik JF, Barker SJ, Tremper KK. Fundamental principles of monitoring instrumentation. In: Miller's anesthesia: 2-volume set (anesthesia). 6th edition. New York: Elsevier/Churchill Livingstone; 2005. p. 1213.
162. Barker SJ, Tremper KK. The effect of carbon monoxide inhalation on pulse oximetry and transcutaneous PO2. Anesthesiology 1987;66:677–9.
163. Barker SJ, Tremper KK, Hyatt J. Effects of methemoglobinemia on pulse oximetry and mixed venous oximetry. Anesthesiology 1989;70:112–7.
164. Blum RH, Coté CJ. Pediatric equipment. In: A practice of anesthesia for infants and children. 4th edition. Philadelphia: Elsevier Health Sciences; 2009. p. 1116–20.
165. Yelderman M, New W. Evaluation of pulse oximetry. Anesthesiology 1983;59:349–52.
166. Chitilian HV, Kaczka DW, Vidal M, et al. In: Miller's anesthesia. 2014. p. 1541–79.e8.
167. Coté CJ, Goldstein EA, Coté MA, et al. A single-blind study of pulse oximetry in children. Anesthesiology 1988;68:184–8.
168. Coté CJ, Rolf N, Liu LM, et al. A single-blind study of combined pulse oximetry and capnography in children. Anesthesiology 1991;74:980–7.
169. Ayas N, Bergstrom LR, Schwab TR, et al. Unrecognized severe postoperative hypercapnia: A case of apneic oxygenation. Mayo Clin Proc 1998;73:51.
170. Gravenstein JS, Paulus DA, Hayes TJ. Gas monitoring in clinical practice. 2nd edition. Boston: Butterworth-Heinemann; 1995.
171. Moon RE, Camporesi EM. Respiratory monitoring. In: Miller's anesthesia: 2-Volume set (Anesthesia). 6th edition. New York: Elsevier/Churchill Livingstone; 2005. p. 1456.
172. American Society of Anesthesiologists. Standards for basic anesthetic monitoring. Standards and Practice Parameters Committee (approved by the ASA House of Delegates on October 21, 1986, and last amended on October 20, 2010, with an effective date of July 1, 2011). Available at: http://www.asahq.org/For.../Standards-Guidelines-and-Statements.aspx. Accessed October 16, 2012.
173. American Heart Association. 2005 American Heart Association (AHA) guidelines for cardiopulmonary resuscitation (CPR) and emergency cardiovascular care (ECC) of pediatric and neonatal patients: pediatric basic life support. Pediatrics 2006;117:e989–1004.

174. Baudendistel L, Goudsouzian N, Coté CJ, et al. End-tidal CO2 monitoring: its use in the diagnosis and management of malignant hyperthermia. Anaesthesia 1984;39:1000–3.

175. Slesnick TC, Gertler R, Miller-Hance WC. Essentials of cardiology. In: A practice of anesthesia for infants and children. 4th edition. Philadelphia: Elsevier Health Sciences; 2009. p. 309.

176. Goldberger AL. Basic ECG waves. In: Clinical electrocardiography: a simplified approach. 6th edition. St Louis (MO): Mosby; 1999. p. 9–29.

177. Hillel Z, Thys DM. Electrocardiography. In: Miller's anesthesia: 2-volume set (anesthesia). 6th edition. New York: Elsevier/Churchill Livingstone; 2005. p. 1397, 1399–1403.

178. Angelini L, Feldman MI, Lufschonwski R, et al. Cardiac arrhythmias during and after heart surgery: diagnosis and management. Prog Cardiovasc Dis 1974;16:469.

179. Alexander JP. Dysrhythmia and oral surgery. Br J Anaesth 1971;43:773.

180. Slapa WJ. The sick sinus syndrome. Am Heart J 1976;92:648.

181. Skeehan TM, Thys DM. Monitoring the cardiac surgical patient. In: Hensley FA, Martin DE, editors. The practice of cardiac anesthesia. Boston: Little, Brown; 1990. p. 123.

182. Goldberger AL. Myocardial ischemia and infarction section 1. In: Clinical electrocardiography: a simplified approach. 6th edition. St Louis (MO): Mosby, Inc; 1999. p. 87.

183. Lee HH, Milgrom P, Starks H, et al. Trends in death associated with pediatric dental sedation and general anesthesia. Paediatr Anaesth 2013;23(8): 741–6.

184. Coté CJ, Karl HW, Notterman DA, et al. Adverse sedation events in pediatrics: analysis of medications used for sedation. Pediatrics 2000;106(4):633–44.

185. Jimenez N, Posner KL, Cheney FW, et al. An update on pediatric anesthesia liability: a closed claims analysis. Anesth Analg 2007;104(1):147–53.

186. Coté CJ, Notterman DA, Karl HW, et al. Adverse sedation events in pediatrics: a critical incident analysis of contributing factors. Pediatrics 2000;105(4 Pt 1): 805–14.

187. Domino K. Office-based anesthesia: lessons learned from the closed claims project. ASA Newsl 2001;65(6):9–11.

188. American Academy of Pediatric Dentistry. Guideline for monitoring and management of pediatric patients during and after sedation for diagnostic and therapeutic procedures. Adopted 2006, reaffirmed 2011. Available at: http://www. aapd.org/media/Policies_Guidelines/G_Sedation.pdf. Accessed July 15, 2015.

189. Bull M, Agran P, Laraque D, et al. American Academy of Pediatrics, Committee on Injury and Poison Prevention. Transporting children with special health care needs. Pediatrics 1999;104:988–92.

190. Malviya S, Voepel-Lewis T, Tait AR. Adverse events and risk factors associated with the sedation of children by non-anesthesiologists. Anesth Analg 1997;85: 1207–13.

191. Asprey DP. Evaluation of children with heart murmurs. Lippincotts Prim Care Pract 1998;2(5):505–13.

192. Guideline for monitoring and management of pediatric patients during and after sedation for diagnostic and therapeutic procedure. Am Acad Pediatr Dentistry 2006;36(6):209–25.

193. Kang J, Vann WF Jr, Lee JY, et al. The safety of sedation for overweight/obese children in the dental setting. Pediatr Dent 2012;34(5):392–6.

194. Kinder KL, Lehman-Huskamp KL, Gerard JM. Do children with high body mass indices have a higher incidence of emesis when undergoing ketamine sedation? Pediatr Emerg Care 2012;28(11):1203–5.

195. Goodson JM, Moore PA. Life-threatening reactions after pedodontic sedation: An assessment of narcotic, local anesthetic, and antiemetic drug interaction. J Am Dent Assoc 1983;107:239–45.

196. Jastak JT, Peskin RM. Major morbidity or mortality from office anesthetic procedures: A closed-claim analysis of 13 cases. Anesth Prog 1991;38:39–44.

197. American Academy of Pediatric Dentistry. Guideline on appropriate use of local anesthesia for pediatric dental patients. Pediatr Dent 2005;27(Suppl):101–6.

198. Scherrer PD, Mallory MD, Cravero JP, et al. The impact of obesity on pediatric procedural sedation-related outcomes: results from the Pediatric Sedation Research Consortium. Paediatr Anaesth 2015;25(7):689–97.

199. Bimstein E, Katz J. Obesity in children: a challenge that pediatric dentistry should not ignore–review of the literature. J Clin Pediatr Dent 2009;34(2):103–6.

200. McNab S, Ware RS, Neville KA, et al. Isotonic versus hypotonic solutions for maintenance intravenous fluid administration in children. Cochrane Database Syst Rev 2014;12:CD009457.

201. Blount RL, Loiselle KA. Behavioural assessment of pediatric pain. Pain Res Manag 2009;14(1):47–52.

202. Avidan MS, Zhang L, Burnside BA, et al. Anesthesia awareness and the bispectral index. N Engl J Med 2008;358:1097–108.

203. Conway A, Sutherland J. Depth of anaesthesia monitoring during procedural sedation and analgesia: a systematic review protocol. Syst Rev 2015;4:70.

Update on Analgesic Medication for Adult and Pediatric Dental Patients

 CrossMark

Constantinos Laskarides, DMD, DDS, PharmD

KEYWORDS

- Analgesic medications • Opioid analgesics • Nonsteroidal antiinflammatory drugs
- Acute oral pain • Pain control for dental patients • Pediatric dental pain

KEY POINTS

- This is an update on analgesia for acute oral pain.
- Analgesic medications in the dental setting are reviewed.
- The article includes updates for nonsteroidal anti-inflammatory drugs (NSAIDs) for dental pain.
- The article includes updates for opioid analgesics for dental pain.
- A review of analgesia for pediatric dental pain is presented.

One of the most important criteria that patients appreciate and rank a dental care provider for, far beyond knowledge and academic background, skills, and professional accolades, is effective pain management. Pain and analgesia are subjects often inherent (the former) and imperative (the latter) to oral health care. Today, despite the great scientific advances and breakthroughs in dentistry (and in its specialties) there are no real "game changers" in the world of analgesia; this fact calls for meticulous knowledge, by the clinician, of the current armamentarium and techniques to provide optimal pain control. This article navigates through this vast subject, limiting and filtering the information as to what is pertinent and useful in the dental care setting and the dental patient, adult and pediatric.

Three types of pain can be distinguished:

- Acute physiologic nociceptive pain that is generated by acute noxious stimuli and forms a protection from tissue damage (needle injection, incision);
- Pathophysiologic nociceptive pain that accompanies tissue inflammation or injury in absence of intentional stimuli (burn, postincision, local inflammation); and

Disclosure Statement: The author has nothing to disclose.
Advanced Residency Program, Oral & Maxillofacial Surgery, Tufts Medical Center, Tufts University, One Kneeland Street, Boston, MA 02111, USA
E-mail address: constantinos.laskarides@tufts.edu

- Neuropathic pain that is elicited from either peripheral or central disease, or injury, of neurons. It is not related to noxious stimuli and it is perceived as unnatural (diabetic neuropathy, trigeminal neuralgia).[1]

This classification may be oversimplified because new types of pain have been described and in many cases different types coexist. A more fundamental distinction, one that is recognized even by the general public and our patients, is the one between acute and chronic pain. Chronic pain has been described as one that lasts longer than 6 months.[2] Recently, state boards have adapted the following time frames regarding pain, to form guidelines for controlled substances:

- Acute pain: up to 4 weeks from onset;
- Postoperative pain: up to 4 weeks from date of surgery;
- Subacute pain: 4 to 12 weeks from onset; and
- Chronic pain: greater than 12 weeks from onset.

Chronic pain is more complex and the relation between nociception and pain is not linear. It may be affected by neuroendocrine dysregulation and impaired physical or mental status.[2] Chronic pain frequently has significant effects on psychological health. Frequently, there is a direct association of chronic pain with depression and anxiety that in turn can profoundly affect pain perception.[3]

It is beyond the purpose of this article to analyze the complex mechanisms of pain and describe the nociceptive system, yet we must recognize that a thorough understanding of those parameters will form a better and more comprehensive appreciation and selection of analgesic medications in the clinical setting.

We can consider 3 main categories of analgesics medications in the clinical dental setting:

1. Opioids,
2. NSAIDs, and
3. Nonopioid, non-NSAID drugs.

Of course there are other categories used in the broader sense of head and neck analgesia like:

- Triptans (serotonin receptor agonists) that are mainly indicated for acute migraines and cluster headaches;
- Anticonvulsants and antidepressants that target mainly neuropathic pain that follows nerve injury; and
- Local anesthetics used, not for common local anesthesia, but to treat symptoms of chronic pain. Intravenously administered local anesthetics have shown remarkable results for neuropathic pain. This indication is not relevant to the usual dental clinical setting.[4]

Different classes of analgesic medications modulate different mechanisms and vary in their effectiveness in managing different pain states in adults (**Table 1**). Significant pharmacodynamic and pharmacokinetic differences also exist between the adult and the pediatric populations that need to be recognized by clinicians.[5] Here's an outline of few differences, perhaps oversimplified:

- Immature blood–brain barrier in neonates may facilitate drug delivery to the brain.
- Lower plasma levels of albumin in neonates will result in less protein binding of drugs thus increasing action potential or even toxicity.

Table 1
Classes of analgesic medications and their effectiveness in managing different pain states in adults

Medication Class	Relative Effectiveness in Pain States
Nonsteroidal antiinflammatory drugs	Tissue injury >> acute stimuli = nerve injury = 0
Opioids (μ agonists)	Tissue injury = acute stimuli > nerve injury > 0
Anticonvulsants	Nerve injury > tissue injury = acute stimuli = 0
Antidepressants	Nerve injury > tissue injury >> acute stimuli = 0

- Neonates and infants have higher body water content and thus a greater volume of distribution of water-soluble drugs, which will extend the duration of action.
- There are fewer pharmacodynamically inactive tissues, like muscle and adipose tissue, so there is less drug uptake by that tissue. The consequence is higher plasma concentrations.
- Hepatic clearance of drugs in children 2 to 6 years old may be greater compared with adults because of a larger hepatic mass relative to body weight. This may result in adjusting for relatively higher doses and shorter intervals.
- Renal function and excretion of drugs is reduced in neonates.

Another important, yet understated, factor in pediatric patients is pain assessment and evaluation. Older children (school age) can usually perceive and convey an adequate pain self-assessment especially with the help of visual analog scales. The challenge lies with younger children and children with cognitive delay. For those children, third-party assessment tools are necessary. To add to the challenge, it is documented that third-party assessment is inferior to self-assessment of pain intensity.[6] There are many pain scales that can be used by parents or clinicians. One example is the FLACC (face, legs, activity, cry, consolability) scale shown in **Table 2**. It is designed for children between 2 months and 7 years of age and can be used even in children who are unable to speak. The range is 0 to 10 with 0 representing no pain.[7]

Table 2
FLACC pain scale (face, legs, activity, cry, consolability)

Parameters	Score 0	Score 1	Score 2
Face	No particular expression or smile	Occasional grimace or frown, withdrawn, uninterested	Frequent to constant quivering chin, clenched jaw
Legs	Normal position or relaxed	Uneasy, restless, tense	Kicking, or legs drawn up
Activity	Lying quietly, normal position, moves easily	Squirming, shifting back and forth, tense	Arched, rigid, or jerking
Cry	No cry (awake or asleep)	Moans or whimpers: occasional complaint	Crying steadily, screams or sobs, frequent complaints
Consolability	Content, relaxed	Reassured by occasional touching, hugging, or being talked to, distractible	Difficult to console or comfort

Copyright © 2002, The Regents of the University of Michigan. Used with permission.

The major categories of analgesics are presented next. In this article, only drugs currently approved by the US Food and Drug Administration, for use in United States, are discussed.

OPIOID ANALGESICS

When it comes to severe pain the most effective and broadly used drugs are opioids. Three classes of true opioid receptors (μ, δ, and κ) have been described with multiple receptor subtypes.

μ (mu) - The μ opioid receptors produce the most profound analgesia, and can cause euphoria, respiratory depression, physical dependence, and bradycardia. They are responsible for most of the analgesic effect of the opioid.

κ (kappa) - The κ opioid receptors contribute to analgesia at the spinal level. These receptors trigger a lesser analgesic response, and may cause miosis, sedation, and dysphoria.

δ (delta) - The δ opioid receptors modulate μ receptor activity and are more important in the periphery.

Additionally, the following receptors have been associated with opioids but are not consider as true opioid receptors:

σ (sigma) - The σ opioid receptors can be stimulated by opioids and may account for the excitatory actions of opioids; however, these excitatory effects probably are produced by an interaction with the phencyclidine binding site on ionotropic glutamate receptors.

Orphan opioid receptor-like receptors are structurally similar to the μ opioid receptor, but are insensitive to opioid ligands.

The pathways of opioid receptor signaling are multiple, like G-protein coupling, cyclic adenosine monophosphate inhibition, and Ca^{++} channel inhibition; a detailed analysis of these agents is beyond the purpose of this article. The opioid effect is a selective one on nociception. Touch, pressure, and other sensory modalities are generally unaffected.

All known use of opioid medications goes back in history thousands of years and it starts with the plant *Papaver somniferum.* The dry exudate of the plant's seed pod is *opium*, which is a complex mix that includes alkaloids like morphine, codeine, noscapine, papaverine, and thebaine. These alkaloids have been used traditionally in medicine to treat pain, cough, and visceral spasms. Morphine is recognized as the standard opioid.

Opioids can be used in both acute and chronic severe pain. Acute situations include intraoperative, postoperative, and posttraumatic pain. The application can be preemptive, before the noxious stimulus, like the administration of intravenous (IV) opioids with anesthetic agents before surgery, or therapeutic after the noxious stimulus. Chronic conditions where opioids can be considered should be divided into:

A. Malignant (cancer pain) that is responsive to opioids.
B. Nonmalignant (like neuropathic or inflammatory pain). This type will be better addressed in a multidisciplinary way with both pharmacologic and nonpharmacologic treatments.

In general, long-term use of opioids for chronic conditions falls outside of the subject matter of most dental care facilities.

Opioid Pharmacodynamics

Opioids can be agonists, partial agonists, or antagonists (**Fig. 1**). Drug A is a drug that binds and produces a concentration-dependent activation of the receptor is an agonist. Drug B is a partial agonist in relation to drug A. Drug C binds to the receptor yet elicits no effect is an antagonist. By far the most efficacious and widely used clinically drugs are the μ-receptor agonists.

Opioid Pharmacokinetics

Absorption after oral administration is rapid and first-pass metabolism at the liver is significant. Because of the rapid absorption, sustained-release opioid formulations have been developed to achieve adequate duration of analgesia. The lipophilicity of the formulation also increases the bioavailability. Lipophilic drugs can be absorbed from mucosal surfaces into the bloodstream; hence, opioids are now available commercially in buccal, intranasal, and transdermal formulations. Distribution is speedy throughout the body. In the case of peripheral tissue injury, like surgical trauma, up to 80% of an analgesic effect after systemic opioid administration may be mediated by peripheral opioid receptors.[8]

All clinically available opioids undergo extensive hepatic metabolism to metabolites that are excreted by the kidneys. The only exception is remifentanil (not available for oral administration), which is rapidly hydrolyzed by esterases in peripheral tissues and plasma.[9]

Side Effects

- Cardiovascular: bradycardia in high doses.
- Respiratory: dose-dependent respiratory depression. This is a direct effect on the respiratory center in the medulla.[10] High doses can produce apnea.
- Gastrointestinal: opioids cause inhibition of normal intestinal secretions and peristalsis that can lead to increased water absorption and constipation.
- Central: nausea and vomiting stimulation by a direct effect in the brainstem.
- Central: cough suppression by direct effects on medullary cough centers.

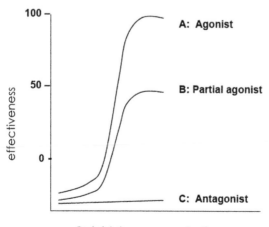

Fig. 1. Opioid pharmacodynamics.

- Central: pupil constriction (miosis) by a direct effect on the autonomic nucleus (Edinger–Westphal) of the oculomotor nerve.
- Central: euphoria and sedation in higher doses.
- Histamine release from tissue mast cells is usually associated with IV administration. Local itching, redness, or hives are observed near the site of injection and do not represent an allergic reaction because true allergy to opioids is extremely rare.
- Tolerance after repeated or prolonged exposure. This affects more the analgesic effect.
- Physical dependence: abrupt discontinuation of opioids causes a stereotypical withdrawal syndrome. Another dimension to this phenomenon is the psychological dependence. Addiction liability is apparently very low in chronic pain patients.

Management suggestions for some of those side effects are illustrated in **Table 3**.

Opioid agents can be used for pain experienced as moderate to severe. In this article, agents that are administered orally and/or may be considered for analgesia in the dental care setting are highlighted. A few others are listed as honorable mentions. A comparison of various pharmacokinetic parameters can be found in **Table 4**. Adult dosing is found in **Table 5**.

Regarding the pediatric patient population, in the dental care setting there are few and distinct instances where the need for opioids would emerge to manage moderate to severe nociceptive pain. In such cases careful titration is required to obtain the desired level of analgesia while monitoring side effects. **Table 6** provides dosing for children.

Morphine

Morphine is the quintessential opioid, the drug that best represents the aforementioned pharmacology. Generic and multiple trade formulations are available and it can be also given by mouth usually as an elixir. Bioavailability is approximately 30%. Larger oral doses are needed to produce equivalent analgesia with parenteral administration with the ratio being 3:1. The pharmacokinetics of morphine in children are comparable with those in adults. Neonates, however, differ, because morphine doses need to be reduced owing to hepatic immaturity. Examples of brand names are MS Contin, Avinza, Kadian, and Roxanol.

Table 3
Management suggestions for opioid side effects

Side Effects of Opioids	Examples of Pharmacologic Management
Constipation	Osmotic laxative: magnesium citrate Softening agent: sodium docusate Cathartic: bisacodyl, senna
Nausea and vomiting	Neuroleptic: prochlorperazine Antihistamines: promethazine, diphenhydramine, meclizine Prokinetics: metoclopramide
Pruritus, hives	5-HT3 receptor antagonist: ondansetron Antihistamines: diphenhydramine

Adapted from McCarberg B, Pasternak G, Fine PG, et al. Opioid analgesics for pain management. Critical thinking to balance benefits & risk. Stamford, CT: PharmaCom Group; 2007.

Table 4
Opioid pharmacokinetics

Opioid	Route	Onset of Action (min)	Time to Peak Effect (min)	Duration of Action (h)
Morphine	Oral	60	60–120	4–5
Fentanyl	Intravenous	1–2	3–5	0.5–1
Hydromorphone	Oral	30	90–120	4
Levorphanol	Oral	10–60	90–120	4–5
Meperidine	Oral	15	60–90	4–6
Codeine	Oral	30–40	60–120	4
Hydrocodone	Oral	10–30	30–60	4–6
Oxycodone	Oral	10–30	60	3–4
Pentazocine	Oral	15–30	30–60	2–3
Tramadol	Oral	30–40	120	6

Methadone

Methadone is best known for its use in treating narcotic addiction. It is not recommended in the dental care setting and without significant expertise.

Meperidine

Meperidine or pethidine is well-absorbed from gastrointestinal track with a bioavailability reaching 50% to 60%. It crosses the placenta and also enters breast milk. It has fallen out of favor, in relation with past use, mostly because of its neurotoxic metabolite, norpethidine, Meperidine has demonstrated local anesthesia ability, particularly in spinal anesthesia, so local administration has being explored intraorally for anesthesia and analgesia without encouraging outcomes.[11,12] Examples of brand names are Demerol and Meperitab.

Table 5
Opioid pharmacokinetics for dosing in adults

Opioid	Oral Dose for Severe Pain in Adults
Morphine (MS Contin, Avinza, Kadian)	15–30 mg q3-4 h (short acting) Dosages may vary for long-acting formulations
Codeine (generic)	15–60 mg q4 h
Codeine (with acetaminophen) (Tylenol #3)	15–60 mg q4 h
Hydrocodone (with acetaminophen) (Vicodin)	5–7.5 mg q4-6 h
Oxycodone (Oxycontin)	5–15 mg q4-6 h
Oxycodone (with acetaminophen) (Percocet)	2.5–10 mg q4-6 h
Hydromorphone (Dilaudid)	2–8 mg q3-6 h
Levorphanol (Levo-Dromoran)	2–3 mg q6-8 h
Meperidine (Demerol)	50–150 mg q3-4 h
Pentazocine (Talwin NX)	50 mg q3-4 h (contains also naloxone)
Tramadol (Ultram)	50–100 mg q4-6 h. MAX 400 mg/d

Note: For formulations containing acetaminophen: MAX 4000 mg acetaminophen/24 h.

Table 6
Opioid dosages for children

Opioid Medication	Starting Dose for Children (Oral)
Morphine Oral - immediate release	1–2 y: 200–400 µg/kg q4 h 2–12 y: 200–500 µg/kg q4 h (max 5 mg)
Morphine Oral - prolonged release	200–800 µg/kg q12 h
Hydromorphone Oral - immediate release	30–80 µg/kg q3–4 h (max 2 mg/dose)
Oxycodone Oral - immediate release	125–200 µg/kg q4 h (max 5 mg/dose)
Oxycodone Oral - prolonged release	5 mg q12 h
Hydrocodone	100–200 µg/kg q4 h
Codeine	0.5–1 m/kg q4 h
Tramadol	1–2 mg/kg q6 h (max per dose: 100 mg max per day 400 mg)

mcg = µg; 1 mg = 1000 µg
Adapted from World Health Organization (WHO). WHO guidelines on the pharmacological treatment of persisting pain in children with medical illnesses. Geneva (Switzerland): World Health Organization; 2012.

Fentanyl

Fentanyl is available in transdermal extended release formulation and sublingual spray, both prescribed by pain specialists to chronic pain patients. The IV form, however, may be encountered in the dental care outpatient setting because qualified practitioners may administer it during IV sedation.

Remifentanil

Remifentanil is a potent, ultra–short-acting opioid that is also used in the outpatient IV sedation setting. It works best when combined with another agent (like propofol), especially using computer controlled infusion pumps.

Naloxone

Naloxone (Narcan) is an µ-opioid receptor competitive antagonist, and is usually administered parenterally to counter the effects of opioid overdose. It has no analgesic effects.

Codeine

Codeine is a weak µ opioid agonist used as an analgesic and as an antitussive. Codeine is considered a prodrug because it is metabolized in vivo to the primary active compounds morphine and codeine-6-glucuronide. This metabolism of codeine takes place in the liver through the actions of CYP2D6 enzyme. Most patients have normal CYP2D6 activity and their codeine response is normal. A substantial minority of patients, however, expresses genetic polymorphism that is racially and ethnically influenced and has CYP2D6 activity that is higher or lower than normal.[13]

a. Higher activity means increased conversion to morphine and excessive sedation, constipation and side effects. Ultrarapid metabolizers are found in about 1% of people from Finland and Denmark, about 4% in Caucasian North Americans, about

10% of people from Greece and Portugal, about 20% in Saudi Arabia, and almost 30% of people from Ethiopia.
b. Lower activity means that codeine is unlikely to be an effective painkiller. Total CYP2D6 deficiency occurs in about 6% to 10% of Caucasians, 3% to 6% of Mexican Americans, 2% to 5% of African Americans, and about 1% of Asian Americans.

Also, people with normal CYP2D6 activity may be taking drugs that substantially inhibit CYP2D6, rendering codeine ineffective (**Table 7**). Because of case reports involving morbidity and mortality owing to the use of codeine in children with higher enzymatic activity, the European Medicines Agency restricted the use of codeine to children over 12 years of age. Additionally, the US Food and Drug Administration issued a boxed warning in 2012 regarding avoiding codeine for postoperative pain in children undergoing tonsillectomy. The warning says that, "for management of other types of pain in children, codeine should only be used if the benefits are anticipated to outweigh the risks."[14] Dental pain may very well fit into this description.

The most common formulation is in combination with acetaminophen. Examples of brand names are Tylenol #3 and Tylenol #4.

Oxycodone

Oxycodone is a weak opioid agonist used either alone or in combination with NSAIDs or acetaminophen for analgesia. Because oxycodone does not rely on active metabolites there are no considerations regarding enzymatic activity addressed previously for codeine. Examples of brand names include:

- *Plain:* Oxycontin, Roxicodone;
- *With acetaminophen:* Percocet, Roxicet, Narvox;
- *With aspirin:* Percodan, Endodan; and
- *With ibuprofen:* Combunox.

Hydrocodone

Hydrocodone is a weak opioid agonist used in combination with NSAIDs or acetaminophen for analgesia. Hydrocodone shares the same considerations regarding

Table 7
Medications that inhibit CYP2D6 enzyme

Generic Name	Brand Name
Amiodarone	Cordarone
Bupropion	Wellbutrin
Chloroquine	Aralen
Cinacalcet	Sensipar
Diphenhydramine	Benadryl
Fluoxetine	Prozac
Haloperidol	Haldol
Imatinib	Gleevec
Paroxetine	Paxil
Propafenone	Rythmol
Quinidine	Quinidex
Terbinafine	Lamisil
Thioridazine	Mellaril

enzymatic activity addressed previously for codeine. The plain form is formulated as extended release and is used for chronic pain. It can be found also in cough suppressing drug combinations. Examples of brand names include:

- *Plain:* Hysingla extended release, Zohydro extended release;
- *With acetaminophen:* Vicodin, Lorcet, Lortab, Hycet; and
- *With ibuprofen:* Vicoprophen, Ibudone, Reprexain.

Pentazocine

Pentazocine is a κ opioid receptor agonist and a μ opioid receptor antagonist. Its analgesic effects are subject to a ceiling effect. Pentazocine is more likely to cause hallucinations and other psychotomimetic effects. It is provided in combination with naloxone. Naloxone is not orally bioavailable and it produces no effect when administered orally, but it blocks the opioid effects of pentazocine if injected intravenously for recreational purposes. Examples of brand names include Talwin NX.

Hydromorphone

Hydromorphone is a μ-opioid agonist and is better absorbed orally than morphine. It is also faster acting and more potent that morphine. Examples of brand names include Dilaudid and Exalgo.

Propoxyphene (Darvon)

Propoxyphene (Darvon) has been discontinued since 2010.

Tapentadol

Tapentadol is a recently approved medication with a dual mechanism: μ-opioid receptor agonist and norepinephrine reuptake inhibitor. It has equal analgesic effect, with a lower incidence of side effects, when compared with morphine and oxycodone. The potential for dependency is not fully clarified yet emerging data are favorable.[15] Brand names include Nucynta.

Tramadol

Tramadol is a synthetic substance that shows both opioid and nonopioid properties. It is an atypical opioid that structurally is related to codeine, but it is 10 times less potent. Tramadol undergoes hepatic metabolism that is dependent on CYP2D6. It is a weak agonist for μ-opioid and κ-opioid receptors and a norepinephrine and serotonin reuptake inhibitor.[16] Owing to this monoaminergic action, may also exhibit antidepressant and anxiolytic-like effects.[16] The advantage of tramadol is that it displays a lower incidence of side effects and abuse potential. It can be considered a preferable choice for pain relief compared with NSAIDs because their long-term use may lead to impairment of renal function and cause gastrointestinal complications, and with respect to other opioid medications for its low addiction rate and favorable safety profile. The most troubling adverse effect of tramadol is nausea and vomiting, especially with oral administration.[17] Also, caution should be exercised in patients with seizure disorder. Metabolizes in the liver. As of August of 2014 the Drug Enforcement Administration has placed Tramadol into schedule IV of the Controlled Substances Act. Examples of brand name include Ultram, Ryzolt, ConZip, and Ultracet (combined with acetaminophen).

NONSTEROIDAL ANTIINFLAMMATORY DRUGS

Aspirin and other NSAIDs are among the most widely used classes of drugs, with both prescription and over-the-counter sales of the agents contributing to total usage. NSAIDs are a group of chemically heterogeneous compounds with several pharmacologic actions like:

1. Antiinflammatory: to relieve symptoms of inflammation.
2. Analgesic: the alleviation of pain, which is one of the major reasons of patients seeking medical assistance.
3. Antipyretic: the lowering of fever owing to increased prostaglandin levels in the hypothalamic thermoregulatory area. NSAIDs do not decrease normal body temperature and they do not decrease temperature elevated by nonprostaglandin mechanisms (like with exercise).
4. Antiplatelet: inhibition of platelet aggregation and consequent prolongation of bleeding time.

Mechanism of Action

Their principal mechanism involves inhibition of the synthesis of prostaglandins, specifically the action of cyclooxygenase (COX), the initial enzyme in the pathway of prostaglandin synthesis from arachidonic acid. The COX enzyme has 2 isoforms: COX-1 and COX-2. COX-1 is formed continuously without external stimulus in many tissues, including the stomach, platelets, kidney, and synovium. Low levels of expression are found, however, in most cell types. COX-2 is an inducible enzyme; its activity is increased by various physiologic conditions including inflammation. COX-2 is found mostly in the synovium, brain, kidney, and female reproductive tract.

All of the NSAIDs essentially inhibit the COX active site, but subtle mechanism variances in the way in which individual NSAIDs interact and bind with the active site are responsible for some of the differences in their pharmacologic characteristics. Acetylsalicylic acid is the only irreversible inhibitor of COX-1 and COX-2, whereas all of the other NSAIDs are competitive (therefore reversible) inhibitors of arachidonic acid for binding in the active site. More recent studies suggest that there may be other mechanisms of action, like inhibition of free radical formation, cytokine synthesis, or major cellular signaling pathways mediating inflammatory responses.[18]

NSAIDs generally are grouped according to their chemical structure, plasma half-life, and COX-1 versus COX-2-selectivity (**Table 8**). Some pharmacodynamics and pharmacokinetics parameters for representative NSAIDs are illustrated in **Table 9**.

Side Effects

Gastrointestinal
Products of normal COX activity (mainly COX-1) include inflammatory mediators but also prostanoids that are critical to the maintenance of the gastric mucosal lining and certain renal functions. Therefore, inhibition of COX may lead to gastric ulceration and renal damage.

Renal
The renal effects include sodium retention and peripheral edema, increase in mean arterial pressure, attenuation of antihypertensive medications effects, and an idiosyncratic reaction accompanied by massive proteinuria and acute interstitial nephritis. The relatively recent development of selective COX-2 inhibitors introduced a class of NSAIDs with gastrointestinal-protective properties[19] but evidently not completely renal safe.[20]

Table 8
Classification of common nonsteroidal antiinflammatory drugs

Category	Subclass	Generic	Brand
Carboxylic acid	Salicylic acids	Acetylsalicylic acid	Aspirin
		Diflunisal	Dolobid
		Salsalate	Disalcid, Salflex, Amigesic
	Acetic acids	Diclofenac	Voltaren, Cataflam, Solaraze, Rexaphenac
		Etodolac	Lodine
		Indomethacin	Indocin
		Sulindac	Clinoril
		Tolmetin	Tolectin
		Ketorolac	Toradol, Acular
	Proprionic acids	Ibuprofen	Advil, Motrin, Caldolor, Bufen, Genpril
		Ketoprofen	Orudis, Oruvail
		Flurbiprofen	Ansaid, Ocufen
		Naproxen	Naprosyn, Aleve, Anaprox, Naprelan
		Oxaprozin	Daypro
		Fenoprofen	Nalfon
	Fenamic acids	Meclofenamate	—
Enolic acids	Oxicames	Piroxicam	Feldene
		Meloxicam	Mobic
Non-acid	—	Nabumetone	Relafen
Cyclooxgygenase-2 selective	—	Celecoxib	Celebrex

Cardiovascular

Recently, there has been increasing evidence of cardiovascular risk elevation by all NSAIDs (apart from aspirin [ASA]), whether COX selective or not. It is understood that modulation of the COX pathways leads to important physiologic changes in cardiovascular homeostasis and that presents a concern specifically regarding chronic use. Recent metaanalyses[21] concluded that the risk for major cardiovascular events is small (lower that suggested by earlier studies) in low cardiovascular risk patients. In high-risk patients, both short- and long-term administration of NSAIDs not only increases the risk of major cardiovascular events and death, but also that risk persists for 5 years or longer.[22] Therefore, a patient's medical history and cardiovascular risk assessment should be thorough and NSAIDs selection should be tailored.

Studies suggest that naproxen has the best safety profile compared with other NSAIDs in relation to cardiovascular risk.[23] Diclofenac, instead, and a couple of recently discontinued COX-2 inhibitors, demonstrated consistently higher cardiovascular risk.[24]

The long-term administration of NSAIDs for chronic pain can be challenging. If desired, then patients will require laboratory monitoring for gastrointestinal complications, as well as renal and hepatic impairment. Baseline values should be established and, depending also on medical comorbidities and other concomitant medications, laboratory studies at regular intervals should be instituted.

Pediatric Use

In children, the main risk in taking NSAIDs is dosage errors resulting in overdose, which can cause substantial morbidity, or even death. Among NSAIDs, the most

Table 9

Pharmacodynamics and pharmacokinetics of some representative nonsteroidal antiinflammatory drugs

Medication	Onset of Action (h)	Duration of Action (h)	Bioavailability (%)	Time to Peak Concentration (h)	Protein Binding	Metabolism	Elimination Half-life
ASA	0.5	4–6	50–75	1–2	75–90	Hepatic	3–10
Diflunisal	1	8–12	80–90	2–3	99	Hepatic	8–12
Diclofenac	1–4.5	12–24	100	1–2	99	Hepatic	1–2
Ibuprofen	0.5–1	4–6	85	1–2	90–99	Hepatic	2–4
Naproxen	1	6–7	95	1–2	99	Hepatic	12–17
Indomethacin	0.5	4–6	100	2	99	Hepatic and enterohepatic recirculation	4–5
Piroxicam	1	Variable	n/a	3–5	99	Hepatic and enterohepatic recirculation	40–50
Celecoxib	0.75	4–8	n/a	3	97	Hepatic	11
Ketorolac	0.2	6–8	100	0.75	99	Hepatic	5

popular in pediatrics are ibuprofen followed by naproxen. Overall, between all analgesics, acetaminophen (nonopiod non-NSAID, reviewed further elsewhere in this paper) is the most broadly used drug in children and consists the preferred first-line agent because of its superior tolerability profile.

Although the magnitude and extend of gastrointestinal complications of NSAIDs in children is not thoroughly documented, yet is perceived to be less than the one on adults.[25] Gastroprotective medications are usually not necessary. Food is recommended with administration of NSAIDs to reduce risk.

In general NSAIDs should be avoided in:

- Children currently treated for asthma;
- Children who have history of asthma, urticaria, rhinitis, or sinusitis precipitated by NSAIDs;
- Children with impaired renal function;
- Children with impaired coagulation mechanism;
- Children on anticoagulation medications; and
- Children on nephrotoxic medications, like aminoglycoside antibiotics (eg, gentamycin, neomycin, and amicasin).

Tolerance of NSAIDs in pediatric patients has been reported as excellent for up to 3 weeks of use, yet administration should be limited to the first few days after the procedure.

There has been a lot of interest and discussion regarding preemptive use of analgesics in children to reduce intraoperative pain and need for postoperative analgesia. The outcomes, so far, are not encouraging; a large recent metaanalysis could not determine whether or not preoperative analgesics are of benefit in pediatric dental patients for procedures under local anesthetic.[26] Pediatric dosage suggestions for most common NSAIDs and acetaminophen are illustrated in **Table 10**.

The following is a further discussion on the 2 most popular NSAIDs in the dental care setting.

Acetylsalicylic acid (aspirin, ASA), the prototype NSAID, deserves special discussion. One of the most noteworthy reports of the use of salicylic acid comes from the father of modern medicine, Hippocrates, the Greek physician (c. 460–377 BC), who wrote that willow leaves and bark relieved pain and fever. Later, Dioscorides (c. 40–90 AD) a Greek physician and author of the precursor to all pharmacopeias ("Περί ύλης ιατρικής" or "De Materia Medica" in Latin) described willow bark (derived from the plant Salix alba) as an antiinflammatory agent. In high doses (3-4 g/d), it is used for inflammatory conditions such as osteoarthritis, rheumatic fever, rheumatoid

Table 10 Dosages for common analgesics in children			
Medication	Dose (mg/kg)	Frequency (h)	Max per day (mg/kg/d)
Aspirin	10–15	4–6	90
Ibuprofen	5–10	6–8	40
Naproxen	5–10	12	20
Acetaminophen children	10–15	4–6	Children: 100
Acetaminophen infants	10	4–6	Infants: 75

Adapted from World Health Organization (WHO). WHO guidelines on the pharmacological treatment of persisting pain in children with medical illnesses. Geneva (Switzerland): World Health Organization; 2012.

arthritis, and dysmenorrhea. ASA use is also popular for symptomatic relief of fever, headaches, and muscular and joint pains.

In low doses (80–325 mg/d), it is well-established that ASA, owing to the antiplatelet action, is the only NSAID used for prevention and treatment for cardiovascular disease, transient ischemic attacks and stroke either in primary or secondary prophylaxis. ASA reduces the risks of cardiovascular events by around 15% and myocardial infarction by around 30%.[27,28]

ASA mainly, and other NSAIDs, may exacerbate respiratory disease in a small percentage of patients with asthma by COX-1 inhibition–driven bronchoconstriction. This is often referred to as aspirin-induced asthma.[29] Also, these medications may cause rhinitis and sinusitis symptoms in patients with nasal polyps. Various desensitization protocols have been developed to treat aspirin-induced asthma, especially in patients who need to continue using ASA.[30]

ASA is contraindicated in pregnancy at high (analgesic) doses because it crosses the placenta and may harm the fetus.

In children, ASA use is not recommended particularly for undiagnosed fever when influenza is suspected, owing to risk of Reye syndrome (a rare disorder presented by symptoms of encephalitis combined with evidence of liver failure). This potentially fatal condition occurs after certain viral infections like chickenpox, or those accompanied by minor fever. It is characterized by vomiting and lethargy, which may progress to delirium and coma. Acetaminophen should be used instead. There are certain exceptions in using ASA for children, like rheumatologic conditions, but will not usually involve the dental care provider.

Ibuprofen is a well-proven and popular analgesic. Metaanalyses show that ibuprofen produces greater analgesia than acetaminophen/codeine combinations.[31] Ibuprofen was found, with high-quality evidence and in relation to oral surgery, to be a superior analgesic to plain paracetamol, at doses of 200 to 512 mg and 600 to 1000 mg, respectively.[32] This analgesia is dose dependent over the range of 200 to 800 mg. Obviously, alleviation of pain and side effects should be balanced. Maximum daily dose for adults is 3200 mg. Ibuprofen follows the broad pharmacologic principles outlined earlier and it is used effectively also in combination with other analgesics like oxycodone and hydrocodone.

NONOPIOID, NON-NSAID DRUGS

Acetaminophen (paracetamol), like ASA, is an analgesic with equal efficacy for mild to moderate pain and an antipyretic.

Mechanism of Action and Pharmacokinetics

Unlike ASA, acetaminophen does not have a significant effect on platelets or on inflammation. It has no effect on gastric mucosal lining therefore cannot produce the gastric ulceration, common with NSAIDs. Acetaminophen does not inhibit COX-1 or COX-2 enzymes like NSAIDs do. In contrast with NSAIDs, the mechanism of action of acetaminophen includes blockade of prostaglandin and substance P production and modulation of nitric oxide production. Details of the mechanism still need further elucidation.

The gastrointestinal tract, after oral administration, rapidly absorbs acetaminophen. The binding to plasma proteins is dose dependent and ranges between 5% and 50%. It reaches maximum plasma concentration after oral administration in 30 to 90 minutes. The terminal half-life of elimination is 1.5 to 2.5 hours, and the usual dosage is 325 to 1000 mg every 4 to 6 hours as needed and maximum daily dose for adults is 4 g that must not be exceeded. In a large metaanalysis evaluating the effectiveness of acetaminophen alone in controlling pain after oral surgery (third molar removal), it was found both effective and safe.[33] The most effective scheme was 1000 mg every 6 hours.

Side Effects

A small proportion of acetaminophen is metabolized to the highly toxic nucleophilic N-acetyl-benzoquinoneimine that is usually inactivated by reaction with sulfhydryl groups in glutathione. However, ingestion of large doses of acetaminophen, and consequent hepatic depletion of glutathione, may result in potentially fatal hepatic necrosis. At early stages, overdose can be antagonized within the administration of N-acetylcysteine. It is thus essential to assess patient's liver function and avoid acetaminophen in patients with liver impairment or history of alcohol abuse. Recently, the US Food and Drug Administration recognized the potential hepatotoxicity of acetaminophen and reduced its strength in prescription drugs (like opioid/acetaminophen combinations) to 325 mg per dosage unit. Also, because of the hepatotoxicity, very careful calculation of appropriate dosages is necessary for administration in children.

Pediatric Use

Regarding use in children, recent studies of acetaminophen, when used in association with NSAIDs, have demonstrated real and significant reductions in opioid requirements in children after surgery.[34] Thus, opioid use to control moderate to severe pain after oral surgery in children should always be accompanied by acetaminophen and NSAIDs, unless they are contraindicated.

Use during pregnancy used to be considered absolutely safe. This concept is under scrutiny and our former beliefs may be soon questioned and administration guidelines altered.[35,36] Examples of brand names include Tylenol, Aminophen, Feverall, Genapap, and Ofirmev.

Interesting Facts and Suggestions

- Generally and from a strictly clinical point of view, there are no clear algorithms to assist in selecting the most appropriate NDAID for a patient. No definite evidence specifies that a particular NSAID is more effective, or safer, than other members of this drug group. The basis for selection depends on clinical experience, patient convenience, side effects, and cost.
- Most cases of postprocedural dental pain will respond well to NSAIDs as a first-line approach. If NSAIDs are contraindicated, then acetaminophen is the choice. Furthermore, combination of an NSAID with acetaminophen provides greater analgesic efficacy than does either agent alone.[37]
- Regarding opioid medications, different agents will have equal analgesic effect if given at equipotent doses. Effective pain control is established on selecting an optimal dose, rather than selecting a particular agent. Patient-specific variables, however, may direct toward choosing a specific opioid.
- Use of NSAIDs within 3 to 6 months of an acute cardiovascular event, or procedure, is contraindicated.
- NSAIDs may increase the activity or toxicity of sulfonylurea, hypoglycemic agents, oral anticoagulants, phenytoin, and sulfonamides by displacing these medications from their protein binding sites and increasing the plasma level of the free form of those medications. A clinician should be vigilant on appreciating the patient's medication list.

- There is an increased risk of gastrointestinal toxicity when NSAIDs and selective serotonin reuptake inhibitors are taken concomitantly compared with taking either medication alone.[38] Thus, patients taking serotonin reuptake inhibitors for depression or for anxiety and eating disorders may be considered high risk for gastrointestinal complications.
- For patients with history of gastric ulcers or at high risk for gastrointestinal complications choose a COX-2 inhibitor at lowest effective dose or a nonselective NSAID with a proton pump inhibitor (like omeprazole)for protection. The prior eradication of *Helicobacter pylori* also decreases the risk.
- In high-risk patients for complications, choose the lowest dose of a short-acting NSAID for the shortest time required and titrate.
- For chronic management of painful peripheral neuropathies, like trigeminal neuropathy, NSAIDs should not be used as primary therapy owing to lack of evidence-based support.
- Ketorolac is the only NSAID available, apart from oral, also for intramuscular administration. It can be used for moderate to severe pain (like postoperative pain) because it has an analgesic potency equal to a moderate dose of morphine.
- For analgesia of musculoskeletal pain in patients at high risk for cardiovascular events the American Heart Association recommends as first preference: acetaminophen, tramadol, and short-term opioid analgesics.[39]
- The World Health Organization has introduced an analgesic ladder (**Fig. 2**) and some fundamental recommendations regarding use for analgesics for cancer patients that essentially have being applied for all patients with either acute or chronic pain who require analgesics.[40,41]
  - Oral administrations should be preferred when possible.
  - Analgesics should be given at regular intervals. The dosage is calculated according to patients' pain level and adjusted until pain dissipates.
  - Analgesic schemes should match pain intensity. Pain intensity can be determined after clinical examination and adequate pain assessment. The patient's input is very important.
  - Dosages should be adapted to the individual, balancing adequate analgesia and side effects. There are no standardized recipes.

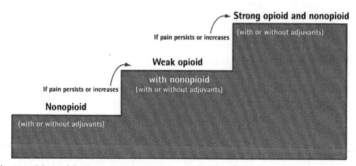

Fig. 2. The World Health Organization analgesic ladder for treating chronic pain. Adjuvant medications include steroids, anxiolytics, antidepressants, hypnotics, anticonvulsants, antiepileptic-like gabapentinoids (gabapentin and pregabalin), membrane stabilizers, sodium channel blockers, cannabinoids and N-methyl-D-aspartate receptor antagonists for the treatment of neuropathic pain. (*From* Vargas-Schaffer G. Is the WHO analgesic ladder still valid? Twenty-four years of experience. Can Fam Physician 2010;56(6):515; with permission.)

○ Prescriptions should be tailored. That dictates customization depending fluctuations of level of pain and time of day.

- Based on consensus guidelines by the American Academy of Pediatrics, ibuprofen, indomethacin, and naproxen are safe to use in breastfeeding women.[42]
- Use of ASA and NSAIDs in patients taking anticoagulants requires caution from prescribers. If concurrent NSAID and anticoagulant (like warfarin) use is necessary, an increase in International Normalized Ratio should be anticipated. There should be appropriate monitoring of the International Normalized Ratio.
- When prescribing combination products containing acetaminophen, the prescriber needs to calculate and inform the patient not to exceed 4 g of acetaminophen daily because of serious concerns for hepatotoxicity.
- In most cases where a patients' condition requires analgesia and there is an inflammatory component, NSAIDs will be the rational first-line agents.
- As research progresses, controlled-released formulations using microparticles or nanoparticles may soon improve sustainability of analgesia, tissue targeting, avoidance of side effects, and patient compliance.

REFERENCES

1. Cervero F, Laird JM. One pain or many pains? A new look at pain mechanisms. News Physiol Sci 1991;6:268–73.
2. Russo CM, Brose WG. Chronic pain. Annu Rev Med 1998;49:123–33.
3. Chapman CR, Gavrin J. Suffering: the contributions of persistent pain. Lancet 1999;353:2233–7.
4. Stein C, editor. Analgesia. Berlin; Heidelberg (Germany): Springer-Verlag; 2007. p. 31–145.
5. Brislin RP, Rose JB. Pediatric acute pain management. Anesthesiol Clin North Am 2005;23:789–814.
6. Brasher C, Gafsous B, Dugue S, et al. Postoperative pain management in children and infants: an update. Paediatr Drugs 2014;16:129–40.
7. Merkel SI, Voepel-Lewis T, Shayevitz JR, et al. The FLACC: a behavioral scale for scoring postoperative pain in young children. Pediatr Nurs 1997;23(3):293–7.
8. Labuz D, Mousa SA, Schäfer M, et al. Relative contribution of peripheral versus central opioid receptors to anti-nociception. Brain Res 2007;1160:30–8.
9. Servin F. Remifentanil; from pharmacological properties to clinical practice. Adv Exp Med Biol 2003;523:245–60.
10. Goodman LS, Gilman A, Brunton LL, et al. Anti-inflammatory, antipyretic, and analgesic agents. In Goodman & Gilman's. The pharmacological basis of therapeutics. Chapter 34. 11th edition. New York, NY: McGraw-Hill; 2006.
11. Bigby J, Reader A, Nusstein J, et al. Anesthetic efficacy of lidocaine/meperidine for inferior alveolar nerve blocks in patients with irreversible pulpitis. J Endod 2007;33(1):7–10.
12. Goodman A, Reader A, Nusstein J, et al. Anesthetic efficacy of lidocaine/meperidine for inferior alveolar nerve blocks. Anesth Prog 2006;53(4):131–9.
13. Haufroid V, Hantson P. CYP2D6 genetic polymorphisms and their relevance for poisoning due to amfetamines, opioid analgesics and antidepressants. Clin Toxicol (Phila) 2015;53(6):501–10.
14. Safety review update of codeine use in children; new Boxed Warning and Contraindication on use after tonsillectomy and/or adenoidectomy. U.S. Food and Drug

Administration. Drug Safety Communication; 2012. Available at: http://www.fda.gov/Drugs/DrugSafety/ucm313631.htm.

15. Tzschentke TM, Christoph T, Kogel B, et al. A novel m-opioid receptor agonist/norepinephrine reuptake inhibitor with broad-spectrum analgesic properties. J Pharmacol Exp Ther 2007;323(1):265–76.

16. Vazzana M, Andreani T, Fangueiro J, et al. Tramadol hydrochloride: pharmacokinetics, pharmacodynamics, adverse side effects, co-administration of drugs and new drug delivery systems. Biomed Pharmacother 2015;70:234–8.

17. Verghese ST, Hannallah RS. Postoperative pain management in children. Anesthesiology Clin N Am 2005;23:163–84.

18. Fernandes E, Costa D, Toste SA, et al. In vitro scavenging activity for reactive oxygen and nitrogen species by nonsteroidal anti-inflammatory indole, pyrrole, and oxazole derivative drugs. Free Radic Biol Med 2004;37:1895–905.

19. Jarupongprapa S. Comparison of gastrointestinal adverse effects between cyclooxygenase-2 inhibitors and non-selective, non-steroidal anti-inflammatory drugs plus proton pump inhibitors: a systematic review and meta-analysis. J Gastroenterol 2013 Jul;48(7):830–8.

20. Akhund L, Quinet RJ, Ishaq S. Celecoxib-related renal papillary necrosis. Arch Intern Med 2003;163:114–5.

21. Coxib and traditional NSAID Trialists' (CNT) Collaboration, Bhala N, Emberson J, Merhi A. Vascular and upper gastrointestinal effects of non-steroidal anti-inflammatory drugs: meta-analyses of individual participant data from randomized trials. Lancet 2013;382:769–79.

22. Anwar A. Elevation of cardiovascular risk by non-steroidal anti-inflammatory drugs. Trends Cardiovasc Med 2015;25(8):726–35.

23. Curiel RV, Katz JD. Mitigating the cardiovascular and renal effects of NSAIDs. Pain Med 2013;14(Suppl 1):S23–8.

24. McGettigan P, Henry D. Cardiovascular risk with non-steroidal anti-inflammatory drugs: systematic review of population-based controlled observational studies. PLoS Med 2011;8(9):e1001098.

25. Kokinsky E, Thornberg E. Postoperative pain control in children. Paediatr Drugs 2003;5(11):751–62.

26. Ashley PF, Parekh S, Moles DR, et al. Preoperative analgesics for additional pain relief in children and adolescents having dental treatment. Cochrane Database Syst Rev 2012;(9):CD008392.

27. Antithrombotic Trialists' Collaboration. Collaborative meta- analysis of randomized trials of antiplatelet therapy for prevention of death, myocardial infarction, and stroke in high risk patients. Br Med J 2002;324:71–86.

28. Botting RM. Vane's discovery of the mechanism of action of aspirin changed our understanding of its clinical pharmacology. Pharmacol Rep 2010;62:518–25.

29. Babu KS, Salvi SS. Aspirin and Asthma. Chest 2000;118:1470–6.

30. Park H, Kowalski ML, Sanchez-Borges M. Hypersensitivity to aspirin and other nonsteroidal antiinflammatory drugs. In: Adkinson Jr NF, Busse WW, Bochner BS, et al. Middleton's allergy. Principles and practice, vol. 80. 8th edition. Philadelphia, PA: Elsevier Science; 2014. p. 1296–309.

31. Ahmad N, Grad HA, Haas DA, et al. The efficacy of nonopioid analgesics for postoperative dental pain: a meta-analysis. Anesth Prog 1997;44:119–26.

32. Bailey E, Worthington HV, van Wijk A, et al. Ibuprofen and/or paracetamol (acetaminophen) for pain relief after surgical removal of lower wisdom teeth. Cochrane Database Syst Rev 2013;(12):CD004624.

33. Weil K, Hooper L, Afzal Z, et al. Paracetamol for pain relief after surgical removal of lower wisdom teeth. Cochrane Database Syst Rev 2007;(3):CD004487.
34. Wong I, St John-Green C, Walker SM, et al. Opioid-sparing effects of perioperative paracetamol and nonsteroidal anti-inflammatory drugs (NSAIDs) in children. Paediatr Anaesth 2013;23(6):475–95.
35. Liew Z, Ritz B, Rebordosa C, et al. Acetaminophen use during pregnancy, behavioral problems, and hyperkinetic disorders. JAMA Pediatr 2014;168:313–20.
36. Brandlistuen RE, Ystrom E, Nulman I, et al. Prenatal paracetamol exposure and child neurodevelopment: a sibling-controlled cohort study. Int J Epidemiol 2013;42:1702–13.
37. Hyllested M, Jones S, Pedersen JL, et al. Comparative effect of paracetamol, NSAIDs or their combination in postoperative pain management: a qualitative review. Br J Anaesth 2002;88:199–214.
38. Mort JR, Aparasu RR, Baer RK. Interaction between selective serotonin reuptake inhibitors and nonsteroidal anti-inflammatory drugs: review of the literature. Pharmacotherapy 2006;26:1307–13.
39. Antman EM, Bennett JS, Daugherty A, et al. Use of nonsteroidal anti-inflammatory drugs: an update for clinicians: a scientific statement from the American Heart Association. Circulation 2007 Mar 27;115(12):1634–42.
40. World Health Organization. Traitement de la douleur cancéreuse. Geneva (Switzerland): World Health Organization; 1997.
41. Vargas-Schaffer G. Is the WHO analgesic ladder still valid? Twenty-four years of experience. Can Fam Physician 2010;56(6):514–7.
42. American Academy of Pediatrics Committee on Drugs. The transfer of drugs and other chemicals into human milk. Pediatrics 1994;93(1):137–50.

Pharmacologic Treatment for Temporomandibular Disorders

Harry Dym, DDS[a],*, Dustin Bowler, DDS[b], Joseph Zeidan, DMD[b]

KEYWORDS

- Pharmacologic treatment • Temporomandibular disorders • Pain

KEY POINTS

- Temporomandibular disorders and its associated pain and dysfunction are known to be multifactorial in cause with many contributing causes, and consequently, the treatment of this condition is varied.
- Pharmacologic agents play an integral role in the overall management of temporomandibular joint disorder.
- A thorough knowledge of the various pharmacologic agents used in the treatment of temporomandibular dysfunction/temporomandibular joint disorders and pain is essential for the dentist or oral surgeon who wish to manage this segment of his or her clinical practice.

The use of drug therapy in the treatment of temporomandibular dysfunction/temporo-mandibular joint disorders (TMD/TMJ) should be viewed as merely adjunctive treatment as opposed to definitive treatment of this disorder. Temporomandibular disorders and its associated pain and dysfunction are known to be multifactorial in cause with many contributing causes, and consequently, the pharmacologic therapy used in treatment of this condition is varied (**Box 1**).

Most often,[1] inflammation is present either in the joint and its surrounding capsule or within the muscles of mastication. In addition, like many chronic facial pain conditions, anxiety and possibly depression may also contribute to the patient's symptoms. In addition, muscle spasms are often found to be associated with TMD/TMJ disorders caused by chronic clenching and hyperactivity of the masticatory musculature.

Finally, like many chronic facial pain conditions, there may over time develop a neuropathic cause for the patient's TMD/TMJ pain as well. Clearly with these varied

[a] Department of Dentistry/Oral & Maxillofacial Surgery, The Brooklyn Hospital Center, 121 Dek-alb Avenue, Box 187, Brooklyn, NY 11201, USA; [b] Division of Oral and Maxillofacial Surgery Residency Training Program, The Brooklyn Hospital Center's, Brooklyn, NY, USA
* Corresponding author.
E-mail address: hdymdds@yahoo.com

Dent Clin N Am 60 (2016) 367–379
http://dx.doi.org/10.1016/j.cden.2015.11.012
0011-8532/16/$ – see front matter Published by Elsevier Inc.

dental.theclinics.com

Box 1
Drugs used in the treatment of temporomandibular dysfunction/temporomandibular joint disorders

- NSAIDs
- Opioids
- Corticosteroids
- Antidepressants
- Muscle relaxants
- Sedative, hypnotics

---

etiologic factors, a clinician should be familiar with the different drug therapies noted in the literature to treat the various underlying etiologic condition associated with TMD disorders.

Certainly, as stated earlier, one must first perform a thorough physical/diagnostic survey of the patient with TMD/TMJ to determine the primary reason for the patient's presenting condition and address those concerns by instituting a variety of possible therapeutic interventions in addition to drug treatment:

- Muscle trigger point injections
- Fabrication of a splint/stent
- Instituting physical therapy
- Heat/cold applications to the involved muscles
- Arthrocentesis/arthroscopy
- Open joint surgery

However, medication management will often and should play a role in the overall management of the patient with TMD/TMJ. This article reviews the common types and categories of such drugs commonly in use and also discusses techniques and drugs used to perform intramuscular and intra-articular injections to treat temporomandibular disorders.

ANTIDEPRESSANTS

The biomedical literature supports the use of antidepressants to treat chronic nonmalignant (such as TMD/TMJ) pain, and multiple reviews of controlled studies of the use of antidepressants for pain management indicate that their analgesic effects are largely independent of their antidepressant activity.[2]

Studies in patients with nondental chronic pain also indicate that antidepressant medications, such as Amitriptyline, that inhibit both the reuptake of serotonin and norepinephrine, are more efficacious than drugs that are selective for either neurotransmitter.[3–5]

Analgesia occurs well before the antidepressant effect and at lower doses that are not effective for management of depression in many patients with chronic pain. This finding was confirmed in a study by Sharav and colleagues,[6] who showed that a low dose of Amitriptyline (mean dose 23–6 mg) was as effective for chronic orofacial pain as a higher dose (mean = 129 mg). The usual daily antidepressant dose of Amitriptyline is 75 mg to 150 mg daily.

The current biomedical literature supports the use of tricyclic antidepressants, such as Elavil (amitriptyline hydrochloride), which contains both serotonergic and noradrenergic effects in low doses of 25 mg to 75 mg for the treatment of chronic nonmalignant pain, such as TMD/TMJ conditions, when other treatments have failed or if depression accompanies the pain.

The dose of antidepressants will usually be limited by anticholinergic side effects, such as dry mouth, urinary retention, and blurred vision, and should be adjusted according to analgesic effects and side effects.

SPASMOLYTIC

Spasmolytics are drugs that eliminate muscular spasms and are often used in conjunction with physical therapy, heat, rest, and analgesics in treating patients with TMD/TMJ disorders (**Table 1**).

A drug in this category that has been demonstrated[7] to be effective in the treatment of chronic musculoskeletal disorders is cyclobenzaprine (Flexeril).

Although this drug has not been directly assessed for TMD, the scientific studies available suggest the efficacy of this drug in the treatment of muscle relaxation in the orofacial region.

Cyclobenzaprine acts primarily within the central nervous system (CNS) at the brainstem, as opposed to the spinal cord levels, and does not act directly on skeletal muscles.

It is recommended that Flexeril be used only for short periods of time (2 weeks) and should not be used in patients on monoamine oxidase inhibitors because it can, in such cases, lead to a hyper pyretic crisis, convulsions, or both.

ADVERSE EFFECTS OF CYCLOBENZAPRINE

Potential side effects include drowsiness, malaise, tachycardia, and dysrhythmia and may enhance effects of other CNS depressants, such as alcohol and barbiturates. This drug may also cause xerostomia.

DOSAGE

The usual dose for adults is 5 to 10 mg 3 times a day. The authors prefer to use 10 mg at bedtime so that the patient will not be very sluggish during the workday.

BENZODIAZAPINES

Drugs of the benzodiazepine class have been prescribed to patients who suffer from chronic orofacial pain of myogenic origin; they have been shown to be helpful in

Table 1 Muscle relaxants (spasmolytic)	
Drugs	**Dosage**
Chlorzoxazone (Parafon Forte)	250–500 mg 3 times daily Poorly tolerated in elderly
Cyclobenzaprine (Flexeril): do not use with monoamine oxidase inhibitors	10 mg at bedtime initially; 10 mg 3 times daily (usual adult dosage): do not use longer than 2–3 wk
Methocarbamol (Robaxin)	1500 mg 4 times daily for 2–3 d then decreased to 1000 mg 3 times daily
Orphenadrine (Norflex)	100 mg 2 times daily

multiple studies, especially when combined with Ibuprofen (**Table 2**). Although the use of Benzodiazepines in the treatment of chronic TMD pain has been discouraged by many because of the depression seen in some patients who take this class of drugs, it is thought by some authors[8] that the depression seen in these patients is not due to the Benzodiazepines themselves but rather due to some type of depressive symptom often seen in patients who suffer from chronic pain status.

NONSTEROIDAL ANTI-INFLAMMATORY DRUGS

The use of nonsteroidal anti-inflammatory drugs (NSAIDs) has been developed as a first-line treatment for TMD. NSAIDs have a multifactorial influence on the TMJ and its function. TMD disorders have 2 separate and distinct physical causes: internal joint derangement and dysfunction associated with activity of the muscles of mastication. NSAIDs help address these noted causes of TMD pain.

NSAIDs' anti-inflammatory properties can help alleviate pressure and pain within the joint. In addition, the analgesic effects can give the patient respite from the often constant and potentially debilitating pain associated with acute and chronic TMJ pain of both the masticatory muscles and the involved TMJs.

Prescribers tend to be inclined to prescribe naproxen as the first-line treatment for patients with TMJ disorders, although many NSAID options exist. Lists of the most commonly prescribed NSAIDs are found in **Tables 3** and **4**.

Naproxen has been shown to produce more pain relief than celecoxib and placebos.[9] Typical doses used for treatment of acute and chronic TMJ pain are 500 mg twice daily, a dose similar to those recommended for treatment of osteoarthritis. The dosages may be increased to a maximum of 750 mg twice daily as needed. The prescribed NSAIDs can be used in conjunction with muscle-relaxant medications. When multiple pharmaceuticals are prescribed, it is common practice to initiate treatment with the more conservative doses and advance as necessary on an individual basis depending on patient response.

Additional NSAIDs, including ibuprofen, celecoxib, piroxicam, and diclofenac, have been used with varying frequency and effectiveness (see **Table 4**). Ibuprofen (400 mg) has been referred to as the gold standard for pain control and is a popular choice among prescribers for the alleviation of TMD pain symptoms.

NSAIDs are widely used with few and typically minor side effects. NSAIDs inhibit cyclo-oxygenase (COX) in 2 forms: COX-1, which is found in the stomach, kidneys, and platelets; and COX-2, which functions as part of the inflammatory process. The inhibition of COX-2 is beneficial in the treatment of TMD, and COX-1 functions as a protective agent for the gastrointestinal tract. Prescribers can use proton pump inhibitors, H2 antagonists, and prostaglandin E1 analogues, such as Nexium, Ranitidine, and Misoprostol, respectively, in concert with NSAIDs to minimize the gastrointestinal side effects of NSAID use during TMD treatment.

Prescribers must be aware, as with any prescriptions, whether patients are healthy enough and do not display any medical comorbidities that could lead to the

Table 2 Tranquilizers/anxiolytics/benzodiazepines	
Drugs	**Dosages**
Alprazolam (Xanax)	0.25–0.5 mg 3 times daily; maximum dose 4 mg/d
Diazepam (Valium)	2–10 mg 2–4 times daily
Lorazepam (Atavan)	1–2 mg 2 times daily

Table 3	
Commonly prescribed nonsteroidal anti-inflammatory drug groups	
Drug Group	**Example**
Propionic acid	Flurbiprofen, ibuprofen, ketoprofen, naproxen
Fenamic acid	Menfenamic acid
Salicylic acid	Aspirin, diflunisal, salsalate
Acetic acid	Diclofenac, etodolac, indomethacin, ketorolac, sulindac, tolmetin

From Laskin DM, Giglio JA. The use of steroids and nonsteroidal anti-inflammatory drugs in oral and maxillofacial surgery. Oral Maxillofac Surg Clin North Am 2001;13(1):38; with permission.

contraindication of use of the medications. Prescribers should be specifically cognizant of any past medical history that includes gastrointestinal tract dysfunction, including ulcers and/or bleeding. Additional care should be used when prescribing to patients with compromised liver or renal function because the concentrations of active NSAID metabolites may reach increased levels, resulting in significant side effects even with the use of normal recommended doses.

It is unrealistic and illogical to treat all forms and stages of TMJ pain and TMD with one modality. Notwithstanding, many patients can benefit from treatment of TMJ pain and TMD with pharmaceuticals in concert and as an intermediate intervention to more invasive or surgical treatment.

Table 4		
Commonly used NSAIDs in treatment of temporomandibular dysfunction		
	Brand Name	**Dosage**
Diclofenac	Voltaren	50 mg 3 times/d
Diflunisal	Dolobid	250 mg 2 times/d
Etodolac	Ultradrol	300 mg 2 times/d
Fenoprofen	Nalfon, Naprofen	200–600 mg 3–4 times/d
Flurbiprofen (systemic)	Ansaid	100 mg 2 times/d
Ibuprofen	Motrin, Advil	600 mg 3 times/d
Indomethacin	Indocin	25 mg 3 times/d
Ketoprofen	Orudis	50 mg 3 times/d
Ketorolac	Toradol	10 mg 4 times/d (po)
Meclofenamate	Meclomen	50 mg 4 times/d
Mefenamic acid	Ponstel	250 mg 4 times/d
Nabumetone	Relafen	1 g 4 times/d
Naproxen	Aleve	200–500 mg every 12 h (po)
Oxaprozin	Daypro	600 mg
Piroxicam	Feldene	20 mg 4 times/d
Sulindac	Clinoril	150 mg 2 times/d
Tolmetin	Tolectin	200–600 mg 3 times/d

From Dym H, Isreal H. Diagnosis and treatment of temporomandibular disorders. Dent Clin N Am 2012;56(1):156; with permission.

Corticosteroids in Intra-Articular Injections

Different therapeutic solutions can be administered by intra-articular injection into the TMJ space to allow for targeted treatment of inflammation and joint degeneration. Administration of medications into the TMJ space is commonly performed in conjunction with arthrocentesis or arthroscopy. The superior joint space is commonly used; however, recent evidence suggests that administration of medications into the inferior joint space, or in combination of the superior and inferior joint spaces, is more effective in increasing incisal opening and decreasing TMJ pain.[10]

Corticosteroids are powerful anti-inflammatory agents that can be administered orally or intra-articularly. There are multiple mechanisms of action, such as the blockade of phospholipase A_2, which decreases the production of proinflammatory prostaglandins and leukotrienes, as well as a decrease in the number and activity of proinflammatory cells, including lymphocytes, eosinophils, basophils, and macrophages. There are multiple well-documented clinical trials demonstrating the therapeutic benefit of corticosteroids in patients with TMD.[11] A variety of corticosteroids and doses has been reported in the literature. In uncontrolled case studies of arthritic TMJs, intra-articular steroids have been used, such as 0.7 mL methylprednisolone acetate 40 mg/mL (Depo-Medrol) combined with local anesthetics in children, or 1 mL triamcinolone acetonide (Kenalog-40), or 1 mL triamcinolone hexacetonide (THA; Aristospan-20) in adults.[11] The intra-articular injection is also performed with prednisolone trimethylacetate 25 mg.[12] Intra-articular steroid injections can be performed in the superior joint space using THA with either 5 or 10 mg per TMJ with or without a local anesthetic, such as 1% lidocaine, in patients with juvenile idiopathic arthritis. THA has been found to be superior to triamcinolone acetonide, betamethasone, and methylprednisolone acetate in the treatment of arthritis in patients with non-TMJs.[13]

Concerns exist regarding the use of corticosteroids in TMJ arthritis, with one animal model in rabbits demonstrating arrest of the mandibular growth plate, although this was not noted in other animal models or in human studies. Documented adverse effects from intra-articular steroid injections include a case report of ankylosis in an adult with a trauma-related TMJ disorder and a case series of osteoarthritis in adults who suffered damage to the condylar head (fibrous layer, cartilage, bone), hypopigmentation, facial swelling, and lipoatrophy.[13] One investigator reported repeated injections with betamethasone; however, the injections did not improve or worsen radiologic signs of joint inflammation over a 6-month period, but did improve pain scores.[14] Others have reported intra-articular destruction, infection, and disease progression due to overly aggressive intra-articular corticosteroid injections and recommend that this treatment should only be administered in severe cases and that frequent injections must be avoided.[10] Repeated intra-articular injections of corticosteroids are of limited use in other joints in the body due to risk of infection, and destruction of articular cartilage, tendon, or ligament attachments.[12] Repeated intra-articular corticosteroid injections into the TMJ have been implicated in the chemical condylectomy phenomenon. Intra-articular injections of steroids are not routinely recommended in patients who have low inflammation arthritic conditions and should only be considered in patients with acute high inflammation of the TMJ and be limited to 2 injections in 6 months. After injections, decreased activities within pain-free limits should be recommended to prevent acceleration of the degenerative process.[12]

Corticosteroids in intramuscular injections

TMD can be divided into articular and nonarticular disorders. Most nonarticular disorders are related to myofascial pain of the muscles of mastication. In addition to myofascial pain, nonarticular pain disorders include chronic conditions such as fibromyalgia, muscle strain, and myopathies. Myofascial pain is theorized to arise from clenching, bruxism, or other parafunctional habits with resulting masticatory musculature strain, spasm, pain, and functional limitation. Myofascial pain can be treated with several modalities, including combinations of nonsteroidal anti-inflammatory medications, occlusal guards, physical therapy, muscle relaxants, and injectable local anesthetic/steroid combinations into the masticatory muscle insertion points[10] (**Fig. 1**).

Fibromyalgia is a common condition of muscle aching, stiffness, generalized fatigue, and nonrestorative sleep pattern with multiple myofascial tender points. Although there is no universally definitive treatment for fibromyalgia, treatment programs rely on pain management counseling for patient self-management and lifestyle modification. Medical treatments depend on nonsteroidal analgesics and low-dose tricyclic antidepressants to increase pain tolerance and normalize sleep. Tender-point injections with local anesthetics combined with corticosteroids along with spray and stretch physical therapy may bring about sustained remissions.[15] Temporomandibular myofascial pain and dysfunction (TMD) is distinguished from primary fibromyalgia by pain being confined to the head and neck, the pattern of referred pain, and specific trigger points. Musculoskeletal tender-point block therapies using local anesthetics with adrenocorticosteroids such as bupivacaine-dexamethasone have proven to be valuable. Blocks may reduce pain for 1 to 3 months and can be combined with physical therapy programs.[15] When chronic pain is localized, it can be relieved temporarily with local anesthetic blocks, sometimes for a prolonged duration. Infiltration of a local anesthetic/glucocorticoid with adjunctive therapies, such as stretching, cold, massage, or exercise, may prolong the benefits. Patients with uncomplicated myofascial pain are likely to benefit from this treatment, but those with more complex chronic pain conditions will need a more comprehensive approach.[16]

Local anesthetic administration of a long-acting agent such as bupivacaine combined with a corticosteroid is also used for treatment of trigeminal neuralgia. Although this technique is used empirically by many practitioners, there is a lack of definitive support from controlled studies in the literature.[15]

Hyaluronic acid
What is it? Hyaluronic acid (HA) or its salt, sodium hyaluronate (SH), is a glycosaminoglycan found in epithelial, neural, and connective tissue. It is a highly viscous

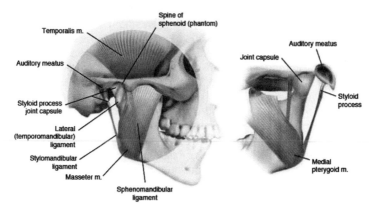

Fig. 1. Musculoskeletal structures of TMJ (lateral and medial views). m., muscle. (*From* Liu F, Steinkeler A. Epidemiology, diagnosis, and treatment of temporomandibular disorders. Dent Clin North Am 2013;57(3):465–79; with permission.)

high-molecular-weight substance that plays an important role in joint lubrication and protection of cartilage.[17] HA is also involved in buffering, nutrition, anti-inflammation, and cartilage repair.[18] In double-blind studies in hips, shoulders, and knees, HA has been shown to provide significantly better sustained results for 1 year than saline.[12] Studies support the efficacy of HA injections to treat TMJ internal derangements, with more recent evidence suggesting that it may be effective in inflammatory-degenerative disorders as well, especially if combined with joint lavage.[19] Injection of exogenous HA can stimulate endogenous HA, regulate the property of the synovial fluid, form a protective barrier on the joint surface, decrease the joint friction coefficient, and decrease the risk of damage.[18] High-molecular-weight HA improves cartilage integrity and decreases osteophyte formation in experimental osteoarthritis.[18] Intra-articular injection of either corticosteroid or SH has a significant long-term effect on chronic arthritis of the TMJ.[18] SH may be the best alternative due to the lower risk of side effects.[17]

How it is used or injected? HA has the potential to alleviate pain, decrease joint noise, and increase maximum incisal opening and lateral mandibular movements when injected following arthrocentesis. In one study consisting of patients with internal derangement, the patients were treated with arthrocentesis alone or arthrocentesis with SH administration into the superior joint space.[18]

Evaluation was performed immediately after the procedure, on postoperative day 1, and was followed at 1, 2, 3, 4, 5, 6, 9, 12, and 24 months. Maximal mouth opening increased in both arthrocentesis and arthrocentesis with SH groups for both closed lock and anterior disc displacement with reduction (ADDR), but the results were only significant for the latter with closed lock. Lateral movements increased in both groups but only significantly for the arthrocentesis with SH group. Intensity of pain decreased significantly for the arthrocentesis with SH group. Clicking disappeared significantly in patients receiving SH for closed lock and ADDR but not in the arthrocentesis-only groups. Both groups showed an improvement in jaw function, but the arthrocentesis with SH group improved irrespective of diagnosis, whereas the arthrocentesis-only group only showed statistical significance in the ADDR subgroup.[17]

Technique for intra-articular injections with arthrocentesis The operative site was prepared aseptically and isolated with sterile drapes. A 20-gauge needle was inserted at a point 10 mm in front of the tragus and 2 mm below the canthal-tragal line. An auriculotemporal nerve block was achieved by administering 0.3 to 0.5 mL of anesthetic. The needle was then advanced into the superior joint space and 3.5 mL of anesthetic was deposited. After this, a second needle attached to a syringe and filled with sterile saline solution was introduced 2 mm anterior to the former and the upper joint compartment was irrigated with 200 to 300 mL of sterile saline. Following the procedure, 1 mL of SH was injected into the upper joint space in 26 of the joints, leaving 15 not injected. Maximal mouth opening and range of lateral jaw movement were measured and recorded at each appointment. Intensity of pain, mandibular function, and presence of TMJ sounds were recorded on 100-mm visual analogue scales.[18]

HA, when injected into the superior and inferior joint spaces of patients with disc displacement without reduction and osteoarthritic changes, has shown a radiographic reversal of the degenerative changes. In a study by Long and colleagues,[20] patients with osteoarthritis or disc displacement without reduction received injections into the superior or inferior joint spaces with 1 mL of HA at 2-week intervals for a total of 3 injections. Follow-ups were completed at 3 and 9 months.[20]

One hundred thirty-six patients presented for a 3-month follow-up and 74 returned for the 9-month follow-up. Reparative remodeling of the condyle was observed in 44 and 51 patients in the superior and inferior groups, respectively. Severe degenerative changes were observed in 13 patients in the superior group and 6 patients in the inferior groups. Eight patients in the superior group and 4 patients in the inferior group showed no changes. Most patients at 3 months showed improvement of mandibular movement, pain relief, and an increase of maximal opening. At 9-months follow-up, most patients had better condylar morphology. Condylar remodeling was found in most patients at follow-up, exhibiting a rounded contour of the condyle, formation of new bone, osteophyte dissolution, decrease of sclerosis, and decrease of cysts.

Cone-beam computed tomography assessment showed a better effect of osteoarthritic changes after the inferior joint space injection and that patients with HA injections into the inferior joint space in patients with disc displacement without reduction had significantly less pain, a lower clinical dysfunction index, and a greater maxillomandibular opening compared with those with HA injections into the superior joint space.[20]

Technique

Superior space injection technique The preauricular area is disinfected with povidone iodine and ethanol. A 5-mL syringe with 4 mL of 2% lidocaine and a 22-gauge needle are used for the joint injection. The entry point of the needle is approximately 10 mm anterior to the tragus. The needle is directed anteriorly, superiorly, and medially until the tip of the needle reaches the glenoid fossa. One milliliter of 2% lidocaine is injected and aspirated to confirm the intracapsular position of the needle. A successful aspiration without difficulty confirmed the correct needle position. The 5-mL syringe is removed while the needle remains in place, and 1 mL of SH is connected to the needle and injected into the joint space. The patient is instructed to move the lower jaw actively but without operator manipulation.[20]

Inferior joint space injection technique After disinfection of the preauricular area with povidone iodine and ethanol, the lateral pole of the condyle is palpated. A 5-mL syringe with 4 mL of 2% lidocaine and a 22-gauge needle are used for the injection. The area over the condyle is infiltrated with 1 mL of 2% lidocaine. The needle is advanced medially to contact the lateral aspect of the condyle head. The patient is instructed to open his or her mouth to an incisal distance of 1 cm, while the operator moves the needle in a posteromedial direction to enter the inferior joint space along the posterior surface of the condylar head. One milliliter of 2% lidocaine is injected into the inferior joint space and aspirated to confirm the correct position of the needle within the inferior joint space. After exchanging the anesthetic containing syringe with one with SH, 1 mL of SH is injected. The patient is instructed to open to a maximum mouth opening. The operator can apply downward force on the lower anterior teeth if the patient is unable to open actively; however, no vigorous manipulation of the mandible is applied.[20]

The role of opioids for chronic nonmalignant pain

Oral and maxillofacial surgery, by its nature, is oriented toward the short-term needs of patients in a primarily surgical manner. Since the 1970s, it has become clear that differences exist between acute and chronic pain, and that the surgeon can have a major impact toward the cause, prevention, and treatment of both. To successfully manage chronic pain, the surgeon must identify the underlying cause of the pain, assess the peripheral and central nervous systems, and be prepared to use the full spectrum of surgical, pharmacologic, physical, and behavioral therapies that are available. Although some patients may be managed by a single clinician, oftentimes a multidisciplinary team or pain clinic is required.[15]

The use of opioids in chronic nonmalignant pain when managed by experts is not only considered acceptable, but is warranted treatment in the carefully selected patient.[11] Although there are many patients whose pain is well controlled and functional status improved by daily use of long-acting narcotic and sedative agents without habituation, the use of narcotics and muscle relaxants for chronic myofascial pain remains controversial.[15] The long-term use of opioids in patients with chronic TMJ dysfunction can neither be supported nor refuted.[15] Most state dental boards consider the routine prescribing of chronic opioid therapy in TMD patients to be a red flag and discourage its use as a first-line therapy.[11] This topic has historically been controversial with literature against the use of opioids.[3] The lack of clinical trials evaluating opioids in the treatment of chronic orofacial pain compounds this problem.[11] Despite this, the extended use of opioids for intractable TMD pain seems reasonable when managed by a skilled provider.[11]

Chronic pain has been defined as pain persisting for at least 3 months. The treatment of patients with chronic TMJ pain can be challenging. The pathophysiology of pain, especially chronic pain, is poorly understood. The biopsychosocial model has been used to explain chronic pain in patients with TMD, which includes a biologic, psychological, and social component. Pain is perceived by the sufferer and influenced by cognitive, behavioral, environmental, and cultural factors.[11] Although chronic pain does not follow a specific demographic, the patient's general health and psychosocial factors influence the severity of pain reported, pain tolerance, and responses to therapy. Chronic pain is influenced by the patient's age, gender, socioeconomic status, education level, family and marital status, religious and cultural background, previous life experience with chronic disease, the presence of litigation, levels of daily exercise, and avocation satisfaction.[15]

The pathophysiology of pain is conceptually divided into the central and peripheral nervous systems that interact in a complex manner in response to painful stimuli. Peripheral neurotransmitters and the axonal influx of calcium ions results in the transmission of pain impulses to the CNS. The modulation of pain occurs at many levels and is influenced by the receptor type and presence of norepinephrine, serotonin, opioids, and γ-aminobutyric acid.[21]

Peripheral sensitization occurs in response to the noxious stimuli and the mix of inflammatory mediators at the site of injury, leading to the upregulation and increased sensitivity of peripheral nociceptors, which can result in allodynia. Central sensitization is often triggered by the constant activity of primary afferent fibers and is characterized by central neuronal plasticity. Sensitization of both the peripheral and the central nervous systems can increase and prolong the pain experience.[21]

The contribution of psychological factors to chronic pain is significant. It is often not possible to determine whether these factors were present before the development of the chronic pain or are present as a result of it. Factors such as anxiety and depression are known to adversely affect pain perception and influence chronic pain states. Somatization within patients with chronic pain, including TMD, is also thought to be an influencing factor in pain. The use of cognitive therapy, hypnosis, and other psychological treatments has been shown to reduce chronic pain in both the short and the long term. Treating chronic pain without consideration to the psychological and emotional aspects is fraught with danger and is discouraged. A multidisciplinary team approach is preferable, and if not possible, then a referral to a counselor, psychiatrist, or psychologist is advised.[21]

The use of opioids in the management of chronic cancer-related pain has been well defined and accepted, and the efficacy of opioids for managing chronic non-cancer pain has also been reported. The outcomes typically measured include pain, function, quality of life, and sleep. The published data support the efficacy of opioids for chronic non-cancer pain, but the choice between short-acting and long-acting opioids has been controversial. Short-acting opioids have a more rapid onset, easier titration, and a better ability to manage pain in those whose pain intensity fluctuates throughout the day. The main concern has been the dosing frequency, compliance, and potential for adverse drug-related behavior (ADRB). Long-acting opioids provide a more reliable and consistent plasma level, improved pain control, better compliance, and less ADRB. Chronic TMJ pain that has not responded to other treatments can be thought of as a form of chronic non-cancer pain.[21]

The potential for ADRB is a concern for all patients using opioids for pain management. ADRB is best defined as addiction, abuse, or diversion, and its behaviors should be recognized early. Opioid-naïve patients should be screened for potential ADRB before beginning opioid therapy. There are several assessment tools available, such as the Screener and Opioid Assessment for Patients with Pain (SOAPP), revised SOAPP, and the Opioid Risk Tool. Patients currently on opioid therapy can be evaluated by the Current Opioid Misuse Measure. Patients at a high risk for abuse should be monitored in dedicated pain clinics, where monitoring is more stringent and a referral to addiction medicine is readily available.[21]

Treating patients with long-term opioid therapy must be considered carefully. A history and physical examination along with screening or monitoring tools will allow for risk stratification. A referral to a chronic pain specialist may be required. Moreover, patients must have a clear understanding of the goals of treatment, their responsibilities, and the monitoring plan. A verbal and written informed consent should be implemented with clearly defined physician and patient responsibilities, and possible sanctions or discontinuation of treatment should ADRBs develop.[21] The contract should stipulate a daily dosage schedule, avoidance of duplicate medications from other physicians, careful combinations of other CNS agents such as alcohol, and the maintenance of nonpharmacologic activity known to aid in the patient's pain management.[15] The monitoring process for patients with chronic non-cancer pain should involve monthly visits to assess the level of analgesia, activities of daily living, ADRB, and any adverse effects.[21]

The ideal opioid for any patient is determined by many factors, such as the efficacy of the drug, dosing requirements, use of adjunctive medications, adverse effects, and risk for ADRB. Fentanyl and morphine are supported by cohort or case-controlled analytical studies, whereas hydrocodone and methadone are supported only by opinions of respected authorities or based on experience. Transdermal fentanyl should be titrated slowly, with 12.5 or 25 μg/h. The titration process is more difficult than oral opioids due to the extended half-life of the fentanyl patch and the need for oral opioids for breakthrough pain, which is typically managed by the use of transmucosal fentanyl or immediate-release morphine. Commonly administered oral opioids include morphine, oxycodone, tramadol, hydrocodone, and methadone. Oxycodone is a reasonable choice for chronic non-cancer pain, being easier to titrate and having fewer side effects than morphine. Tramadol, despite being a μ-, κ-, and γ-agonist as well as an inhibitor of norepinephrine and serotonin reuptake, has not been found to be effective for patients with TMD and chronic pain. Methadone may be another choice and has been shown to reduce pain, although its highly variable bioavailability, time to peak concentration, volume of distribution, and half-life make it unpredictable. Sleep disturbances and torsades de pointes are other concerns with methadone and an

Table 5
Equi-analgesic conversion table (oral)

Drug	Dose (mg)
Morphine	30
Oxycodone	20
Hydrocodone	30
Hydromorphone	7.5
Methadone	2–4
Meperidine	300
Codeine	200

Courtesy of the Oregon Health Sciences Center; and *Data from* Bouloux GF. Use of opioids in long-term management of temporomandibular joint dysfunction. J Oral Maxillofac Surg 2011;69: 1889–91; with permission.

electrocardiogram before and after treatment is initiated is recommended to verify that the QT interval is not greater than 500 ms.[21]

Adverse effects to opioid therapy are common, especially at the initiation of treatment, and include respiratory depression, nausea, emesis, constipation, pruritis, delayed gastric emptying, sexual dysfunction, sleep disturbance, and sedation. Nausea and sedation typically improve with time but can remain problematic for some patients. Constipation typically persists, and treatment with stool softeners or laxatives may be required.[21]

The chronic use of opioids can cause the development of tolerance to a particular drug or an increase in the severity of adverse effects, creating a need to rotate opioid medications. Cross-tolerance to opioids does exist, but it cannot be predicted. Conversion to another opioid requires knowledge of an equi-analgesic conversion table (**Table 5**). Once the equi-analgesic dose is calculated, it should be reduced by 25% to 50%, and a short-acting opioid should be made available for breakthrough pain.

SUMMARY

A thorough knowledge of the various pharmacologic agents used in the treatment of TMD/TMJ dysfunction and pain is essential for the dentists or oral surgeon who wishes to manage this segment of his/her clinical practice.

REFERENCES

1. Dym H, Israel H. Diagnosis and treatment of temporomandibular disorders. Dent Clin North Am 2012;56(1):149–61.
2. Magni G. The use of antidepressants in the treatment of chronic pain. A review of the current evidence. Drugs 1991;42:730–48.
3. Dionne RA. Pharmacologic treatments for temporomandibular disorders. Oral Surg Oral Med Oral Pathol Oral Radiol Endod 1997;83(1):134–42.
4. Max MB, Culnane M, Schafer SC, et al. Amitriptyline relieves diabetic neuropathy pain in patients with normal or depressed mood. Neurology 1987;37:589–96.
5. Onghena P, Van Houdenhove B. Antidepressant-induced analgesia in chronic non-malignant pain: a meta-analysis of 39 placebo-controlled studies. Pain 1992;49:205–19.

6. Sharav Y, Singer E, Schmidt E, et al. The analgesic effect of amitriptyline on chronic facial pain. Pain 1987;31:199–209.
7. Elenbaas JK. Centrally acting oral skeletal muscle relaxants. Am J Hosp Pharm 1980;37:1313–23.
8. Dellemijn PL, Fields HL. Do benzodiazepines have a role in chronic pain management? Pain 1994;57:137–52.
9. Ta LE, Dionne RA. Treatment of painful temporomandibular joints with a cyclooxygenase-2 inhibitor: a randomized placebo-controlled comparison of celecoxib to naproxen. Pain 2004;111:13–21.
10. Liu F, Steinkeler A. Epidemiology, diagnosis, and treatment of temporomandibular disorders. Dent Clin North Am 2013;57(3):465–79.
11. Hersh EV, Balasubramaniam R, Pinto A. Pharmacologic management of temporomandibular disorders. Oral Maxillofac Surg Clin North Am 2008;20(2):197–210.
12. Mercuri LG. Osteoarthritis, osteoarthrosis, and idiopathic condylar resorption. Oral Maxillofac Surg Clin North Am 2008;20(2):169–83.
13. Carrasco R. Juvenile idiopathic arthritis overview and involvement of the temporomandibular joint prevalence, systemic therapy. Oral Maxillofac Surg Clin North Am 2015;27(1):1–10.
14. Cairns BE. Pathophysiology of TMD pain—basic mechanisms and their implications for pharmacotherapy. J Oral Rehabil 2010;37(6):391–410.
15. Gregg JM. Chronic maxillomandibular head and neck pain. In: Fonseca RJ, editor. Oral and maxillofacial surgery. Saunders; 2009. p. 136–63.
16. Breivik H. Local anesthetic blocks and epidurals. In: FM, McMahon SB, editors. Wall & Melzack's textbook of pain. Saunders; 2013. p. 523–37.
17. Alpaslan GH, Alpaslan C. Efficacy of temporomandibular joint arthrocentesis with and without injection of sodium hyaluronate in treatment of internal derangements. J Oral Maxillofac Surg 2001;59(6):613–8.
18. Li C, Long X, Deng M, et al. Osteoarthritic changes after superior and inferior joint space injection of hyaluronic acid for the treatment of temporomandibular joint osteoarthritis with anterior disc displacement without reduction: a cone-beam computed tomographic evaluation. J Oral Maxillofac Surg 2015;73(2):232–44.
19. Guarda-Nardini L, Olivo M, Ferronato G, et al. Treatment effectiveness of arthrocentesis plus hyaluronic acid injections in different age groups of patients with temporomandibular joint osteoarthritis. J Oral Maxillofac Surg 2012;70(9):2048–56.
20. Long X, Chen G, Cheng AH, et al. A randomized controlled trial of superior and inferior joint space injection with hyaluronic acid in treatment of anterior disc displacement without reduction. J Oral Maxillofac Surg 2009;67(2):357–61.
21. Bouloux GF. Use of opioids in long-term managment of temporomandibular joint dysfunction. J Oral Maxillofac Surg 2011;69(7):1885–91.

Orofacial Pain

Pharmacologic Paradigms for Therapeutic Intervention

Leslie Halpern, MD, DDS, PhD, MPH[a],*, Porchia Willis, DDS[b]

KEYWORDS

- Episodic/continuous pain • Anticonvulsants • Antidepressants • SSRIs • Antivirals
- Botox • Topical medicaments

KEY POINTS

- Orofacial pain (OFP) is a complex process whose causes originate from the trigeminal nociceptive reflex arcs within the central and peripheral nervous systems.
- The primary management of intraoral, neuropathic, and neurovascular OFP within the soft and hard tissues of the head, face, and neck is based on sound and rational pharmacotherapy.
- The current perspectives of OFP management require the clinician to be cognizant of comorbid conditions and apply balanced pharmacologic paradigms for optimal outcomes. Many of the drugs in combination can elicit both beneficial and adverse effects in patients treated.
- Evidence-based clinical trials characterize opioids, tricyclic antidepressants, selective serotonin reuptake inhibitors, anticonvulsants, and several topical medicaments as viable choices in the pharmacologic management of pain associated with OFP syndromes.
- New innovations in routes of pharmacotherapy will augment not only the efficacy of medication but allow for combination therapy that has fewer adverse effects and greater prolongation of relief in patients who have OFP.

INTRODUCTION

The definition of pain according to the International Association for the Study of Pain is "an unpleasant sensory and emotional experience associated with actual or potential tissue damage, or described in terms of such damage."[1–3] Pain is a universal experience that has profound effects on the physiology, psychology, and sociology of the population. The World Health Organization (WHO) has estimated that more than

[a] Residency, Oral and Maxillofacial Surgery, Meharry Medical College, 1005 TB Todd Jr. Boulevard, Nashville, TN 37208, USA; [b] Oral and Maxillofacial Surgery, Meharry Medical College, 1005 TB Todd Jr. Boulevard, Nashville, TN 37208, USA
* Corresponding author.
E-mail address: lhalpern@mmc.edu

Dent Clin N Am 60 (2016) 381–405
http://dx.doi.org/10.1016/j.cden.2015.11.011
0011-8532/16/$ – see front matter © 2016 Elsevier Inc. All rights reserved.

dental.theclinics.com

one-third of the population has some form of acute or chronic pain.[1,2] Within the United States, the health care costs of diagnoses and treatment of pain exceed several billion dollars annually.[1]

Orofacial pain (OFP) refers to pain associated within the head and neck regions, soft and hard tissues, both extraorally and intraorally. Okeson[3] divides OFP into physical (axis 1) and psychological (axis 2) conditions. Physical conditions comprise temporomandibular disorders (TMD), which include disorders of the temporomandibular joint (TMJ) and disorders of the musculoskeletal structures (eg, masticatory muscles and cervical spine); intraoral dental and pulpal pain of somatic origin; neuropathic pain (NP), which include episodic (eg, trigeminal neuralgia [TN]) and continuous (eg, peripheral/centralized mediated) characteristics; and neurovascular disorders/headaches (eg, migraine and temporal arteritis). OFP can often be a presenting symptom for systemic illnesses, such as chronic pain seen in fibromyalgia, gastroesophageal reflux disease (GERD)/irritable bowel disease, posttraumatic stress disorder (PTSD)/other psychological disorders, myocardial ischemia, and cancerous lesions in other parts of the body.[4] Therefore, the evaluation of patients presenting with OFP accounts for a cornucopia of diagnostic possibilities. The oral health care clinician must be judicious in diagnosing clinical presentations as odontogenic and other dental conditions as a primary versus secondary cause of OFP.[4,5] A careful deciphering of signs and symptoms will set the foundation for specific treatment to improve long-term prognosis and resolution of most OFP syndromes.

Evidence-based observational and controlled experimental clinical trials suggest that pharmacologic therapy may significantly improve patient outcomes either alone or when used as a part of a comprehensive treatment plan for OFP.[6–8] The aim of this article is to provide the practitioner with therapeutic options from a pharmacologic perspective to treat a broad spectrum of both acute and chronic OFP syndromes. The epidemiology and neurophysiology/pathophysiology of OFP are introduced with respect to the most common treated areas of the head and neck followed by the latest in pharmacologic management strategies for pain management.

EPIDEMIOLOGY

Demographic studies have determined that greater than 39 million people, 22% of US citizens, report pain in the orofacial region.[8] Studies by Turp and colleagues[5] report that greater than 80% of patients presenting with OFP symptoms had concomitant pain systemically, that is, fibromyalgia, panic disorders, multiple chemical sensitivities, and PTSDs.[1,4,5,8] The classification and epidemiology of OFP are quite challenging because of a lack of consensus regarding diagnostic criteria. Lancer and Gesell[5] has coined the phrase "Pain management: the fifth vital sign" because patient sex, age, and psychosocial factors seem to be a prominent risk predictor for chronic facial pain.[9] Evidence-based studies have been published at a greater pace over the past decade in OFP, and there are still many questions unanswered with respect to the dynamics of this disease process.[1,8] Many drugs used to treat the symptoms are usually prescribed over an extended period of time necessitating careful monitoring for adverse effects and potential drug interactions. In addition, the latest experimental evidence demonstrates gender/sex differences in causes and clinical presentation of pain, that is, pharmacogenetic-specific responses to different analgesics and other medications to treat OFP. Future research in this area is ongoing and will continue to affect the epidemiologic criteria with respect to diagnoses and treatment options. A thorough understanding of the epidemiology/cause of OFP is essential to the practice of evidence-based oral health care.[9]

NEUROPHYSIOLOGY

OFP can arise from different regions and causes within the head and neck. The clinician who treats OFP must have a clear understanding of the neuroanatomy/physiology of these regions. Most of these pathways communicate with cranial nerve (CN) V that forms the trigeminal nociceptive system. This complex network of reflex arcs function based on the properties of trigeminal afferents innervating distinct target tissues.[8,10] Most are transmitted by somatic, motor and autonomic nerve networks. These target tissue interactions with trigeminal neuron terminals contribute to the awareness and degree of pain perceived.[1]

Trigeminal pain conditions can arise from injury secondary to dental procedures, infection, neoplasia, or other diseases/dysfunction within the peripheral and/or central nervous system (CNS). TMDs, for example, are one of the most prevalent OFP conditions for which patients seek treatment. Neurovascular disorders, such as primary headaches, can present as chronic OFP, such as in the case of facial migraine, whereby the pain is localized in the second and third division of the trigeminal nerve. CNs VII, IX, and X also contribute to afferent input of the head and neck precipitating/exacerbating OFP. Their afferent pathways converge on the trigeminal system at the level of the brainstem. This complex network can cause dilemmas with respect to origin of pain. The clinician must differentiate *heterotopic pain* (source of pain not localized at site of pain) from *referred pain* (pain at one area that is supplied by afferents from another source of nociception). The latter explains and why a patient complains of shoulder and neck pain when describing pain intraorally.

The trigeminal system has provided a model for studying how pharmacologic therapy contributes to the resolution of inflammatory cascades and their effect on pain pathways.[8,11] The dental impaction model of Cooper and Desjardins[11] characterizes a standard clinical method for evaluating a variety of analgesic medications for acute inflammation: the use of preemptive analgesia, activation of opioid CNS pathways, and the association of sexually dimorphic pain pathways.[12] Studies on chronic trigeminal myofascial pain syndromes demonstrate that sex/gender and exposure to sex steroids are risk predictors for developing chronic OFP conditions.[12–14] Additional studies have characterized morphologic changes in trigeminal neurons exposed to injury-induced inflammatory insult to tissue innervated by afferents from peripheral and central pathways[8] that are further modulated by sex steroids, prolactin and estradiol.[8] Further studies are examining sex-dependent differences in pain pathways with respect to the biological basis for pharmacogenetic responses: genetic variations that affect an individual's response to medications for pain.[14] Together, the aforementioned disorders of the trigeminal system impact the quality of life of the sufferer dramatically.

PATHOPHYSIOLOGY/PHARMACOLOGIC MANAGEMENT

The pathophysiology of OFP forms a segue for different algorithms of pharmacologic therapeutics in the treatment of OFP syndromes. **Box 1** depicts the most common differential of acute and chronic OFP according to the American Academy of Orofacial Pain.[1,7,15] For the purposes of this article, only NP, headaches, and intraoral pain are included with respect to pathophysiology and pharmacologic management.[1,7] It is further discussed in this article and in this issue (See Dym H, Bowler D, Zeidan J: Pharmacological Treatment for Temporomandibular Disorders).

Neuropathic Pain (NP)

NP is defined as pain caused by a lesion or disease of the somatosensory nervous system.[1] NP is diagnosed quite commonly with up to 25% to 35% presenting to facial

Box 1
Differential diagnosis of OFP

Intraoral pain

Dental caries

Dental abscess

Dentin sensitivity

Dry socket

Periodontal disease

Pericoronitis

Cracked tooth

TMD

Myofascial pain

Internal derangement of TM joints

Muscles of mastication

Eagles syndrome

Intracranial pain

Intracranial

Hemorrhage

Aneurysm

Tumor/cyst

Abscess

NP (Neuropathic pain)

Trigeminal neuralgia

Glossopharyngeal neuralgia

Postherpetic neuralgia

Atypical odontalgia

Burn mouth syndrome

Atypical facial pain, idiopathic

Headaches

Migraine

Tension-type headache

Cluster headache

Paroxysmal hemicrania

Temporal arteritis

Trigeminal autonomic C

Cervical pain

Myalgia

Neck

Degenerative joint disease

Referred pain

Cardiac

Renal

Gastrointestinal

Jaw

Data from Refs.[1,7,15]

---

pain centers across the United States and Europe.[16–18] Causes of NP include trauma, infection, chemotherapy, surgery, neurotoxins, inflammation, and tumor infiltration. Studies have equated NP to a dysfunctional pain due to afferent stimulation that can be both spontaneous and stimulus dependent.[16] The trigger can be perioral stimuli and/or triggers that are intraoral or environmental like cold and touch. **Box 2** lists the clinical presentation/features that patients present with who exhibit orofacial NP. Further classification separates NP into episodic and continuous. Episodic is characterized by sudden episodes that are electriclike shooting pains and can last seconds to minutes. It is preceded by a perioral/intraoral trigger. Continuous NP is pain originating in neural structures that is constant and varies in intensity without total remission. Episodic disorders include TN and glossopharyngeal neuralgia, whereas continuous pain disorders can arise from injury of nerves in both the peripheral and CNS, that is, neuromas and atypical odontalgia.[16–18]

An understanding of the pathophysiology of episodic and continuous NP provides the clinician with a strong rationale for choices of pharmacologic therapy. **Box 3** lists most agents broken into 3 main tiers that vary in mechanism of action because of site of neurologic innervation, synapses, membrane stabilizing agents, receptor agonists/antagonists, administered either by topical application or systemically. Studies have suggested using local anesthesia as a diagnostic aid before choosing one or more pharmacologic agents for treatment because it exerts its effect by membrane stabilization and suppression of pain transmission peripherally.[17–20]

Box 2
Typical clinical presentation of patients with OFP

Acute presentation due to trauma or disease, trigger points

Delayed/chronic occurrence over days/months, trigger points

Pain described as burning, lancinating, sharp, dull, episodic or unremitting

Local pathophysiology due to invasive procedures, abnormal nerve healing

Paresthesia, dysesthesia, hypesthesia, allodynia, phantom tooth pain

Neurosensory loss, anesthesia dolorosa, hypoesthesia

Parafunctional habits: bruxism, clenching

Facial nerve weakness, loss of taste to anterior two-thirds of tongue

Headaches, tinnitus, vertigo, photophobia, phonophobia, dysgeusia

Psychosocial issues, referred pain, heterotopic pain

Box 3
Pharmacologic agents by location/cause of drug action

Synaptic cleft

Benzodiazepines

Clonidine

Tricyclic antidepressants:
  Amitriptyline
  Nortriptyline
  Imipramine

Serotonin reuptake inhibitors/norepinephrine selective reuptake inhibitors:
  Venlafaxine
  Duloxetine
  Trazodone
  Milnacipran

Membrane stabilizing drugs

Anticonvulsants:
  Carbamazepine
  Oxcarbazepine
  Phenytoin
  Gabapentin
  Pregabalin
  Lamotrigine
  Valproic acid
  Topiramate
  Tiagabine
  Zonisamide

Other drugs

Opioids

Local anesthetics

Corticosteroids

Nonsteroidal antiinflammatory drugs

Aspirin

Acetaminophen

Antifungal agents

Antiviral

Botox

Antioxidants: alpha lipoic acid

Salivary stimulants: pilocarpine, cevimeline

Topical agents

Lidocaine patches

Proparacaine

Streptomycin/lidocaine

Capsaicin

Topical nonsteroidal antiinflammatory drugs

Antidepressants

Anticonvulsants

Botulinum toxins

Other agents

Analgesic drugs are usually the number one choice for relief in patients with NP.[21] Morphine, for example, can interact with endorphins, the natural opioid of CNS. Tricyclic antidepressants (TCAs) act to increase catecholaminergic analogues that travel systemically to targets for relief by both acting as membrane stabilizers and trans-synaptic effects.[16,17] The salicylates act as antiinflammatory agents that inhibit cyclooxygenase pathways with inhibition of prostaglandins. The anticonvulsant medications act as membrane stabilizers because they suppress hyperexcitability of the axonal membrane.[20] When the drugs in addition to others are used together they can either potentiate or inhibit each other's actions. Pharmacokinetics and dynamics should be considered, especially if an effect is to be prolonged as well as side effects, allergic reactions, and dependence. Therefore, the pharmacotherapy is eclectic based on a diversity of analgesics whose dosing and concentrations vary with the type of NP being treated (see later discussion).

Episodic neuropathic pain

Trigeminal neuralgia TN is an episodic, unilateral pain that consists of brief shocking pains that can be sudden in onset and termination. It originates from one or more divisions of CN V, usually V2 and V3. There exists pain-free periods between attacks. The most common trigger zones of the face is the ala of nose and commissure of lip, both innervated by V2 and V3 divisions of CN V. The pain can refer to the teeth, making diagnoses difficult. Many clinicians have treated teeth with endodontic therapy without considering a neuropathic origin, such as TN.[1,5,8] The etiologic mechanism is often a result of vascular compression and focal demyelination both peripherally and centrally. MRI is usually a reliable imaging strategy because these findings may also be related to a neoplasm/tumor impinging on the nerve.[5] Vascular brainstem lesions, angiomas, or arteriovenous (AV) malformations are further causes of TN.[22,23] Fifteen percent to 20% of patients also exhibit a sensory loss along the distribution of CN V2/V3.[23] The differential for demyelination should also include multiple sclerosis because symptoms and demographics are within this patient population.[22,23] The pharmacologic paradigms for TN typically consist of first- and second-line therapies.[9,15,17,19] Each group of agents is described as well as dosing recommendations:

Anticonvulsive agents First-line therapy consists of antiepileptic medications, such as carbamazepine, oxcarbazepine, and gabapentin.[22–25] Systematic reviews have supported the use of carbamazepine (200–1200 mg/d) as a prognostic marker for definitive therapy because when it eliminates the symptoms, the clinician has successfully diagnosed TN.[21] Carbamazepine inactivates voltage-gated sodium channels and depresses postsynaptic reflex arcs in the spinal cord. Although it is very effective in resolving pain, it does not address the cause of this neuralgia. The use of carbamazepine requires judicious because this medicine has numerous side effects: leukopenia, agranulocytosis, aplastic anemia, drowsiness, and ataxia. Therapeutic levels must be followed to avoid adverse events, especially thrombocytopenia. Oxcarbazepine is a newer agent that has been used that has fewer side effects and has become the drug of choice for treating TN unless it fails.

Another group of anticonvulsive agents, gabapentin and pregabalin, are now being used to treat NP with even less side effects.[26] The mechanism of action resides in their ability to increase γ-aminobutyric acid (GABA) in the CNS and, therefore, increase the inhibition of pain sensors.[27] The main side effect of this group is drowsiness and the requirement of good kidney function. Baclofen and lamotrigine are two other agents that have fewer side effects and are used for treatment of TN. Baclofen has less of an effect on blood cells but does have gastrointestinal (GI) sequelae: vomiting and cramping. Lamotrigine is a phenothiazine derivative and also acts by stabilizing sodium channels and inhibiting the release of neurotransmitters.[21,26] Caution must be used when this agent is chosen because it elicits Steven-Johnson syndrome and, if present, must be discontinued at a tapering dose. Topiramate is another agent that can act at the voltage-sensitive sodium channels as well as modulating GABA. It is derived from the sulfonamide group and has side effects, such as nephrolithiasis, somnolence, anxiety, and drowsiness. This agent must also be tapered if discontinuing its use. **Table 1** depicts the dosing and daily administration of the anticonvulsant medications for TN.

Antidepressants The use of the TCAs in the treatment of NP has met with some debate because of their anticholinergic and cardiac side effects: xerostomia, constipation, urinary retention, and anesthetic drug interactions. Amitriptyline has been used at doses that elicit a membrane stabilizing effect.[20,21,27] A 10-mg dose of this agent can have a profound effect because of their mechanism of increasing the load of biogenic serotonin and norepinephrine at the synaptic cleft and relieving tension headaches and NP. TCAs are first-line agents in the treatment of musculoskeletal pain associated with fibromyalgia.[21,27]

More recently, the selective serotonin reuptake inhibitors have been applied for treatment of not only NP but also other OFP syndromes such as chronic pain.[28] Selective serotonin reuptake inhibitors (SSRIs) (fluoxetine and paroxetine) as well as serotonin-norepinephrine reuptake inhibitors (duloxetine/milnacipran) have been successfully used for fibromyalgia and other centrally mediated pain syndromes (see section on neurovascular pain later). **Table 1** lists the dosing schedule for the antidepressants.

The benzodiazepines have been used in combination with the aforementioned groups of agents for TN (see section on TMD and neurovascular pain management for further use).

Glossopharyngeal neuralgia Glossopharyngeal neuralgia is another episodic form of NP. It is unilateral with electric shock–like episodes localized to the tongue, throat, ear, and under the mandible. It is usually provoked with swallowing or speech and can occur concurrently in 10% of patients with TN.[21,23] Its incidence rate is 0.2 per 100,000 patients seen yearly and is also seen in patients with multiple sclerosis. Often there are other symptoms, such as syncope and cardiac arrhythmias, as well as poor nutrition because swallowing food or liquids precipitate severe attacks. Pharmacologic therapeutics are similar to TN. First-line therapy is the use of carbamazepine or oxcarbazepine with second-line therapy use of local anesthetics to direct sites of pain. If medical treatment is unsuccessful, then surgical procedures are warranted.[19,23,29]

Occipital neuralgia Occipital neuralgia presents as a unilateral pain in the posterior scalp area innervated by the greater and lesser occipital nerves. It must be distinguished from referred pain from the neck. It is treated with corticosteroids and local anesthesia.[30]

Continuous neuropathic pain As stated earlier, continuous NP has its origin in neural regions, constant in awareness and unremitting. There may be refractory periods but never totally gone. Okeson's[21] classification of facial pain axis 1 maps the 3 types of continuous NP: centrally mediated, peripherally mediated, and metabolic polyneuropathies.[20] Several examples are described:

Peripheral trigeminal neuritis This type of neuritis is a unilateral facial/OFP that manifests itself as a burning sensation following trauma of the trigeminal nerve. The latency period is about 3 to 6 months and is preceded by allodynia and hyperalgesia. The cause is often an exposure to dental work like a root canal or dentoalveolar trauma. Chronic pain will persist in 5% of patients who report this event.[31] Pharmacologic

Table 1
Pharmacologic agents for NP: dosing schedule episodic: trigeminal neuralgia/ glossopharyngeal neuralgia/occipital neuralgia

	Dosing Per Day
First line:	
Carbamazepine	200–1200 mg/d
Oxcarbazepine	600–1800 mg/d
Second line:	
Combination of the aforementioned agents +	
Lamotrigine	400 mg/d
Baclofen	40–80 mg/d
Third line:*	
Phenytoin	—
Gabapentin	600 mg, 3 times a day to maximum of 1800 mg per day
Pregabalin	Vary based upon individual practitioner
Valproate	Vary based upon individual practitioner
Tizanidine	Vary based upon individual practitioner
Tocainide	Vary based upon individual practitioner
Local anesthetics	Vary based upon individual practitioner

Continuous NP: Peripheral Neuritis/Postherpetic Neuralgia/Atypical Odontalgia/Burning Mouth Syndrome	
	Dosing Per Day
Peripheral neuritis	
NSAIDs	Vary as per practitioner preference
Corticosteroids	Vary as per practitioner preference
Postherpetic neuralgia	
Antivirals	Vary as per practitioner preference
Acetaminophen	Vary as per practitioner preference
NSAIDs	Vary as per practitioner preference
Opioids	Vary as per practitioner preference
TCAs	Vary as per practitioner preference
Anticonvulsants	Vary as per practitioner preference
Atypical odontalgia	Vary as per practitioner preference
Burning mouth syndrome:	
Benzodiazepines:	
Clonazepam	0.5–2.0 mg/d
Chlordiazepoxide	10–30 mg/d
Anticonvulsants:	
Gabapentin	300–1600 mg/d; dosing varies depending on side effects seen; can start with 100 mg at night and the increase to 3×/d
Pregabalin	25–300 mg/d: start with 25 mg at night and then increase by 25 mg over 7 days to 3×/d
Antidepressants:	
Amitriptyline	10–150 mg/d: 10 mg at night and increase by 10 mg over 7 d not exceeding 4×/d

(continued on next page)

Table 1 (continued)	
Continuous NP: Peripheral Neuritis/Postherpetic Neuralgia/Atypical Odontalgia/Burning Mouth Syndrome	
	Dosing Per Day
Nortriptyline	10–150 mg/d: 10 mg at night and increase as needed 10/d over 7 d not exceeding 4×/d
Selective serotonin reuptake inhibitors:	
Paroxetine	20–50 mg/d
Sertraline	50–200 mg/d: 50 mg initially and can increase by 25 mg every 7 d; max 200 mg/d
Trazodone	100–400 mg/d: 5–0 mg initially and increase by 50 mg 4–7 d; max 400 mg/d
Selective norepinephrine reuptake inhibitors:	
Milnacipran	100 mg/d: 50 mg BID; 12.5 initially then BID; max 200 mg/d
Duloxetine	60–120 mg/d; PO QID
Antioxidants:	
Alpha lipoic acid	600–1200 mg/d; 300–600 mg BID

Abbreviations: max, maximum; NSAIDs, nonsteroidal antiinflammatory drugs.
  * Dosing is based upon individual practitioner preference.

management consists of antidepressant therapy and anticonvulsants to control explosive periods of burning and stabbing in the area traumatized. In addition, diagnostic blocks with local anesthetics can be applied as immediate relief followed by topical medicaments (discussed later) to both alleviate pain and reduce adverse systemic events.[15,32] The use of capsaicin at a concentration of 0.05% with benzocaine 20% can be applied on a stent. Other topical agents have compounded several drugs, such as ketamine, nonsteroidal antiinflammatory drugs (NSAIDs), and anticonvulsants for relief (see section on the use of topical medicines).

Peripheral neuritis Peripheral neuritis describes neuropathy secondary to inflammation usually mediated by the production of cytokines. Perineural inflammation occurs in the orofacial cavity because of dental procedures, such as implant placement. Other causes include chronic sinusitis, TMJ joint degeneration, and malignant neoplasms that spread on the nerve trunk.[15,23] Pharmacologic intervention consists of antiinflammatory agents, such as NSAIDs, Corticosteroids and topicals.[6,15]

Herpes zoster/postherpetic neuralgia Postherpetic neuralgia (PHN) originates after the outbreak of herpes zoster (HZ) virus. The virus undergoes a dormant period within the dorsal root ganglia: 55% of the time in the thoracic spine and associated with the CNs, most often CN V and CN VII.[17,33] Ten percent to 15% of cases are recorded in CN V3 and 80% of cases are recorded in CN V1. The incidence of disease is greater in the elderly and begins with significant prodromal symptoms: headache, malaise, abnormal skin sensation, and fever. Once reactivated the condition is referred to as shingles. The goals of pharmacologic management are to eliminate pain and accelerate healing. Several prescribed modalities exist to address these concerns (refer to **Table 1** for dosing schedule):

1. Antivirals: These agents are applied within several days of symptoms in order to decrease the rash and pain severity. Examples are acyclovir, valacyclovir, and famciclovir.

2. Opioids: These agents are used for severe pain.
3. Nonopioids: Acetaminophen or NSAIDs are used to control inflammation, pain, and fevers.
4. Corticosteroids: These agents are added to antivirals to relieve pain.
5. Antidepressants: Amitriptyline, desipramine, and nortriptyline are often used in small doses, and the gabapentin group has been recently approved by the Food and Drug Administration (FDA) to treat PHN.[34]

Both HZ and PHN are preventable with vaccinations. The Centers for Disease Control and Prevention recommends patients 60 years or older receive vaccinations regardless of exposure risk.[19]

Table 1 characterizes the respective dosing for all of the aforementioned agents in treating PHN.

Atypical odontalgia/nonodontogenic toothache Atypical odontalgia is a centralized trigeminal neuropathy characterized by an idiopathic pain that is throbbing or burning and misdiagnosed as dental in origin resulting in unnecessary treatment. The age range is usually from 25 to 65 years, and the most common tooth is the molar > premolar > incisor with the maxilla as site of origin greater than the mandible. Diagnostic imaging shows no pathology, but the teeth can elicit a hyperesthetic response to percussion. Diagnostic blocks with local anesthetics may either relieve the pain temporarily or be equivocal in response. Associated symptoms include depression, oral dysesthesia, and problems with oral hygiene.[3,7,19,21] Studies have suggested that vascular mechanisms as well as sympathetic system imbalance may play a role in the neuropathology of atypical odontalgia. Patients will be frustrated because they may want the specific tooth to be treated in a case of a nonodontogenic toothache.[21,35]

Pharmacologic therapy is challenging because both central and peripheral mechanisms are misaligned. The TCAs are first-line agents because at low doses they exhibit their analgesic action: 25 to 50 mg. The reuptake inhibition of serotonin and norepinephrine increase the effectiveness of inhibitory pathways of pain perception.[21,36] The anticonvulsant gabapentin at a moderate dosing of 3600 mg is effective, with drowsiness as a side effect. Pregabalin can also be a drug of choice to relieve continuous NP.[21,36] Peripheral components of atypical odontalgia may be treated with topical agents and stent placement. Benzocaine mixed with carbamazepine and/or ketamine may provide a true benefit. Topical agents dosed in patches are now being studied to reduce the symptoms of continuous NP (see section later on pharmacology of topical agents).

Burning mouth syndrome Burning mouth syndrome (BMS)/burning mouth disorder presents as burning sensations within the oral cavity (ie, tongue, lips, and oral mucosa) that are continuous with an increase in intensity throughout the day.[37] The epidemiology of BMS varies from 1% to 3%. Women are predisposed (6:1 male) to BMS during their perimenopausal to postmenopausal years, and up to 50% report a concomitant xerostomia and dysgeusia.[21,38] The greatest frequency of BMS occurs on the anterior one-third of the tongue followed by the gingiva and palate. It is most often a diagnosis of exclusion. As to a definitive cause, an in-depth history of present illness (HPI) is essential before management because BMS can manifest itself in a variety of systemic diseases (ie, GERD, diabetes, hypertension, and autoimmune) (see **Table 1**). Deficiencies in certain vitamins (ie, iron, vitamin B12, and folic acid) can exacerbate BMS-induced xerostomia, and the clinician may consider saliva flow studies as a prerequisite to treating BMS.[39,40]

Pharmacologic strategies for treatment must begin with establishing a definitive diagnosis, followed by a well-tailored treatment schedule that accounts for the multifactorial risk factors. Treatment can be palliative, symptomatic, and combinations of both in order to reach a therapeutic range of relief. It is judicious for the clinician to explain why therapy is complex so patient compliance can be achieved. The mainstay of treatment is with the use of topical medications. Random control trials have established that benzodiazepines; clonazepam should be considered first at a dosing of 0.25 mg to 2.0 mg/d in wafer or oral disintegrating tablet forms.[41,42] Other topical agents include capsaicin (1:2 dilutions), doxepin (5% cream), and 2% viscous lidocaine, every 4 to 6 hours or as needed. Other topical agents include artificial sweeteners providing mucosal relief; antimicrobials, such as lactoperoxidase rinses using swishing and expectorating 3 times a day; and, when candidiasis is the cause per culturing, the use of antifungal medications.[41,42] Systemic medications are the next choice. As with NP management, opioids and the TCAs amitriptyline and nortriptyline at dosing of 10 to 150 mg maximum (because of side effects) over 5 to 7 days have met with relief in population studies.[42–44] The use of SSRIs paroxetine, sertraline, and trazodone and the anticonvulsants pregabalin and gabapentin as combination therapy have had variable success[43–45] (see **Table 1** for summary of pharmacologic agents for BMS).

The management of BMS is, therefore, quite challenging.[46] Studies of clinical outcomes in large populations conclude that only 3% to 5% of patients reach a complete resolution of their symptoms.[47] Better strategies for definitive diagnoses will aid clinicians in choosing more efficacious pharmacology in order to better manage their patients presenting with BMS.

Neurovascular Pain

Neurovascular pain is episodic and based on disturbances of the trigeminovascular system and often presents clinically as a headache in patients with OFP.[48] The WHO characterizes headache disorders as the 10th disability in women, and the cost of care exceeds $27 billion globally.[21,49,50] The International Headache Society divides primary headaches into 4 categories: (1) migraines; (2) tension-type headaches (TTH), cluster headaches (CHs), and paroxysmal hemicranias; (3) trigeminal autonomic cephalgias; and (4) other headaches.[3,21,49]

Migraines

Migraine is a common primary headache that affects 10% to 12% of the adult population: 6% of men and 18% of women, which peaks between 35 and 45 years of age. The cost of treatment can exceed $19.6 billion per year.[50,51] Symptoms are preceded by triggers, such as stress, foods, loss of sleep, and menstruation. Clinical presentation is separated into 4 phases: (1) prodromal, (2) an aura or without aura, (3) the actual headache, and (4) postdrome phase.[15,21] A careful differential diagnosis includes tension headache, oro-dental pain, other vascular disorders, and intracranial tumors.[52] Although the pathophysiology is not completely clear, it originates form the trigeminovascular system that receives nociceptive afferents from the dura, meningeal blood vessels, and innervation from V1. Cervical innervation also forms part of this network, and migraine pain is most often referred to the neck. These afferents cause release of inflammatory mediators (substance P, calcitonin-gene-related peptide, and neurokinin) that facilitate the pain transmission.[15,53]

The therapeutic interventions of migraine headaches are either nonpharmacologic (biofeedback, hypnosis, and psychological therapies) or pharmacologic and are predicated on whether the migraine has an aura phase or not (WA).[15,21,50–53] Facial migraines (WA) present with a typical migraine that is localized to the face and is unilateral, associated with nausea, phonophobia, and photophobia.[15,21] Once diagnosed, pharmacologic treatment can be either abortive or preventive based on the timeline of the headache symptoms. Migraines that occur less than 2 times per month can be treated with abortive medications, whereas those that occur more frequently need preventive therapy.

Abortive medications Abortive treatment is for acute symptomatic events as well as supplemental therapy for preventive medications during a migraine event. NSAIDs and selective Cox-2 inhibitors, naproxen sodium, ibuprofen, and rofecoxib, are effective but not over an extended daily regimen because of adverse systemic effects.[15,21] Ergotamine derivatives (DHE) have been quite effective for severe acute migraine episodes because of their significant effect on vasoconstriction of blood vessels. Dihydroergotamine (DHE) can be administered intranasally, intravenously, and subcutaneously.[21,54] Another group, the triptans, has replaced DHE derivatives because of better tolerability and efficacy. Serotonin 5-hydroxytryptamine (5-HT) receptor agonists are very specific for inhibiting the release of calcitonin gene related peptide (CGRP) as well as acting at the receptors of meningeal blood vessels and desensitizing the trigeminovascular system by decreasing neurogenic inflammation.[15,21,55] The SSRIs sumatriptan, rizatriptan, and almotriptan, although quite effective, must be carefully tailored to patients who do not have cardiovascular and cerebrovascular anomalies.[56] Combination therapy using sumatriptan with naproxen sodium have been shown to elicit additive effects; another 5-HT receptor agonist, lasmiditan, was quite effective in randomized controlled trials (RCTs) for acute migraine relief. Future research is examining CGRP antagonists as well as other neurogenic inflammatory antagonists in relieving symptoms with minimal side effects.[57]

Preventive medications More frequent migraine episodes (ie, greater than 5 headaches per month) are treated with preventive medications that aim to reduce the severity, duration, and frequency. When taken on a regular basis, the frequency of attacks is least likely. Their mechanism of action may be different than for acute episodes; but medications that are beneficial include the beta-adrenergic blockers (propranolol and atenolol), calcium channel blockers (verapamil), and the TCAs (amitriptyline and serotonin antagonists). The comorbidity of migraines and depression support the use of these medications.[58] In addition, the TCAs increase the availability of serotonin and norepinephrine by inhibiting their reuptake.[21,55–57]

The antiepileptic agents (gabapentin, pregabalin) are equivocal in their ability to exert a prophylactic effect on prevention of frequency of attacks.[21] Topiramate and valproate may be beneficial as a prophylactic approach for chronic migraines.[15,21] More recent treatment strategies include the use of botulinum toxin injections for the treatment of migraine headaches (see section on botulinum later).[59] Outcome studies do support a 50% reduction in headache frequency with preventive therapies and hold promise for chronic migraine sufferers.[60]

Tension-type headache
TTHs are the most common type of headache in the population, with a 1-year prevalence rate of 80%.[15,19,21] The age range is from 20 to 30 years, and they can be episodic or chronic (<12 or >100 per year). Episodic forms are brought on by stress, fatigue, loss of sleep, and alcohol, whereas chronic TTHs can be preceded by depression, anxiety, or episodic periods. The probable mechanism involves an interaction among the limbic system and peripheral afferents form the intracranial vasculature and skeletal musculature (myofascial input).

The headache is bilateral, dull, and nonpulsating; patients complain of a tight band around the head with myofascial trigger points, most often seen with TMD.

The duration can last from 30 minutes to 72 hours; there may be associated photophobia, phonophobia, nausea, and parafunctional habits. Pharmacologic management includes the use of NSAIDs as well as low dosing of TCAs. Newer methods for chronic TTH relief include the use of onabotulinum toxin injections because the pain associated with muscle contraction is resolved with the paralytic effect of botulinum toxin.[61]

Trigeminal autonomic cephalalgias

Trigeminal autonomic cephalalgias (TACs) are a group of headache disorders that are not only associated with a headache/facial pain but also manifest themselves with parasympathetic autonomic sequelae. TACs are classified as (1) CHs, (2) paroxysmal hemicranias, (3) unilateral neuralgiform, and (4) hemicrania continua type. They are located in the orbital, temporal, supraorbital, orofacial regions, TMJ and intraorally. A careful differential diagnosis must be made since misinterpretation of clinical symptoms can result in unnecessary treatment interventions.

Cluster headaches A CH is the most common headache in the TAC classification with up to 300 cases per 100,000 patients, aged 20 to 30 years, and affecting men more than women (6:1).[62] Most occurrences are usually 2 clusters over several months to a chronic form with greater frequency and no remissions.[21,62]

Headaches are unilateral with ipsilateral autonomic features: conjunctival injection, miosis, ptosis, rhinorrhea, and facial sweating. The intensity of autonomic sequela potentiate the need for an MRI to rule out any organic anomalies as well as sleep studies because many who have CHs also have obstructive sleep apnea.[63]

Pharmacologic therapeutics are again either abortive, that is, oxygen and sumatriptan at dosing of 6 mg subcutaneous, or 10 to 20 mg intranasal (IN), DHE 0.5 to 1.0 mg (IN), and lignocaine 1.0 mL 4% to 10% solution IN.[21,60]

Preventive pharmacologic treatment includes verapamil 360 to 720 mg/d, lithium 300 to 1200 mg/d, and/or prednisone 60 to 80 mg and tapers over 4 weeks. Anticonvulsants, such as valproic acid 600 to 2000 mg/d, gabapentin 900 mg/d, and topiramate 25 to 200 mg/d, can contribute to a remission based on the individual. The clinician must advise that adverse reactions can occur based on the specific drugs as well as drug-drug interactions.[21,60–63]

Paroxysmal hemicranias Paroxysmal hemicranias (PHs) present as a unilateral headache with ipsilateral autonomic sequelae, that is, nasal congestion, lacrimation, and facial flushing. It affects 1 per 50,000 patients presenting for OFP evaluation and is often elusive in diagnosing because of localization in the face. It can be episodic or chronic and is triggered by alcohol and head/neck pain.[63,64] Pharmacologic intervention involves the use of indomethacin, a well-used antiinflammatory for PH and whose side effect is dyspepsia and whose symptoms are controlled with an H2 blocker.[65] The dosage can vary from 25 to 250 mg/d. If symptoms resolve within 24 hours, it is definitively diagnosed as PH. For further interest in the treatment of TAC, the reader is referred to references.[21,64,65]

Vascular Headaches

Vascular headaches have their cause within the veins and arteries of the head and neck that are somatic in origin. Inflammatory cascades will precipitate either a phlebitis or arteritis in the veins or arteries, respectfully. Several vascular pains *refer* to the orofacial region, that is, cranial arteritis and carotidynia.

Cranial arteritis

The most common artery inflamed within the head and neck is the temporal artery. Temporal arteritis (TA), giant cell arteritis, and/or polymyalgia rheumatica are common diagnostic terms.[21,66] TA is diagnosed during the sixth decade, and Caucasian women are at greatest risk. As one ages, the risk for TA increases. Symptoms include a headache in the temporal region with throbbing, burning, and lancinating sequelae. It can occur bilaterally, and palpating the region elicits a severe tenderness that is exacerbated by constant jaw movement: jaw claudication.[67] Pain is referred to the shoulder and hip, with other symptoms, such as malaise, poor eating, and diplopia 30% of the time leading to a loss of vision. Blood work-up of the erythrocyte sedimentation rate (ESR) shows a value greater than 100 mm/h. The definitive diagnosis is obtained with an incisional biopsy of the artery that identifies multinucleated giant cells.[67,68] This inflammatory sequelae contributes to a granulomatous reaction and resultant optic neuropathy.[67,68] TA is considered a medical emergency.[67,68] Treatment with high doses of glucocorticoids should be initiated as early as possible to rapidly control inflammatory symptoms and prevent inflammatory manifestations, such as jaw claudication, visual loss, and stroke. The burden of high-dose glucocorticoids is, however, considerable, especially in the elderly, with more than 80% of the patients experiencing significant treatment-related side effects.[67–69] Studies reported a high number of major adverse advents related to long-term glucocorticoid use in giant cell arteritis (GCA): posterior subcapsular cataract (41%), bone fractures (38%), infections (31%), hypertension (22%), diabetes mellitus (9%), and GI bleeding (4%).[69] The dosing schedule is 40 to 60 mg of prednisone daily that is gradually tapered based on symptoms and decreased ESR. The timeline for treatment will vary based on the individual.[66–69]

Carotidynia

Carotidynia is a unilateral vascular pain that originates from the cervical carotid artery and radiates to the ipsilateral side of origin, that is, the ear and face. Facial pain is reported with overlying edema at the site affected, and palpation at the common carotid bifurcation elicits a severe pain. Pain is referred to the eye, malar region, and back of the ear. Two types, acute and chronic, are diagnosed. The acute form can manifest itself over several weeks as a result of a single illness, whereas the chronic form may be a variant of the acute episode. Women are predisposed with a 4:1 ratio, and diagnosis is during middle age.[21,70] The mechanism may be similar to TA, and it resolves over several weeks. Pharmacologic therapy is similar to TA. A dosage of 30 mg/d of prednisone can be followed by a tapering dose over 4 days. Chronic therapy mimics pharmacologic prescribing for chronic migraines (see section on migraine pharmacologic treatment earlier).[21,70]

TOPICAL MEDICATIONS FOR OROFACIAL PAIN

Topical medications offer distinct advantages over systemic agents: greater safety, rapid onset of action, and low side-effect profile.[70,71] The targeted disorders, however, should be regional and demonstrate a pain relief response locally. Complete cessation of pain on application of topical anesthetic may not, however, be possible, as some of the neuronal changes may be central or due to neuropathic changes not easily reached by most topical anesthetics. Nevertheless, topical medications are useful for NP because of peripheral nerve sensitization as well as for centralized neuropathy that is accompanied by local allodynia. In the latter situation, the topical medication is used over the trigger site to reduce the ongoing neural stimulation that maintains the central sensitization. In cases of mild to moderate pain, the local therapy might be the sole intervention. For moderate to severe pain, the use of systemic medications as well as local topical medications is more appropriate. A locally applied medication can offer faster relief, whereas a centrally acting medication is being titrated up to effective levels.[71-73]

Clinicians can manage OFP by applying topical medications that are formulated according to accepted clinical indications; that is, the composition can be modified for individual patient requirements. These medications should be compounded by a pharmacy known to have high standards of quality, manufacturing technique, and reproducibility of compounded products. Topical medications can be applied directly to mucosa, skin, as well as a custom-made stable intraoral carrier referred to as a neurosensory stent to ensure adequate drug delivery at the site of NP. Examples of the most commonly used medicaments are as follows (also refer to **Table 2**).

Topical Anesthetics

Lidocaine patches
The 5% lidocaine transdermal patch (Lidoderm) is currently FDA approved for the treatment of pain associated with PHN.[74,75] The patch is 10 to 14 cm in area and contains 700 mg of lidocaine, although only about 3% of this dose is absorbed resulting in peak blood levels of 130 ng/mL during the recommended 12-hour application, slightly more than that achieved following an injection of one-half cartridge of 2% lidocaine with epinephrine.[76-78] According to the manufacturer, the patch can be cut into smaller sizes with scissors before removal from the release liner. In addition to placebo-controlled trials in PHN, the drug has also proven efficacious in other NP states, that is, in patients who have chronic lower back pain and osteoarthritis.[79,80] The systemic absorption of lidocaine from the patch is minimal in healthy adults even when 4 patches are applied for up to 24 hours per day, and lidocaine absorption is even lower among patients with PHN than healthy adults at the currently recommended dose. Because of its proven efficacy and safety profile, the lidocaine patch 5% has been recommended as a first-line therapy for the treatment of the NP of PHN.[81]

Proparacaine
The benefit of the topical anesthetic proparacaine in TN was investigated in a randomized double-blind placebo-controlled trial of 47 patients.[82] The patients were assigned randomly to either 2 drops of 0.5% proparacaine or buffered saline into the eye on the side of the trigeminal neuralgia. The results showed no benefit from proparacaine delivered in this way.

Streptomycin and lidocaine
Seventeen patients with TN were entered into a randomized double-blind study involving weekly injections of 2 mL of 2% lidocaine with or without 1 g streptomycin. The investigators concluded that, although effective initially, streptomycin is not responsible for any pain relief in the long-term.[83]

Vanilloid Compounds (Capsaicin)
Capsaicin is a derivative of the chili pepper. Its proposed mechanism of action involves a depletion of substance P and calcitonin gene–related peptide from peripheral afferent nerve endings. Several randomized double-blind trials in osteoarthritis and NP have demonstrated efficacy in these chronic pain populations.[84-86] The recently characterized capsaicin receptor is known as the transient receptor potential channel-vanilloid subfamily 1 whose activation is thought to be necessary for the release of these inflammatory and pain-provoking compounds.[72] Although the use of topical capsaicin has been proposed in patients who have TMD, surprisingly there are no clinical trials or even case-controlled studies evaluating its therapeutic effect in

Table 2
Topical medicaments: pharmacologic groups and dosing schedule

Group	Generic/Name Brand	Dosage Form	Dosing
Topical anesthetic	Lidocaine (Xylocaine, Lidoderm, Akten, AneCream)	2% (lidocaine gel, viscous solution, ointment, spray, lozenge); 5% adhesive patch	Apply topically 2–4 times daily; lozenge: take to every 2 h; patch: place for up to 12 h in any 24-h period
Topical anesthetic	Benzocaine (Anbesol, Cepacol)	20% (aerosol, gel, liquid, lozenge, ointment, solution, mouth strip, mouth swab)	Aerosol: apply for ≤1 s; gel, ointment: apply topically 2–4 times daily; lozenge: can be taken up to every 2 h
Topical anesthetic	Lidocaine/prilocaine (EMLA, Oraqix)	2.5% lidocaine/2.5% prilocaine (cream, periodontal gel)	Apply to skin for 10 min to 2 h
Neuropeptide	Capsaicin	0.025% and 0.075% (cream, gel, liquid, patch, lotion)	Topical: apply to affected area 3–4 times per day; patch: apply to affected area up to 3–4 times a day up to 8 h for 7 d
NSAID	Ketoprofen	10%–20% (cream, patch)	Cream: apply 2–4 times a day × 7 d; patch: apply once daily
NSAID	Diclofenac (Flector, Pennsaid, Voltaren OTC)	10%–20% (gel, patch, solution)	Apply to affected area 4 times a day; patch: apply 1 patch bid
Antidepressant	Amitriptyline	2% (gel, cream)	Cream: apply 2–3 times a day
Sympathomimetic agents	Clonidine	0.01% (gel, cream, patch)	Cream: apply 2–4 times a day; patch: apply once per week
NMDA antagonist	Ketamine	0.5% (cream)	Cream: apply 2–3 times a day
Anticonvulsant	Carbamazepine	2% (cream)	Cream: apply 2–3 times a day

Abbreviations: EMLA, Lidocaine 2.5% and Prilocaine 2.5%; NMDA, N-methyl-d-aspartate; OTC, over the counter.

the TMD population.[72,86] From a safety profile, the topical application of the drug is devoid of systemic toxicity, although patients must be counseled to expect a burning feeling during the initial applications of the drug; with continued application this unpleasant feeling will dissipate. Combining capsaicin with a topical anesthetic, such as benzocaine 20% in pluronic lecithin organogel (PLO), may help reduce this burning sensation.[87] Capsaicin is probably best used as an adjunct to NSAIDs, benzodiazepines, or other systemic modalities. As well as an effective treatment of the pain of postherpetic neuralgia.

Topical Nonsteroidal Antiinflammatory Drugs

Ketoprofen

Ketoprofen (*Topofen*) is a fast-acting transdermal gel NSAID that possesses analgesic, antipyretic, and antiinflammatory properties. Topical application of the active ingredient is locally effective and at the same time minimizes the risk of systemic adverse events. A study at the University of Zagreb, in Croatia, evaluated the use of topical ketoprofen (called Fastum gel in Croatia) with the concurrent use of physical therapy for the treatment of TMD of 32 patients over an 8-month period. They found that in comparing asymptomatic subjects, their active mouth opening was greater than in patients before ($P<.0001$) and after the treatment ($P<.0011$).[88]

Diclofenac

In patients with painful TMD, topical diclofenac (*Voltaren Gel 1%*) was as effective as 100 mg oral diclofenac in reducing symptoms. Di Rienzo Businco and colleagues[89] reported that topically applied diclofenac and oral diclofenac are equally effective in the treatment of TMD symptoms; however, topical diclofenac did not have had untoward effects on the gastric apparatus as the oral diclofenac.

Antidepressants

Topical amitriptyline alone or combined with ketamine relieves peripheral NP.[90,91] Topical application of doxepin significantly relieves chronic NP, and when mixed with capsaicin the effect was observed significantly earlier.[92] Although it is known that there are serotonin receptors in peripheral nerves residing outside the CNS, it is unclear if this fact is important to the topical effect of TCAs, which are known to block the reuptake of serotonin. Additionally, cyclobenzaprine, a TCA analogue, is used as a muscle relaxant. It has been used for peripheral application for muscle trismus and spasm, but adequate studies supporting this use are lacking.

Sympathomimetic Agents

Sympathomimetic agents may be useful in some forms of chronic NP where nociceptor activity is being stimulated by sympathetic fiber release of norepinephrine in the periphery. It has been shown that injured C fibers express α1 receptors on their peripheral membranes. Sympathetic activity then would excite the C fibers, signaling pain. Clonidine is an α2-adrenergic agonist. Clonidine is thought to relieve pain by decreasing the abnormal excitability of these functional nociceptors. Clonidine is available as a transdermal patch for extraoral use. For intraoral use, it is better to have clonidine compounded into a transdermal penetrating cream and dispensed in a calibrated syringe so that the dose can be better controlled. Epstein and others[93] conducted an open-label study on the use of topical clonidine, in which they assessed 17 patients using clonidine cream (0.2 mg/g) and applied it four times daily to the site of pain. Half of these patients reported clinical improvement; however, no patients reported complete resolution of symptoms. The clinical trial suggests that topical clonidine may be effective in the management of some patients with oral neuralgialike pain, but may have a more limited effect in those patients with oral NP.[93]

N-Methyl-D-Aspartate–Blocking Agents

Recent studies have shown that N-methyl-d-aspartate (NMDA)–receptor antagonists may be useful in the treatment of neurogenic pain.[94–97] Several studies have been conducted in which orally administered ketamine, an NMDA antagonist, has shown effectiveness in alleviating refractory NP. Although this medication has promise for the treatment of neuropathies, it can cause adverse effects, such as hallucinations and dysphoria.[98,99] Topical ketamine may be useful, but specific studies are needed to evaluate this therapeutic alternative. As with clonidine, this medication would be best compounded into a transdermal penetrating cream and dispensed in a calibrated syringe.

Anticonvulsants

Although anticonvulsants are useful for NP, their mechanism of action in this setting is unknown. Anticonvulsants are divided into 2 categories: newer (eg, gabapentin [Neurontin], pregabalin [Lyrica]) and traditional (eg, carbamazepine [Tegretol], valproate [Depacon]). Evidence is lacking for the use of other newer anticonvulsants, such as topiramate (Topamax) and lamotrigine (Lamictal).[100,101] The Department of Diagnostic Sciences, Division of Orofacial Pain, University of Medicine and Dentistry of New Jersey, Newark, conducted a study to evaluate the effect of topical medications alone or in combination with systemic medications in the treatment of orofacial NP conditions. A retrospective chart review was performed for 39 patients who were diagnosed with a NP condition, such as deafferentation pain, traumatic neuroma, or trigeminal or glossopharyngeal neuralgia, and were treated for orofacial NP at the Orofacial Pain Clinic. The review concluded that topical medication as single treatment or in combination with systemic medications can reduce orofacial NP severity. They used a compounding pharmacy to produce a topical medication containing carbamazepine 4%, lidocaine 1%, ketoprofen 4%, ketamine 4%, and gabapentin 4%.[73]

BOTULINUM A TOXIN (BOTOX)

Botulinum A toxin is produced by *Clostridium botulinum*, which affects the presynaptic membrane of the neuromuscular junction where it prevents acetylcholine release and, therefore, muscle contraction. Inactivation persists until collaterals form in junction plates on new areas of muscle cell walls. An investigational use of Botulinum toxin is for pain management; the purported mechanism of action is a reduction in spasticity in both dystonias and migraines.[102]

The FDA says Botox A injections have been shown to be effective in the prevention of migraines, which are debilitating headaches that cause intense pulsing or throbbing pain and affect about 12% of Americans. Headaches must be greater than or equal to 15 days per month with headache lasting 4 hours a day or longer. The Botox A is administered via 31 injections into 7 specific head and neck sites. When injected at labeled doses in recommended areas, it is expected to produce results lasting up to 3 months depending on the individual patient. A meta-analysis by Jackson and colleagues[103] showed that there was a modest benefit for chronic headaches/migraines, but it did not reduce the quantity of headaches and did not help with tension headaches. The side effects of botulinum toxin include pain, erythema, and unintended paralysis of nearby muscles.

Over the past decade there has been an increase in the number of studies investigating the use of Botox A to treat TMDs and bruxism; however, it is not considered a first-line treatment option. Before using Botox A as a treatment modality for bruxism, it is imperative that a definitive diagnosis of bruxism be made and that all other noninvasive and commonly validated methodologies are used in an attempt to manage the condition. The possible clinical effects of Botox A in the treatment of bruxism and TMDs at first seem attractive. However, the long-term efficacy of Botox A underwent Cochrane review by Soares and colleagues[104]; they concluded there was not enough evidence to support Botox use for myofascial pain syndrome and that more RCTs are needed.

SUMMARY/FUTURE DIRECTIONS

OFP comprises a highly extensive spectrum of pain disorders because of their unique anatomic/physiologic and biochemical components. The oral health care clinician must be astute in his or her systematic approach in eliciting a differential diagnosis on a case-specific basis. Once a definitive diagnosis is obtained, the primary approach of pain management is through rational pharmacotherapy. Future directions include innovations in routes of pharmacotherapy that will not only augment the efficacy of medication but also allow for combination therapy with fewer adverse effects and greater prolongation of relief. Future directions will also involve evidence-based interprofessional collaboratives that provide both pharmacologic paradigms as well as nonpharmacologic modalities for optimal treatment success. These therapeutic options will encourage greater choices for oral health care practitioners with respect to patient-centered care of OFP syndromes.

REFERENCES

1. De Rossi SS. Orofacial pain: a primer. Dent Clin North Am 2013;57(3):383–92.
2. Melzack R, Wall PD. Pain mechanisms: a new theory. Science 1965;150(3699): 971–9.
3. Okeson JP. The classification of orofacial pain. Oral Maxillofac Surg Clin North Am 2008;20(2):133–44.
4. Lipton JA, Ship JA, Larach-Robinson D. Estimated prevalence and distribution of reported orofacial pain in the United States. J Am Dent Assoc 1993;124(10): 115–21.
5. Lancer P, Gesell S. Pain management: the fifth vital sign. Healthc Benchmarks 2001;8(6):68–70.
6. Benoliel R, Sharav Y. Chronic orofacial pain. Curr Pain Headache Rep 2010;14: 33–40.
7. De Leeuw R. Orofacial pain: guidelines for assessment, classification, and management. The American Academy of Orofacial Pain. 4th edition. Chicago: Quintessence Publishing Co., Inc; 2008.
8. Hargreaves KM. Orofacial pain. Pain 2011;152:S25–32.
9. Shinal RM, Fillingim RB. Overview of orofacial pain: epidemiology and gender differences in orofacial pain. Dent Clin North Am 2007;51(1):1–18.
10. Bereiter DA, Hargreaves KM, Hu JW. Trigeminal mechanisms of nociception: peripheral and brainstem organization. In: Basbaum AL, Kaneko A, Sheperd GM, et al, editors. The senses: a comprehensive reference. San Diego (CA): Academic Press; 2008. p. 435–60.
11. Cooper SA, Desjardins PJ. The value of the dental impaction pain model in drug development. Methods Mol Biol 2010;617:175–90.

12. Kim H, Ramsay E, Lee H, et al. Genome-wide association study of acute postsurgical pain in humans. Pharmacogenomics 2009;10:171–9.
13. LeResche L, Mancl LA, Drangsholt MT, et al. Predictors of onset of facial pain and temporomandibular disorders in early adolescence. Pain 2007;129:269–78.
14. Schaefer J, Holland N, Whelan JS, et al. Pain and temporomandibular disorders: a pharmaco-gender dilemma. Dent Clin North Am 2013;57(2):233–62.
15. Romeo-Reyes M, Uyanik JM. Orofacial pain management: current perspectives. J Pain Res 2014;7:99–115.
16. Costigan M, Scholz J, Woolf CJ. Neuropathic pain: a maladaptive response of the nervous system to damage. Annu Rev Neurosci 2009;31:1–32.
17. Spencer CJ, Gremillion HA. Neuropathic orofacial pain: proposed mechanisms, diagnosis, and treatment considerations. Dent Clin North Am 2007;51:209–24.
18. Katusic S, Williams DB, Beard CM, et al. Incidence and clinical features of glossopharyngeal neuralgia. Rochester, Minnesota, 1945-1984. Neuroepidemiology 1991;10(5–6):266–75.
19. Balsubramaniam R, Klasser GD. Orofacial pain syndromes: evaluation and management. Med Clin North Am 2014;98(6):1385–405.
20. Stacey BR. Management of peripheral neuropathic pain. Am J Phys Med Rehabil 2005;84(3 Suppl):S4–16.
21. Okeson JP. General considerations in managing oral and facial pain. In: Okeson JP, editor. Bell's oral and facial pain. 7th edition. Hanover Park (IL): Quintessence Publishing Co; 2014. p. 181–232.
22. Mueller D, Obermann M, Yoon MS, et al. Prevalence of trigeminal neuralgia and persistent idiopathic facial pain: a population based study. Cephalalgia 2011; 31(15):1542–8.
23. Rozen TD. Trigeminal neuralgia and glossopharyngeal neuralgia. Neurol Clin 2004;22:185–206.
24. Zakrzewska JM. Medical management of trigeminal neuropathic pains. Expert Opin Pharmacother 2010;11(8):1239–54.
25. Reisner L, Pettengill CA. The use of anticonvulsants in orofacial pain. Oral Surg Oral Med Oral Pathol Oral Radiol Endod 2001;91(1):2–7.
26. Attal N, Crucco G, Baron R, et al. EFNS guidelines on the pharmacological treatment of neuropathic pain: 2010 revision. Eur J Neurol 2010;17:1113-e88.
27. Saarto T, Wiffen PJ. Antidepressants for neuropathic pain. Cochrane Database Syst Rev 2005;(3):CD005454.
28. Lee YC, Chen PP. A review of SSRIs and SNRIs in neuropathic pain. Expert Opin Pharmacother 2010;11:2813–25.
29. Stieber VW, Bourland JD, Ellis TL. Glossopharyngeal neuralgia treated with gamma knife surgery: treatment outcome and failure analysis case report. J Neurosurg 2005;102(Suppl):155–7.
30. Vanelderen P, Lataster A, Levy R, et al. Occipital neuralgia. Pain Pract 2010; 10(2):137–44.
31. Polycarpou N, Ng YL, Canavan D, et al. Prevalence of persistent pain after endodontic treatment and factors affecting its occurrence in cases with complete radiographic healing. Int Endod J 2005;38(3):169–78.
32. Bramwell BL. Topical orofacial medications for neuropathic pain. Int J Pharm Compd 2010;14(3):200–3.
33. Kennedy PG. Varicella-zoster virus latency in human ganglia. Rev Med Virol 2002;12:327–34.
34. Scheinfeld N. The role of gabapentin in treating diseases with cutaneous manifestations and pain. Int J Dermatol 2003;42:491–5.

35. Rees RT, Harris M. Atypical odontalgia: differential diagnoses and treatment. Br J Oral Surg 1978;16:212–8.
36. Graff-Radford SB, Solberg WK. Atypical odontalgia. J Craniomandib Disord 1992;6:260–5.
37. Rhodus NL, Carlson CR, Miller CS. Burning mouth syndrome (disorder). Quintessence Int 2003;34:587–93.
38. Danhauer SC, Miller CS, Rhodus NL, et al. Impact of criteria–based diagnosis of burning mouth syndrome on treatment outcome. J Orofac Pain 2002;16:305–11.
39. Rodriguez-de Rivera –Campillo E, Lopez-Lopez J. Evaluation of the response to treatment and clinical evolution in patients with burning mouth syndrome. Med Oral Pato Oral Cir Bucal 2013;18:e403–10.
40. Sreebny LM, Yu A, Green A, et al. Xerostomia in diabetes mellitus. Diabetes Care 1992;15:900–4.
41. Heckmann SM, Kirchner E, Grushka M, et al. A double-blind study on clonazepam in patients with burning mouth syndrome. Laryngoscope 2012;122(4):813–6.
42. Thoppay JR, DeRossi SS, Ciarrocca KN. Burning mouth syndrome. Dent Clin North Am 2013;57(3):497–512.
43. Patton LL, Siegel MA, Benoliel R, et al. Management of burning mouth syndrome: systematic review and management recommendations. Oral Surg Oral Med Oral Pathol Oral Radiol Endod 2007;103(Suppl):S39.e1–13.
44. deMorales M, do Amaral Bezerra BA, da Rocha Neto PC, et al. Randomized trials for the treatment of burning mouth syndrome: an evidence-based review of the literature. J Oral Pathol Med 2012;41(4):281–7.
45. Gorsky M, Silverman S Jr, Chinn H. Clinical characteristics and management outcome in the burning mouth syndrome. An open study of 130 patients. Oral Surg Oral Med Oral Pathol 1991;72:192–5.
46. Klasser GD, Epstein JB, Villines D, et al. Burning mouth syndrome: a challenge for dental practitioners and patients. Gen Dent 2011;59(3):210–20.
47. Sardella A, Lodi G, Demarosi F, et al. Burning mouth syndrome: a retrospective study investigating spontaneous remission and response to treatments. Oral Dis 2006;12(2):152–5.
48. Franco AL, Goncalves DA, Castanharo SM, et al. Migraine is the most prevalent primary headache in individuals with temporomandibular disorders. J Orofac Pain 2010;24(3):287–92.
49. Olesen J. The international classification of headache disorders. Ed 3 (beta version). Cephalalgia 2013;33:629–808.
50. Hu XH, Markson LE, Lipton RB, et al. Burden of migraine in the United States: disability and economic costs. Arch Intern Med 1999;159:813–8.
51. Stewart WF, Ricci JA, Chee E, et al. Lost productive work time costs from health conditions in the United States: results from the American Productivity Audit. J Occup Environ Med 2003;45(12):1234–46.
52. Karli N, Zarifoglu M, Calisir N, et al. Comparison of pre-headache phases and trigger factors of migraine and episodic tension-type headache: do they share similar clinical pathophysiology? Cephalalgia 2005;25(6):444–51.
53. Durham PL. Calcitonin gene-related peptide (CGRP) and migraine. Headache 2006;46(Suppl 1):S3–8.
54. Silberstein S, Kori S. Dihydroergotamine: a review of formulation approaches for the acute treatment of migraine. CNS Drugs 2013;27(5):385–94.
55. Silberstein SD, Holland S, Freitag F, et al. Evidence-based guideline update: pharmacologic treatment for episodic migraine prevention in adults: report of

the quality standards subcommittee of the American Academy of Neurology and the American Headache Society. Neurology 2012;78:1337–45.

56. Dodick D, Lipton RB, Martin V, et al. Triptan cardiovascular safety expert panel: consensus statement: cardiovascular safety profile of triptans (5-HT agonists) in the acute treatment of migraine. Headache 2004;44(5):414–25.

57. Farkkila M, Diener HC, Gerard G, et al. Efficacy and tolerability of lasmiditan, an oral 5-HT (1F) receptor agonist, fir the acute treatment of migraine: a phase 2 randomized, placebo-controlled, parallel group, dose ranging study. Lancet Neurol 2012;11(5):405–13.

58. Scher AL, Bigal ME, Lipton RB. Comorbidity of migraine. Curr Opin Neurol 2005; 18(3):305–10.

59. Dodick DW, Turkel CC, DeGryse RE, et al, PREEMPT Chronic Migraine Study. Onabotulinum toxin A for treatment of chronic migraine: pooled results from the double blind, randomized, placebo-controlled phases of the PREEMPT clinical program. Headache 2010;50(6):921–36.

60. Benoliel R, Eliav E. Primary headache disorders. Dent Clin North Am 2013;57(3): 513–39.

61. Wheeler A, Smith HS. Botulinum toxins: mechanisms of action, anti-nociception and clinical applications. Toxicology 2013;306:124–46.

62. Leone M, Bussone G. Pathophysiology of trigeminal autonomic cephalalgias. Lancet Neurol 2009;8(8):755–64.

63. Chervin RD, Zallek SN, Lin X, et al. Timing patterns of cluster headaches and association with symptoms of obstructive sleep apnea. Sleep Res Online 2000;3(3):107–12.

64. Balasubramaniam R, Klasser GD, Delcanho R. Trigeminal autonomic cephalalgias: a review and implications for dentistry. J Am Dent Assoc 2008;139(12): 1616–24.

65. Cittadini E, Matharu MS, Goadsby PJ. Paroxysmal hemicranias: a prospective clinical study of 31 cases. Brain 2008;131(Pt 4):1142–56.

66. Ponte C, Rodrigues AF, O'Neill L, et al. Giant cell arteritis: current treatment and management. World J Clin Cases 2015;3(6):484–94.

67. Kraemer M, Metz A, Harold M, et al. Reduction in jaw opening: a neglected symptom of giant cell arteritis. Rheumatol Int 2011;31:1521–3.

68. Redillas C, Solomon S. Recent advances in temporal arteritis. Curr Pain Headache Rep 2003;7:297–302.

69. Proven A, Gabriel SE, Orces C, et al. Glucocorticoid therapy in giant cell arteritis: duration and adverse outcomes. Arthritis Rheum 2003;49:703–8.

70. Comacchio F, Bottin R, Brescia G, et al. Carotidynia: new aspects of a controversial entity. Acta Otorhinolaryngol Ital 2012;32:266–9.

71. Svensson P, Baad-Hansen L, Eliav E, et al, Special Interest Group of Oro-facial Pain. Guidelines and recommendations for assessment of somatosensory function in oro-facial pain conditions: a task force report. J Oral Rehabil 2011;38(5):366–94.

72. Padilla M, Clark GT, Merrill RL. Topical medications for orofacial neuropathic pain: a review. J Am Dent Assoc 2000;131(2):184–95.

73. Heir G, Karolchek S, Kalladka M, et al. Use of topical medication in orofacial neuropathic pain: a retrospective study. Oral Surg Oral Med Oral Pathol Oral Radiol Endod 2008;105(4):466–9.

74. Comer AM, Lamb HM. Lidocaine patch 5%. Drugs 2000;59(2):245–9.

75. Campbell BJ, Rowbotham M, Davies PS, et al. Systemic absorption of topical lidocaine in normal volunteers, patients with post-herpetic neuralgia, and patients with acute herpes zoster. J Pharm Sci 2002;91(5):1343–50.

76. Rowbotham MC, Davies PS, Verkempinck C, et al. Lidocaine patch: double-blind controlled study of a new treatment method for post-herpetic neuralgia. Pain 1996;65(1):39–44.

77. Galer BS, Rowbotham MC, Perander J, et al. Topical lidocaine patch relieves post herpetic neuralgia more effectively than a vehicle topical patch: results of an enriched enrollment study. Pain 1999;80(3):533–8.

78. Galer BS, Jensen MP, Ma T, et al. The lidocaine patch 5% effectively treats all neuropathic pain qualities: results of a randomized, double-blind, vehicle-controlled, 3-week efficacy study with use of the neuropathic pain scale. Clin J Pain 2002;18(5):297–301.

79. Galer BS, Gammaitoni AR, Oleka N, et al. Use of the lidocaine patch 5% in reducing intensity of various pain qualities reported by patients with low-back pain. Curr Med Res Opin 2004;20(Suppl 2):S5–12.

80. Galer BS, Sheldon E, Patel N, et al. Topical lidocaine patch 5% may target a novel underlying pain mechanism in osteoarthritis. Curr Med Res Opin 2004; 20(9):1455–8.

81. Davies PS, Galer BS. Review of lidocaine patch 5% studies in the treatment of postherpetic neuralgia. Drugs 2004;64:937–47.

82. Kondziolka T, Lemley JR, Kestle LD, et al. The effect of single-application topical ophthalmic anesthesia in patients with trigeminal neuralgia: a randomized double-blind placebo-controlled trial. J Neurosurg 1994;80:993–7.

83. Stajcic Z, Juniper RP, Todorovic L. Peripheral streptomycin/lidocaine injections versus lidocaine alone in the treatment of idiopathic trigeminal neuralgia: a double blind controlled trial. J Craniomaxillofac Surg 1990;18:243–6.

84. Kopp S. The influence of neuropeptides, serotonin, and interleukin 1ß on temporomandibular joint pain and inflammation. J Oral Maxillofac Surg 1998;56: 189–91.

85. Sato J, Segami N, Yoshitake Y, et al. Expression of capsaicin receptor TRPV-1 in synovial tissues of patients with symptomatic internal derangement of the temporomandibular joint and joint pain. Oral Surg Oral Med Oral Pathol Oral Radiol Endod 2005;100:674–81.

86. Swift JQ, Roszkowski MT. The use of opioid drugs in management of chronic orofacial pain. J Oral Maxillofac Surg 1998;56(9):1081–5.

87. Epstein JB, Marcoe JH. Topical application of capsaicin for treatment of oral neuropathic pain and trigeminal neuralgia. Oral Surg Oral Med Oral Pathol 1994;77:135–40.

88. Badel T, Krapac L, Savić Pavičin I, et al. Physical therapy with topical ketoprofen and anxiety related to temporomandibular joint pain treatment. Fiz Rehabil Med 2013;25(1–2):6–16.

89. Di Rienzo Businco L, Di Rienzo Businco A, D'Emilia M, et al. Topical versus systemic diclofenac in the treatment of temporomandibular joint dysfunction symptoms. Acta Otorhinolaryngol Ital 2004;24(5):279–83.

90. Lynch ME, Clark AJ, Sawynok J. A pilot study examining topical amitriptyline, ketamine, and a combination of both in the treatment of neuropathic pain. Clin J Pain 2003;19:323–8.

91. Lynch ME, Clark AJ, Sawynok J, et al. Topical amitriptyline and ketamine in neuropathic pain syndromes: an open-label study. J Pain 2005;6:644–9.

92. McCleane G. Topical application of doxepin hydrochloride, capsaicin and a combination of both produces analgesia in chronic human neuropathic pain: a randomized, double-blind, placebo-controlled study. Br J Clin Pharmacol 2000;49:574–9.

93. Epstein J, Grushka M, Le N. Topical clonidine for orofacial pain: a pilot study. J Orofac Pain 1997;11(4):346–52.

94. Karlsten R, Gordh T. How do drugs relieve neurogenic pain? Drugs Aging 1997; 11:398–412.

95. Broadley KE, Kurowska A, Tookman A. Ketamine injection used orally. Palliat Med 1996;10:247–50.

96. Lipman AG. Analgesic drugs for neuropathic and sympathetically maintained pain. Clin Geriatr Med 1996;12:501–15.

97. Mathisen LC, Skjelbred P, Skoglund LA, et al. Effect of ketamine, an NMDA receptor inhibitor, in acute and chronic orofacial pain. Pain 1995;61:215–20.

98. Warncke T, Stubhaug A, Jorum E. Ketamine, an NMDA receptor antagonist, suppresses spatial and temporal properties of burn-induced secondary hyperalgesia in man: a double-blind, cross-over comparison with morphine and placebo. Pain 1997;72(1–2):99–106.

99. Felsby S, Nielsen J, Arendt-Nielsen L, et al. NMDA receptor blockade in chronic neuropathic pain: a comparison of ketamine and magnesium chloride. Pain 1996;64:283–91.

100. Thienel U, Neto W, Schwabe SK, et al, Topiramate Diabetic Neuropathic Pain Study Group. Topiramate in painful diabetic polyneuropathy: findings from three double-blind placebo-controlled trials. Acta Neurol Scand 2004;110(4):221–31.

101. Wiffen PJ, Rees J. Lamotrigine for acute and chronic pain. Cochrane Database Syst Rev 2007;(2):CD006044.

102. Miller RD, Eriksson LI, Fleisher L, et al. Miller's anesthesia. 7th edition. Philadelphia: Churchill Livingstone; 2009. p. 1807.

103. Jackson JL, Kuriyama A, Hayashino Y. Botulinum toxin A for prophylactic treatment of migraine and tension headaches in adults: a meta-analysis. JAMA 2012; 307(16):1736–45.

104. Soares A, Andriolo RB, Atallah AN, et al. Botulinum toxin for myofascial pain syndromes in adults. Cochrane Database Syst Rev 2012;(4):CD007533.

The Pharmacologic Management of Common Lesions of the Oral Cavity

 CrossMark

Mihai Radulescu, DMD

KEYWORDS

- Aphtae • Herpes • Candidas • Lichen planus • Pemphigus • Pemphigoid • Oral
- Treatment

KEY POINTS

- Topical therapy is the first line of treatment of aphtous, herpetic, candida, and lichen planus lesions of the oral mucosa.
- Topical medications can be used in the management of oral pemphigus and pemphigoid lesions.
- Intralesional injections allow maximum local benefit with minimal systemic effect.
- Systemic conditions need to be ruled out in patients with recurrent or persistent oral lesions.

INTRODUCTION

The general dentist should be able to identify the presence of soft tissue lesions in the oral cavity. Some of these lesions may be symptomatic, others could be incidental findings. Their cause could be local or systemic. This article provides an overview of the current pharmacologic modalities available to treat aphthous lesions, herpetic lesions, candidiasis, ulcerative lichen planus, mucous membrane pemphigoid, and pemphigus vulgaris. The emphasis is on local pharmacologic therapies, yet systemic conditions that often present with such oral lesions are briefly reviewed along with the appropriate management.

APHTHOUS LESIONS, ALSO KNOWN AS CANKER SORES

Aphthous lesions are perhaps the most common form of oral ulcerations, the prevalence in the US population being approximately 20%.[1] These lesions can occur as an isolated event or may reoccur at intervals as often as a few days in isolated or multiple foci.[2] In such cases, the condition is known as recurrent aphthous ulcers or

Oral Maxillofacial Surgery, Woodhull Medical Center, 760 Broadway, Brooklyn, NY 11206, USA
E-mail address: miradmd@gmail.com

Dent Clin N Am 60 (2016) 407–420
http://dx.doi.org/10.1016/j.cden.2015.12.003
0011-8532/16/$ – see front matter © 2016 Elsevier Inc. All rights reserved.

dental.theclinics.com

recurrent aphthous stomatitis (RAS) and it seems to be more frequent in women, patients younger than 40 years, white persons, nonsmokers, and those of high socioeconomic status.[3] No precise cause has been identified; the cause is thought to be of genetic predisposition, immune mechanisms, anemia, possible nutritional deficiencies, or stress.[1]

The typical features of aphthous ulcers are their predilection for nonkeratinized mucosa (**Figs. 1** and **2**) and the associated pain. Lesions less than 1 cm usually heal within 1 to 2 weeks and larger lesions may take more than 6 weeks, yet scarring is uncommon.[4] If the patient is immunocompromised, the lesion can become secondarily infected with bacteria or fungi.

The treatment of aphthous ulcers is palliative, the goal being to reduce the duration, size, and recurrence of lesions. First-line treatment options comprise antiseptics, such as chlorhexidine, anti-inflammatory drugs, and analgesics for as long as the lesions persist[5] (**Table 1**).

Topical steroids can decrease the symptoms and improve healing time, but do not affect recurrence rate. If multiple lesions are present, an aqueous solution is preferred. A dexamethasone rinse can be considered.[6] In the case of isolated lesions, a high-potency topical steroid (kenalog, clobetasol, or fluocinomide[6,7]) in an adherent carrier, such as orabase or denture adhesive paste, can be applied in small amount to the specific area.[8] Steroids should not be used for more than 2 weeks and the patient should be monitored for yeast superinfection. Also, topical steroids should not be placed on viral lesions, which could aggravate the lesion.

Minocycline, an antibiotic with immunomodulatory effect suppressing neutrophils, T lymphocytes, and collagenase activity,[4] can also be used. A blind crossover study shows significant reduction in duration and severity of pain compared with placebo.[4]

Intralesional treatment with triamcinolone (0.1–0.5 mL per lesion) can be considered for a painful single aphtha.[9] In case of severe lesions resistant to topical or local treatment, a systemic steroid, such as prednisone, is recommended. It is started at 1 mg/kg/day as a single dose in patients with severe lesions and tapered after 1 to 2 weeks.[10] The recommendation is to use less than 50 mg per day, preferably in the morning, for 5 days.[6]

Severe cases of RAS can be treated with colchicine,[11] pentoxyfiline,[12] dapsone,[13] or infliximab[14] but these modalities should be reserved to oral medicine specialists because of the multiple side effects.

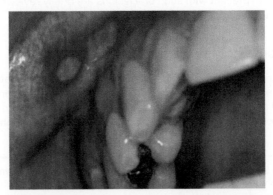

Fig. 1. Single aphthous ulceration of upper lip. (*From* Neville BW, Damm DD, Allen CM, et al. Oral and maxillofacial pathology. 3rd edition. Philadelphia: Saunders/Elsevier; 2016; with permission.)

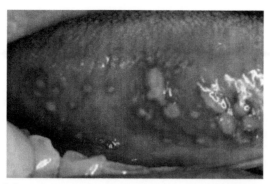

Fig. 2. Multiple aphthous lesions of ventral tongue. (*From* Neville BW, Damm DD, Allen CM, et al. Oral and maxillofacial pathology. 3rd edition. Philadelphia: Saunders/Elsevier; 2016; with permission.)

Additional therapies that have been reported to be effective are chlorhexidine, daily vitamin B_{12} sublingually,[15] and low-level laser therapy.[16] A small study showed lower RAS recurrence in subjects using chewable nicotine tablets.[17]

When treating RAS, the clinician should thoroughly review the medical history of the patient to rule out systemic conditions that are known to cause aphthous ulcers. The most common are Behçet syndrome, cyclic neutropenia, periodic fever with aphthae

Table 1
Topical medications for recurrent aphthous ulcers

Medication	Class	Form	Dispense	Instructions	Notes
Chlorhexidine	Antibiotic	0.12%	480-mL bottle	15-mL rinse and spit tid	Safe
Dexamethasone	Steroid	Elixir 0.05/5 mL	100-mL bottle	5-mL rinse and spit tid	Risk of mucosal atrophy Risk of systemic absorption with prolonged use
Minocycline	Antibiotic	0.2% aqueous solution	200-mL bottle	5-mL rinse and spit qid for 10 d	Safe
Kenalog (triamcinolone)	High-potency steroid	0.1% or 0.5% ointment in Orabase	15-g tube	Apply to affected areas tid	Risk of mucosal atrophy Risk of systemic absorption with prolonged use
Clobetasol	High-potency steroid	0.05% ointment in Orabase	15-g tube	Apply to affected areas tid	Risk of mucosal atrophy Risk of systemic absorption with prolonged use
Fluocinomide	High-potency steroid	0.05% ointment in Orabase	15-g tube	Apply to affected areas tid	Risk of mucosal atrophy Risk of systemic absorption with prolonged use

pharyngitis and adenitis syndrome, Reiter syndrome, and Sweet syndrome (**Table 2**). Other possible conditions are Crohn disease, ulcerative colitis, immune deficiencies, and gluten-sensitive enteropathy.

ORAL HERPES

In oral herpes, the principal symptom is the appearance of vesicles and ulcers that heal spontaneously within 5 to 10 days. The primary cause is often herpes simplex virus type 1 but epidemiology has been changing and herpes simplex virus-2, which was associated with herpes genitalis, can be equally found in herpes labialis.[18]

The primary herpes simplex virus-1 infection can be asymptomatic or can cause gingivostomatitis; the virus then ascends the sensory axons of the trigeminal nerve, establishing latency in the sensory ganglia. It can become reactivated under various stimuli: stress, fever, ultraviolet light, trauma, or mensturation.[19] On reactivation, the patient first experiences the prodromal symptoms of itching, burning, or paresthesia.[20] The lesions first develop as vesicles (**Fig. 3**) that eventually erupt forming ulcerations (**Fig. 4**) and ultimately scabbing. The recurrent herpes labialis occurs typically at the junction of the vermillion and the cutaneous lip. Intraorally, it usually occurs on the keratinized mucosa, which distinguishes it from the recurrent aphthous lesions.[21]

The aim of antiviral therapy is to block viral replication. Peak viral titers occur in the first 24 hours after lesion onset, when most lesions reach the vesicular stage.[19] Thus, for the treatment to be effective, it should be started at the first signs, ideally during the prodromal stage.

For recurrent herpes labialis, the most common topical treatment options are acyclovir[22] and pencyclovir[23] (**Table 3**). Because of the need of frequent applications, oral formulations are available for acyclovir,[24] famciclovir,[25] and valacyclovir.[26] For prophylaxis treatment, such as before dental procedures, valacyclovir (1 g or 2 g twice a day) or acyclovir (400 mg two or three times a day) can be prescribed.[21] Patients with severe recurrent lesions that do not experience prodromal symptoms may be candidates for long-term antiviral therapy.

Table 2
Systemic conditions that would commonly present with oral aphthous lesions

Disease	Specific Characteristics
Behçet syndrome	Severe aphthous ulcers, and recurrent genital ulceration, ocular disease, and a range of neurologic, renal, and hematologic abnormalities
Cyclic neutropenia	Recurrent oral ulcerations, fever, upper respiratory tract infections, and lymphadenopathy caused by cyclic reduction in the circulating levels of neutrophils, about every 21 d
Periodic fever with aphthae pharyngitis and adenitis syndrome	It occurs mostly in children and the condition usually improves with tonsillectomy
Reiter syndrome	Is an uncommon disease characterized by arthritis, urethritis, conjunctivitis, and oral ulcers
Sweet syndrome	Patients have aphthous lesions accompanied by fever, leukocytosis, and well-demarcated, plum-colored skin papules or plaques; there is an associated malignancy (eg, acute myeloid leukemia) in half of patients

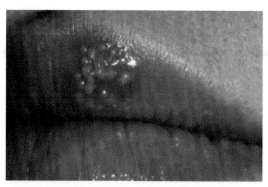

Fig. 3. Herpes labialis. (*From* Neville BW, Damm DD, Allen CM, et al. Oral and maxillofacial pathology. 3rd edition. Philadelphia: Saunders/Elsevier; 2016; with permission.)

For primary herpetic gingivostomatitis, the treatment is systemic and the clinician can choose from acyclovir, famciclovir, and valacyclovir[27] (**Table 4**). For pain management, a topical anesthetic, such as viscous lidocaine or benzocaine, can be administrated.[28] Zilactin, a topical medication containing hydroxypronyl cellulose that adheres to the mucosa, may be used to protect the lesions from irritants.[29]

CANDIDIASIS

Candidiasis is the most common mycosis of the oral cavity. Although *Candida albicans* is a common inhabitant of the oral flora, oral candidiasis is associated with a decrease in the host defense mechanism, which may be local or systemic in nature. Topical or inhaled corticosteroids and systemic medication, such as broad-spectrum antibiotics and immunosuppressive agents (azathioprine and glucocorticoids), are well known to promote candidiasis. Other factors that have been implicated in oral candidiasis are smoking, xerostomia, diabetes mellitus, endocrinopathies, pregnancy, immunosuppressive conditions, malignancies, and nutritional deficiencies.

The pseudomembranous, erythematous (**Fig. 5**), and hyperplastic forms of oral candidiasis are most often treated with topical antifungal agents, such as nystatin

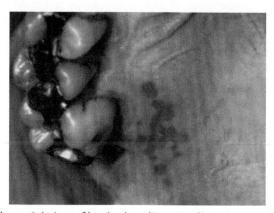

Fig. 4. Recurrent herpetic lesions of hard palate. (*From* Neville BW, Damm DD, Allen CM, et al. Oral and maxillofacial pathology. 3rd edition. Philadelphia: Saunders/Elsevier; 2016; with permission.)

Table 3
Medications for recurrent herpes labialis

Medication	Form	Dispense	Instructions	Notes
Acyclovir	5% ointment	15 g	Every 3–4 h for 4 d	Must be started at first prodromal signs
Pencyclovir	1% ointment	5 g	Every 2 h for 4 d	Must be started at first prodromal signs
Acyclovir	200 mg	25 tablets	1 tablet 5 times daily for 5 d	Must be started at first prodromal signs. Can cause headache, gastrointestinal disturbance, rash
Famciclovir	750 mg	2 tablets	2 tablets as a single dose	Must be started at first prodromal signs. Can cause headache, gastrointestinal disturbance, nausea
Valacyclovir	500 mg	8 tablets	2 g bid for 1 d	Must be started at first prodromal signs. Can cause headache, gastrointestinal disturbance, rash

ointment, and clotrimazole troches (**Table 5**). For patients experiencing xerostomia and having difficulty dissolving the troches, nystatin or amphotericin suspensions can be prescribed. Angular cheilitis (**Fig. 6**) is a mixed infection of *C albicans* and salivary species of streptococci. These lesions respond well to a combination therapy of antifungal and a topical steroid, such as nystatin-triamcinolone acetonide ointment or amphotericin oral suspension.[30]

For patients with refractory candidiasis, muccocutaneous candidosis, women with concurrent candida vaginitis, or patients in whom compliance is a problem, a systemic antifungal therapy with ketoconazole or fluconazole is recommended.[31] Patients should be informed that the systemic use of these drugs can cause hepatotoxicity. Liver function tests should be performed if the medication is used for more than 2 weeks.

LICHEN PLANUS

The most common presentation of oral lichen planus is the reticular form, often asymptomatic, and recognized by the presence of the Wickham striae. There are

Table 4
Medications for acute primary herpetic gingivostomatitis

Medication	Form	Dispense	Instructions	Notes
Acyclovir	400 mg	21 tablets	1 tablet po tid for 7 d	Dosage is for adults and adolescents. For children consult pediatrician about dosage.
Famciclovir	500 mg	21 tablets	1 tablet po tid for 7 d	Must be started at first prodromal signs. Can cause headache, gastrointestinal disturbance, nausea.
Valacyclovir	500 mg	8 tablets	2 tablets po bid for 7 d	Must be started at first prodromal signs. Can cause headache, gastrointestinal disturbance, rash.
Lidocaine	2% viscous	100 mL	2 tsp q 3 h swish and spit	Should not be prescribed to young children who may swallow it.

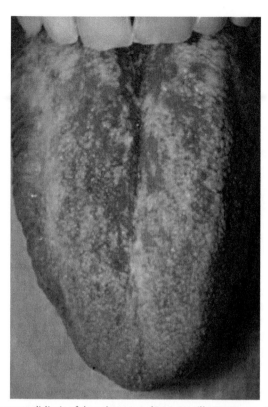

Fig. 5. Erythematous candidiasis of dorsal tongue. (*From* Neville BW, Damm DD, Allen CM, et al. Oral and maxillofacial pathology. 3rd edition. Philadelphia: Saunders/Elsevier; 2016; with permission.)

Table 5
Topical medications for oral candidiasis

Medication	Form	Dispense	Instructions	Notes
Nystatin	Ointment	30-g tube	Apply to affected area or to denture base and insert denture tid.	Safe Inexpensive
Clotrimazole	10-mg troches	70 troches	Dissolve in mouth 5 times daily for 14 d.	Safe High sugar content Expensive
Nystatin	100,000 IU/mL oral suspension	60-mL bottle	Swish with 5 mL qid allowing suspension to be retained in the mouth as long as possible. Continue treatment for 24 h after symptoms disappear.	Safe Inexpensive Poor penetration
Amphotericin	Oral suspension 100 mg/mL	48 mL	Swish with 1 mL for 3 min qid, and swallow.	Topical and systemic effects Expensive
Nystatin-triamcinolone acetonide	Ointment	15-g tube	Apply to corners of mouth after meals and at bedtime for 2 wk.	Safe Inexpensive

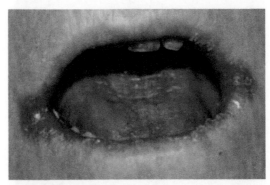

Fig. 6. Angular cheilitis. (*From* Neville BW, Damm DD, Allen CM, et al. Oral and maxillofacial pathology. 3rd edition. Philadelphia: Saunders/Elsevier; 2016; with permission.)

several variations of lichen planus, yet literature agrees that only the erosive (**Fig. 7**), ulcerative, or symptomatic lesions need to be treated. The clinician needs to have in mind that such lesions have a risk of malignant transformation estimated at 0.5% to 2% during lifetime.[32]

The first line of treatment consists of high-potency topical steroids,[33] often coadministred with a topical antifungal to prevent oral candidiasis[32] (**Table 6**). For patients who do not improve or who cannot tolerate topical corticoids for such reasons as allergic contact mucositis or recurrent oropharyngeal candidiasis, the second line of treatment consists of topical calcinerium blockers and intralesional steroids (**Table 7**). Intralesional injections with betamethasone have the advantage of delivering a high local concentration yet repeated injections raises concerns regarding systemic absorption, the potential suppression of the hypothalamic-pituitary-adrenal axis, and resulting side effects.[34] Finally, patients with severe and refractory disease that cannot be managed with topical therapy may be considered for systemic glucocorticoids, such as prednisone, or systemic immunomodulatory agents, such as azathioprine, cyclosporine, methotrexate, thalidomide, mycophenolate, or rituximab.

Additional therapies that have been reported to be effective are topical retinoids,[35] oral retinoids,[36] hydroxychloroquinone,[37] topical rapamycin,[38] oral dapsone,[39] oral metronidazole,[40] and cryotherapy.[41]

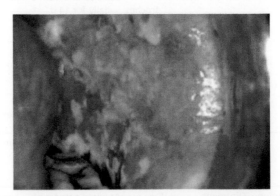

Fig. 7. Erosive lichen planus of the buccal mucosa. (*From* Neville BW, Damm DD, Allen CM, et al. Oral and maxillofacial pathology. 3rd edition. Philadelphia: Saunders/Elsevier; 2016; with permission.)

Table 6
Medications used for lichen planus: first line of treatment

Medication	Class	Form	Dispense	Instructions	Notes
Dexamethasone	Steroid	Elixir 0.5 mg/5 mL	237 mL	5-mL rinse and split 6 times per day	Risk of candidiasis
Clobethasol	High-potency steroid	Ointment 0.05%	15 g	Dry area with gauze and apply tid	Opportunistic candidiasis
Fluocinonide	High-potency steroid	Ointment 0.05%	15 g	Dry area with gauze and apply tid	Eating and drinking should be avoided for 30 min
Bethamethasone	High-potency steroid	Ointment 0.05%	15 g	Dry area with gauze and apply tid	Can be administered in gingival trays or dental base carrier
					Systemic absorption has been documented yet the risk of adrenal suppression seems to be low

Table 7
Medications used for lichen planus: second line of treatment

Medication	Class	Form	Administered	Notes
Pimecrolimus	Topical calcinerium inhibitor	1% cream	Dry area with gauze and apply tid	Concerns of increased risk of cancer
Tacrolimus	Topical calcinerium inhibitor	0.1% ointment	Dry area with gauze and apply tid	Concerns of increased risk of cancer
Triamcinolone	High-potency corticosteroid	10–40 mg/mL	Intralesional injections in submucosa q 2–4 wk	Hypopigmentation Systemic absorption Risk of increased glucose level in diabetics Risk of increased blood pressure

PEMPHIGUS VULGARIS

Pemphigus vulgaris is the most common form of oral mucosal pemphigus. It is an immune-mediated chronic vesicullobullous mucocutaneous disease and almost invariably has oral features. The bullae are formed by the action of antibodies against the desmoglein proteins of the desmosomes, thus causing intraepithelial blisters that eventually rupture, causing the ulcerations (**Fig. 8**). The lesions can be induced clinically on manual pressure or with a cotton swab (positive Nikolsky sign).

The treatment of pemphigus vulgaris is with systemic glucocorticoids (prednisone, prednisolone, methylprednisone) and immunomodulatory agents (azathioprine, mycophenolate mofetyl, cyclosporine).

MUCOUS MEMBRANE PEMPHIGOID

Mucous membrane pemphigoid is chronic autoimmune disease forming subepithelial blisters. It affects the mucous membrane of the mouth (**Fig. 9**), eyes (**Fig. 10**), nose, pharynx, larynx genitals, and anus. The treatment goals are to stop the disease

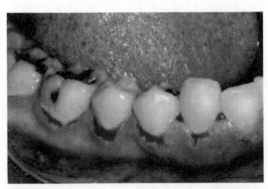

Fig. 8. Pemphigus vulgaris lesions of marginal gingiva. (*From* Neville BW, Damm DD, Allen CM, et al. Oral and maxillofacial pathology. 3rd edition. Philadelphia: Saunders/Elsevier; 2016; with permission.)

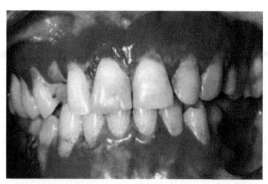

Fig. 9. Mucous membrane pemphigoid of the gingiva. (*From* Neville BW, Damm DD, Allen CM, et al. Oral and maxillofacial pathology. 3rd edition. Philadelphia: Saunders/Elsevier; 2016; with permission.)

progression, improve symptoms, and prevent the sequelae of tissue ulceration and subsequent scarring.

Proper management requires multidisciplinary care. Patients who present with lesions confined to the oral mucosa can be managed with topical corticosteroids, such as 0.1% triamcinolone acetonide, 0.05% fluocinolone acetonide, or 0.005% clobetasol proprionate in oralbase, applied three to four times a day for 9 to 24 weeks.[42] For patients who find the direct application of topical applications difficult to use, gingival trays can be fabricated to ease the drug application and left in place for 10 to 20 minutes per treatment. Alternatively, dexamethasone, 0.1 mg/mL, as a 5-mL swish and spit two or three times a day can be prescribed. When using topical steroids, patients should be monitored for oropharyngeal candidiasis. For lesions that do not respond sufficiently to local measures, intralesional corticosteroid could be used, such as triamcinolone acetonide (10 mg/mL) in 0.1 to 0.5 mL per injection side. The recommendation is to use no more than 20 mL per treatment session.[43]

Patients who do not improve with local therapy for oral mucous membrane pemphigoid or who present widespread disease may be treated with systemic agents, such as glucocorticoids (prednisone, prednisolone, methylprednisone) and immunomodulatory agents (azathioprine, mycophenolate mofetyl, cyclosporine). Dapsone, intravenous immunoglobulin, and rituximab have also been used.

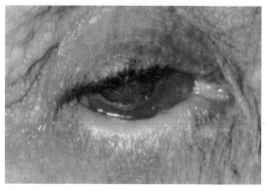

Fig. 10. Conjunctival involvement in mucous membrane pemphigoid. (*From* Neville BW, Damm DD, Allen CM, et al. Oral and maxillofacial pathology. 3rd edition. Philadelphia: Saunders/Elsevier; 2016; with permission.)

SUMMARY

The general dentist has the training to identify and treat a wide variety of oral soft tissue lesions. The first and perhaps most important step when managing such lesions is to take a comprehensive medical history. Based on this, the clinician can decide if the disease is likely of local or systemic origin. The signs and symptoms suggest the most plausible cause: viral, fungal, bacterial, immunologic, or nutritional. This allows the clinician to use the appropriate local or systemic pharmacologic agents, or a combination of both. The medications presented in this article emphasize the multiple treatment modalities available to the general dental practitioner. These pharmacologic interventions are highly effective, yet the clinician should use them accordingly to his or her experience and level of comfort. If in doubt, or if the lesions do not respond to treatment, the patient should be referred to an oral surgeon or oral medicine specialist for further evaluation.

REFERENCES

1. Messadi DV, Younai F. Aphtous ulcers. Dermatol Ther 2010;23:281–90.
2. Porter SR, Hegarty A, Kaliakatsou F, et al. Recurrent aphthous stomatitis. Clin Dermatol 2000;18:569–78.
3. Scully C. Clinical practice. Aphthous ulceration. N Engl J Med 2006;355:165–72.
4. Gorsky M, Epstein J, Raviv A, et al. Topical minocycline for managing symptoms of recurrent aphthous stomatitis. Spec Care Dentist 2008;28:27–31.
5. Belenguer-Guallar I, Jiminez-Soriano Y, Claramunt-Lozano A. Treatment of recurrent aphtous stomatitis. A literature review. J Clin Exp Dent 2014;6(2):168–74.
6. Scully C, Gorsky M, Lozada-Nur F. The diagnosis and management of recurrent aphthous stomatitis. A consensus approach. J Am Dent Assoc 2003;134:200–7.
7. Ship J, Arbor A. Recurrent aphtous stomatitis [review]. Oral Surg Oral Med Oral Pathol 1996;80(2):141–7.
8. Muñoz-Corcuera M, Esparza-Gómez G, González-Moles MA, et al. Oral ulcers: clinical aspects. A tool for dermatologists. Part I. Acute ulcers [review]. Clin Exp Dermatol 2009;34:289–94.
9. Altenburg A, Zouboulis CC. Current concepts in the treatment of recurrent aphthous stomatitis. Skin Therapy Lett 2008;13:1–4.
10. Healy CM, Thornhill MH. An association between recurrent oro-genital ulceration and non-steroidal anti-inflammatory drugs. J Oral Pathol Med 1995;24:46–8.
11. Ruah CB, Stram JR, Chasin WD. Treatment of severe recurrent aphtous stomatitis with colchicine. Arch Otolaryngol Head Neck Surg 1988;114(6):671–5.
12. Thornhill MH, Baccaglini L, Theaker E, et al. A randomized, double-blind, placebo-controlled trial of pentoxifiline for the treatment of recurrent aphtous stomatitis. Arch Dermatol 2007;143(4):463–70.
13. Lynde CB, Bruce AJ, Rogers RS 3rd. Successful treatment of complex aphtosis with colchicine and dapsone. Arch Dermatol 2009;145(3):273–6.
14. Sfikakis PP, Markomichelakis N, Alpsoy E, et al. Anti-TNF 21 therapy in the management of Behçet's disease: review and basis for recommendations. Rheumatology (Oxford) 2007;46(5):736–41.
15. Volkov I, Rudoy I, Freud T, et al. Effectiveness of vitamin B12 in treating recurrent aphthous stomatitis: a randomized, double-blind, placebo-controlled trial. J Am Board Fam Med 2009;22:9–16.
16. Aggarwal H, Singh MP, Nahar P, et al. Efficacy of low level laser therapy in treatment of recurrent aphthous ulcers. J Clin Diagn Res 2014;8(2):218–21.
17. Bittoun R. Recurrent aphthous ulcers and nicotine. Med J Aust 1991;154(7):471–2.

18. Arduino PG, Porter SR. Herpes simplex virus Type 1 infection: overview on relevant clinico-pathological features. J Oral Pathol Med 2008;37:107–21.
19. Cunningham A, Griffiths P, Leone P, et al. Current management and recommendations for access to antiviral therapy of herpes labialis [review]. J Clin Virol 2012; 53:6–11.
20. Fatahzadeh M, Schwartz RA. Human herpes simplex virus infections: epidemiology, pathogenesis, symptomatology, diagnosis, and management. J Am Acad Dermatol 2007;57:737–63.
21. Woo SB, Challacombe SJ. Management of recurrent oral herpes simplex infections. Oral Surg Oral Med Oral Pathol 2007;103:S12.e1–8.
22. Spruance SL, Nett R, Marbury T, et al. Acyclovir cream for treatment of herpes labialis. Antimicrob Agents Chemother 2002;46(7):2238–43.
23. Spruance SL, Rea TL, Thoming C, et al. Penciclovir cream for treatment of herpes labialis. JAMA 1997;227(17):1374.
24. Spruance SL, Stewart JC, Rowe NH, et al. Treatment of recurrent herpes simplex labialis with oral acyclovir. J Infect Dis 1990;161(2):185–90.
25. Spruance SL, Bodsworth N, Resnick H, et al. Single-dose, patient initiated famciclovir: a randomized, double-blind, placebo-controlled trial for episodic herpes labialis. J Am Acad Dermatol 2006;55(1):47–53.
26. Spruance SL, Jones TM, Blatter MM, et al. High-dose, short duration, early valacyclovir therapy for episodic treatment of cold sores. Antimicrob Agents Chemother 2003;47(3):1072–80.
27. Chauvin PJ, Ajar AH. Acute herpetic gingivostomatitis in adults: a review of 13 cases including diagnosis and management. J Can Dent Assoc 2002;68(4):247.
28. Vestey JP, Norval M. Muccocutaneous infections with herpes simplex and their management. Clin Exp Dermatol 1992;17(4):221.
29. Rodu B, Mattingly G. Oral mucosal ulcers: diagnosis and management. J Am Dent Assoc 1992;123(10):83.
30. Sheikh S, Gupta D, Pallagatti S, et al. Role of topical drugs in the treatment of oral mucosal disease. N Y State Dent J 2013;11:58–64.
31. Muzyka BC. Update on fungal infections. Dent Clin North Am 2013;57:561–81.
32. Stoopler E, Sollecito T. Recurrent gingival and oral mucosal lesions. JAMA 2014; 312(17):1794–5.
33. Casparis S, Borm JM. Oral lichen planus, oral lichenoid lesions, oral dysplasia, and oral cancer: retrospective analysis of clinicopathological data from 2002–2011. Oral Maxillofac Surg 2015;19:149–56.
34. Liu C, Xie B, Yang Y, et al. Efficacy of intralesional betamethasone for erosive oral lichen planus and evaluation of recurrence: a randomized, controlled trial. Oral Surg Oral Med Oral Pathol Oral Radiol 2013;116:584–90.
35. Buajeeb W, Kraivaphan P, Pobrurksa C. Efficacy of topical retinoic acid compared with topical fluorocinolone acetonide in the treatment of oral lichen planus. Oral Surg Oral Med Oral Pathol Oral Radiol 1997;83(1): 21–5.
36. Camisa C, Allen CM. Treatment of oral erosive lichen planus with systemic isotretinoin. Oral Surg Oral Med Oral Pathol Oral Radiol 1986;62(4):293–6.
37. Torti DC, Jorizzo JL, McCarty MA. Oral lichen planus: a case series with emphasis on therapy. Arch Dermatol 2007;143(4):511.
38. Soria A, Agbo-Godeau S, Taïeb A, et al. Treatment of refractory erosive lichen planus with topical rapamycin. Dermatology 2009;218(1):22–5.
39. Beck HI, Brandrup F. Treatment of erosive lichen planus with dapsone. Acta Derm Venereol 1986;66(4):366–7.

40. Rasi A, Behzadi AH. Efficacy of oral metronidazole in the treatment of cutaneous and oral lichen planus. J Drugs Dermatol 2010;9(10):1186–90.
41. Amanat D, Ebrahimi H, Zahedani MZ, et al. Comparing the effects of cryotherapy with nitrous oxide gas versus topical corticosteroids in the treatment of oral lichen planus. Indian J Dent Res 2014;15(6):711–6.
42. Ata-Ali F, Ata-Ali J. Pemphigus vulgaris and mucous membrane pemphigoid: update on etiopathogenesis, oral manifestations and management. J Clin Exp Dent 2011;3(3):246–50.
43. Knudson RM, Kalaaji AN, Bruce AJ. The management of mucous membrane pemphigoid and pemphigus. Dermatol Ther 2010;23:268–80.

Review of Top 10 Prescribed Drugs and Their Interaction with Dental Treatment

(●) CrossMark

Robert J. Weinstock, DDS[a,b],*, Michael P. Johnson, DMD[a,b]

KEYWORDS

- Drug interactions with dental treatment • Hypothyroidism • Hypertension • Diabetes
- Hypercholesterolemia • Asthma • Pain management

KEY POINTS

- The top 10 prescribed drugs and their interactions with dental treatment are reviewed.
- This article demonstrates the different ways drugs may interact with dental treatment for example, side effects, drug–drug interactions.
- This article facilitates analysis of any drug and what to seek out when considering relevant drug interactions with dental treatment.

The global proportion of people over the age of 60 is growing faster than any other age group.[1] Chronic medical conditions such as cancer, cardiovascular disease, hypertension, and diabetes are prevalent in this age group and contribute to this group's overall morbidity and mortality.[2] Poor oral health in this cohort is also common and presents in the form xerostomia, tooth loss, periodontal disease, and edentulism.[3] Dental visits by patients over age 65 are also increasing.[4]

Owing to our aging population and their multiple comorbidities, 9 out of 10 patients over age 65 are taking one or more medications (compared with 1 in 4 when compared with children). Because dentists will be seeing an increasing number of patients taking 1 or more medications, it is important for the dentist to become familiar with the interactions between dental treatment and commonly prescribed medications. Elements of dental treatment with potential for interactions with medications include:

1. Local anesthetics;
2. The dental treatment itself; and
3. Medications the dentist may prescribe.

The authors have nothing to disclose.
[a] Private Practice, 87 State Street, Guilford, CT 06437, USA; [b] Oral and Maxillofacial Surgery, Yale-New Haven Hospital, 20 York Street, New Haven, CT 06510, USA
* Corresponding author. 87 State Street, Guilford, CT 06437.
E-mail address: rjw2119@gmail.com

In this article, we review the top 10 prescribed drugs and their interactions with dental treatment. According to the IMS institute national prescriptions audit of January 2015, the following drugs were the top 10 most prescribed drugs in the United States, by number of dispensed prescriptions:

1. Levothyroxine
2. Acetaminophen with hydrocodone
3. Lisinopril
4. Metoprolol
5. Atorvastatin
6. Amlodipine
7. Metformin
8. Omeprazole
9. Simvastatin
10. Albuterol

LEVOTHYROXINE
Background

Levothyroxine is marketed as Synthroid (Abbvie Inc, North Chicago, IL) and is the most commonly prescribed drug in the United States, with 119.9 million prescriptions dispensed in 2014. Levothyroxine is a thyroid hormone supplement.

Pharmacology

The thyroid gland is responsible for synthesizing and releasing the hormones triiodothyronine and tetraiodothyronine (T4). Triiodothyronine is 10 times more potent than T4; however, 80% of triiodothyronine is actually formed by deiodination of T4 in peripheral tissues.[5] Levothyroxine is a synthetic form of T4.

Thyroid hormones are believed to exert their physiologic effect by modulating DNA transcription and promoting protein synthesis. These proteins then act on their target organs to secrete hormones that regulate growth and metabolism.[6]

Supplementing deficient thyroid hormones requires delicate titration because the therapeutic index of levothyroxine is narrow. Excessive thyroid hormone administration can precipitate symptoms of thyrotoxicosis that include adverse cardiac, respiratory, central nervous system, and gastrointestinal, hepatic, and musculoskeletal sequela.

Interactions with Dental Treatment

For the well-controlled hypothyroid patient taking a longstanding stable dose of levothyroxine, there are no specific interactions between levothyroxine and dental treatment. For patients who are recently diagnosed with hypothyroidism and are not yet euthyroid, elective treatment is best deferred and emergent treatment carried out with caution.[7] The concern in the uncontrolled patient is that if the thyroid levels are too high then thyrotoxicosis can ensue. Hypothyroidism rarely results in an emergent situation; however, these patients are at risk for arrhythmias, heart failure, and myxedema coma if severely deficient.[8]

Levothyroxine has several important relevant drugs interactions. Specifically, there are interactions with levothyroxine and warfarin, ketamine, and carbamazepine. Levothyroxine increase the International Normalized Ratio (INR) in patients taking warfarin. It is therefore important, especially when initiating levothyroxine, to monitor INR levels and adjust warfarin dosage until the INR is stable. Levothyroxine may increase the hypertension and tachycardia that occurs with administration of ketamine during parenteral sedation. Carbamazepine may increase thyroid hormone metabolism; thus, patients initiating these medications may need an adjustment of their levothyroxine dose.[7]

ACETAMINOPHEN WITH HYDROCODONE
Background

Opioids are central for pain management of the dental patient, especially when other medications such as nonsteroidal antiinflammatory drugs (NSAIDs) are inadequate. Hydrocodone with acetaminophen (hydrocodone/APAP) is marketed as Vicodin (AbbVie Inc, North Chicago, IL) and Lortab (UCB Inc, Smyrna, GA) and is the second most commonly prescribed drug in the United States, with 119.2 million prescriptions dispensed in 2014.[5] Vicodin is a schedule II semisynthetic narcotic analgesic. All hydrocodone/APAP formulations contain 300 mg of acetaminophen; the hydrocodone contained in the tablet can be prescribed at 5, 7.5, or 10 mg.

Hydrocodone/APAP is an excellent analgesic; however, it is also a drug of abuse with approximately 97,000 drug-related emergency room visits in 2011.[9] Owing to its abuse potential, the US Drug Enforcement Administration in 2014 rescheduled hydrocodone from a schedule III to a schedule II drug.[10]

Pharmacology

Hydrocodone exerts its clinical effects by acting at the central nervous system opiate receptors and at smooth muscle. There are multiple subtypes of opioid receptors; the most commonly referenced are the μ-1, μ-2, δ, κ, and ORL-1 (nociceptin receptor). The clinically useful action of hydrocodone, that is, analgesia, occurs at the μ-1 receptor; however, the other opioid receptors are also activated by hydrocodone with μ-2 activation resulting in respiratory and cardiovascular depression, and constipation.[11] The APAP component acts as an antipyretic by modulating hypothalamic heat regulating centers. The analgesic qualities of APAP are believed to be owing to prevention of prostaglandin synthesis. APAP is also a weak inhibitor of cyclooxygenase (COX)-1, COX-2, and possibly also COX-3.[12] The combination of an opioid with acetaminophen improves the quality of pain relief when compared with APAP or an opioid alone.[13]

Hydrocodone is metabolized by the liver and excreted in the urine. Hydrocodone has not been shown to have adverse effects in patients with renal failure[14]; however, some authors recommend using lower doses in moderate renal failure and longer time intervals in cases of severe renal failure.[15] Acetaminophen has a plasma half-life of 1.25 to 3 hours and is increased in patients with liver damage.[16] There is no ceiling dose with hydrocodone; however, owing to potentially dangerous side effects, particularly respiratory depression, the lowest functional dose should be used. The maximum acetaminophen dose in healthy patients should not exceed 4000 mg because of the risk of hepatotoxicity. Because one can approach toxic levels of APAP by taking opioids in combination with APAP, the US Food and Drug Administration (FDA) recommends discontinuing prescribing and dispensing of combination drugs containing more than 325 mg of APAP.[17]

Interactions with Dental Treatment

There are no specific interactions between hydrocodone/APAP with dental procedures or local anesthetics. Because dentists will be prescribing opioids for perioperative pain management, we will present several pertinent scenarios warranting prudent prescribing of hydrocodone/APAP.

Patients on chronic opioids

Patients visiting the dentist may be taking hydrocodone/APAP for acute or chronic pain. Patients receiving chronic opioid therapy present a unique perioperative dilemma because they experience more severe acute pain and opioid-related complications than the opioid naive patient.[18] It is believed that chronic opioid receptor activity induces a hyperalgesia, thereby decreasing a patient's pain tolerance.[19] When presenting for a procedure that may incur postoperative pain, patients should be encouraged to take their basal opioid the morning of the procedure. Then, using multimodal analgesia, nonopioid analgesics such as NSAIDs, APAP, COX-2 inhibitors, clonidine, and anticonvulsants such as gabapentin and pregabalin, may be added to the perioperative regimen.[20] The use of anticonvulsants preoperatively may help to decrease the amount of postoperative opioid required without increasing the side effects of the opioid.[21]

The dentist is cautioned against prescribing increased doses of opioids for patients on chronic opioids because the incidence of sedation is higher in the chronic opioid group[22] and without frequent clinical monitoring it may be difficult to identify the appropriate postoperative opioid dose. The dentist is encouraged to consider the use of long acting local anesthetics, preemptive analgesia, and perioperative NSAIDs to mitigate the postoperative analgesic requirement required by the patient.

Patients with hepatic impairment

In patients with compromised liver function, peak plasma concentrations of hydrocodone can increase rapidly. The use of APAP in patients with compromised hepatic function is controversial. APAP toxicity has been reported to occur more easily with compromised hepatic function because these patients are more sensitive to the toxic metabolites of APAP and have compromised ability to eliminate the toxic metabolites.[23] Contradictory reports suggest that the impaired liver maintains its capacity to metabolize and clear the toxic metabolites effectively and that APAP remains a safe drug when taken at recommended dosages.[24–26]

It is recommended that patients with cirrhosis not exceed a daily limit of 2000 mg APAP.[20,25,27] Practitioners should exercise caution when prescribing hydrocodone/APAP–containing medications to chronic alcoholics. In chronic alcoholics, the risk of hepatotoxicity actually increase if, owing to the APAP, the alcoholic stops their ethanol consumption.[28] If they maintain their ethanol consumption, the risk of toxicity from APAP decreases but the central nervous system–depressing effects of ethanol and hydrocodone are additive.

Drug–drug interactions

Hydrocodone is metabolized to hydromorphone (active metabolite) by the hepatic cytochrome P450 system, specifically, the CYP2D6 enzyme. Therefore, other medications that a patient is taking that are inducers and inhibitors of CYP2D6 can alter the metabolism of hydrocodone.[29] Patients who are poor metabolizers via CYP2D6 experience no analgesia from hydrocodone.[30] Patients who are concomitantly taking other narcotics, antihistamines, anxiolytics, and other central nervous system depressants should use caution when taking hydrocodone, because the central nervous system depression is additive.[17]

LISINOPRIL
Background

Lisinopril is an antihypertensive drug marketed as Zestril (AstraZeneca, Wilmington, DE) and Prinivil (Merck, Whitehouse Station, NJ). It is the third most commonly prescribed drug with 103.7 million prescriptions dispensed in 2014.[5] Lisinopril belongs to the class of antihypertensive agents called angiotensin-converting enzyme inhibitors (ACEi) and has extensive applications in the management of cardiovascular disease.[31]

Pharmacology

The ACEi reduce blood pressure by modulating the hormones of the renin–angiotensin–aldosterone system. Renin is a hormone released by the juxtaglomerular cells of the kidney in response to decreased renal perfusion and increased sympathetic activity[32]; renin is also produced locally in tissues. Renin cleaves and activates angiotensin I. Angiotensin I is cleaved by the angiotensin-converting enzyme into angiotensin II.[33] Angiotensin II acts centrally and peripherally to increase vascular tone thus elevating blood pressure.[34] Angiotensin II also promotes sodium retention through it effects on aldosterone,[35] and volume expansion through its effects on antidiuretic hormone.[36] In summary, ACEi exhibit their effect by reducing systemic vascular resistance without increasing the heart rate effectively reducing blood pressure.[37]

Interactions with Dental Treatment

Routine dental procedures under local anesthesia can proceed safely in patients taking ACEi. Perioperative modification of lisinopril in patients who are receiving general anesthesia is controversial. Most antihypertensive drugs are continued throughout the perioperative period; however, some data show that continuing ACEi perioperatively can exacerbate the hypotensive effect of anesthetics,[38–40] whereas other data show no relation between continuing ACEi and intraoperative hypotension.[41] Cumulative evidence recommends discontinuation of the ACEi the morning of surgery; however, modification of anesthetic induction technique may possibly ameliorate the hypotensive effects of concomitant ACEi use and anesthetics.[39]

The side effects of ACEi are pertinent to the general dentist potentially affecting the process of care delivery. The specific side effects include postural hypotension, coughing, and angioedema, with angioedema potentially being life threatening.

Postural hypotension is a decrease in blood pressure that occurs when one rises from a supine position to an upright position; this can potentially lead to dizziness and syncope. To prevent issues related to postural hypotension, the patient should be uprighted from the supine position slowly.

Between 10% and 35% of patients taking ACEi develop a dry cough.[42–44] This cough may impact the delivery of dental care. The cough is believed to arise from increase in bradykinin production that stimulates the release of prostaglandins.[45] The cough usually develops within the first month and disappears within 1 week of cessation of the drug.[46]

A rare and potentially life-threatening condition linked to ACEi is the development of angioedema. Oral or perioral angioedema describes a process of rapid swelling of the lips, tongue, mucosal, and submucosal surfaces.[47] The incidence of ACEi induced angioedema is 0.1% to 0.2%.[48] Angioedema can occur in any organ system and at anytime, but more commonly the head and neck are affected typically occurs within the first month of treatment.[49] Patients of African descent are 3 times more likely to be affected.[50] Patients with perioral swelling may present to their dentist thinking they have a tooth infection; therefore, the dentist should recognize the link between ACEi and angioedema, and refer the patient to emergency department for definitive management.

Drug–drug interactions

Patient on ACEi should not take NSAIDs for perioperative pain management for longer than 5 days because NSAIDs may decrease the effectiveness of the antihypertensive effects of the ACEi.[51] It has also been shown that combining NSAIDs and ACEi in susceptible patients may precipitate renal failure and subsequent electrolyte abnormalities.[52] Therefore, caution should be used when prescribing NSAIDs to patients taking ACEi, particularly the elderly, those with congestive heart failure, and those with preexisting renal disease.[53,54]

METOPROLOL

Background

Metoprolol is marketed as Lopressor (Novartis, East Hanover, NJ) and is an antihypertensive, antiarrhythmic drug. It is the fourth most commonly prescribed drug with 83.3 million prescription dispensed in the United States in 2014.[5] The indications for metoprolol include management of hypertension, angina pectoris, and to reduce mortality from myocardial infarction.[55,56]

Pharmacology

Metoprolol is a beta-1 selective (cardioselective) beta-blocker. The beta-1 adrenergic receptor modulates heart rate; the beta-2 adrenergic receptor modulates smooth muscle relaxation. Beta-blockers are used to treat tachycardia and hypertension by blocking the activity of endogenous catecholamines at the cardiac beta-1 receptors and by inhibiting renin secretion by the kidneys.[57] Beta-blockers are also used to treat angina pectoris. The mechanism of action is likely related to reductions in heart rate, myocardial contractility, and cardiac oxygen demand.[58] Beta-blockers have also been shown to improve survival after myocardial infarction.

Beta-blockers may be nonselective and block both the beta-1 and beta-2 receptors or they may be beta-1 selective blockers. Beta-2 antagonism is not well-tolerated in asthmatics; therefore, selective beta-1 blockers are typically used when they are indicated in the asthmatic patient.

Interactions with Dental Treatment

Cardioselective beta-blockers have less dental-related interaction than nonselective beta-blockers. Nonselective beta-blockers can exacerbate bronchoconstriction in asthmatics, and cause hypertension and reflexive bradycardia (severe enough to require atropine) with epinephrine containing local anesthetics.[59] As with ACEi, metoprolol can cause orthostatic hypotension; therefore, patients should be moved slowly from a supine to an upright position. Metoprolol may also cause xerostomia, dysgeusia, and oral lichenoid reactions. NSAIDs taken by those on metoprolol may reduce the antihypertensive effects of metoprolol.[42]

ATORVASTATIN AND SIMVASTATIN

Background

Atorvastatin is the fifth most commonly prescribed drug in the United States with 80.7 million prescriptions dispensed in 2014. Simvastatin is the ninth most commonly prescribed drug in the United States with 72.8 million prescriptions dispensed in 2014.[5] Owing to the many similarities between these 2 drugs of same class, they are discussed jointly herein.

Atorvastatin is marketed as Lipitor (Pfizer, New York, NY). Simvastatin is marketed as Zocor (Merck, Whitehouse Statin, NJ). Atorvastatin and simvastatin belong to the group of cholesterol-reducing drugs known as hydroxymethylglutaryl-coenzyme A reductase inhibitors. Cholesterol reducing medications are designed to reduce the morbidity and mortality of coronary heart disease by reducing total cholesterol, low-density lipoprotein cholesterol, triglycerides, and increasing the high-density lipoprotein cholesterol. By reducing cholesterol, the disease process of atherosclerosis is mitigated, therefore reducing the risk of adverse cardiovascular events such as angina and myocardial infarction.[60–62]

Pharmacology

Atorvastatin and simvastatin reduce cholesterol levels by inhibiting hydroxymethylglutaryl-coenzyme A reductase, an enzyme required for the biosynthesis of cholesterol. Cholesterol is circulated bound to lipoprotein complexes. These complexes are classified by the amount of cholesterol they can carry. Low-density lipoprotein cholesterol carries low quantities of cholesterol and is a major contributing factor to atherosclerosis and cardiovascular disease.[63] Conversely, high-density lipoprotein cholesterol carries large quantities of cholesterol and is associated with decreased cardiovascular risk.[64]

The statins are dependent on the liver for metabolism. The hepatic CYP3A4 enzyme metabolizes atorvastatin and simvastatin. These statins can significantly elevate transaminases therefore these patients require regular hepatic function monitoring. Owing to metabolism by CYP3A4, inducers and inhibitors of this cytochrome P450 system may interact with these statins.[61,62]

Interaction with Dental Treatment

There are no specific interactions between dental treatment and patients taking these statins. Dentists should, however, be cognizant of certain drug–drug interactions with these statins. Patients taking coumadin may have elongation of their INR when starting simvastatin; this interaction is not seen with atorvastatin.[61,62,65] The INR may increase with simvastatin owing to decreased warfarin metabolism and displacement of warfarin from proteins.[66] Therefore, patients starting statins while on coumadin should have their INR closely monitored until a stable coumadin dose and desired INR are reached.

Drugs that alter the activity at the hepatic CYP3A4 site may cause specific well-documented toxicities unique to these statins. Drugs that the dentist may prescribe that interact with atorvastatin and simvastatin include itraconazole, ketoconazole, erythromycin, and clarithromycin. The adverse effects of statins, especially when taken with a CYP3A4 inhibitor, include myopathy and muscle weakness that, if severe, can result in rhabdomyolysis and acute renal failure. Confirmation of statin induced myopathy is confirmed by history and elevation of creatinine phosphokinase.[67]

AMLODIPINE
Background

Amlodipine is an antihypertensive and antianginal drug marketed as Norvasc (Pfizer, New York, NY). It is the sixth most commonly prescribed drug in the United States with 78.3 million prescriptions dispensed in 2014. Amlodipine belongs to the class of antihypertensives referred to as calcium channel blockers (CCB) and is commonly prescribed for the treatment of hypertension and angina without congestive heart failure. Patients with coronary artery disease may be taking amlodipine to treat chronic stable angina and vasospastic angina in patients without heart failure or an ejection fraction of greater than 40%.[67]

Pharmacology

Amlodipine exhibits its effects by inhibiting influx of extracellular calcium across myocardial and vascular smooth muscle cells without disturbing serum calcium concentrations; this inhibits cardiac and vascular smooth muscle contraction thereby dilating coronary and systemic arteries. Amlodipine consequently increases myocardial oxygen delivery in patients with vasospastic angina. Amlodipine is metabolized extensively in the liver by cytochrome p450 enzyme, CYP3A4. Inhibition of this enzyme will increase bioavailability and duration of action.[68]

Interaction with Dental Treatment

Amlodipine-induced gingival enlargement

Drug-induced gingival enlargement has been extensively described in the literature. Kimball,[68] who noted gingival enlargement associated with the use of the antiepileptic drug phenytoin, first reported it in 1939. Since then many drugs, primarily from the 3 classes of drugs (anticonvulsants, CCB, and cyclosporins) have been associated with gingival enlargement.

Despite the association of CCB and gingival enlargement, Amlodipine-associated gingival enlargement is rare.[69,70] Reports of amlodipine associated gingival enlargement has been shown primarily at higher doses (in excess of 10 mg per dose) and in patients with poor plaque control. However, gingival enlargement has also been reported to occur in otherwise healthy patients even at lower doses (ie, 5 mg per dose).[71,72]

Treatment consists of confirmation that the enlargement is in fact drug-induced gingival hyperplasia, and not inflammatory or neoplastic. A discussion with the prescribing physician should explore the possibility discontinuing or substituting the offending medication. With plaque control and drug cessation, most cases respond favorably. Severe cases may require gingivectomy.

Patients on amlodipine should be informed of the potential for gingival enlargement as an unwanted side effect, but should also be advised that it is rare, especially at lower doses.[73] Educating the patient, appropriate recall for prophylaxis, and home plaque control play a critical role in preventing drug-induced gingival enlargement.

Hypotension after coprescription of macrolide antibiotics

Patients taking amlodipine are at increased risk for hypotension after the use of clarithromycin or erythromycin, but not azithromycin.

CCB are extensively metabolized by cytochrome P450 isoenzyme 3A4. This enzyme plays an important role in the metabolism of many medications. It is strongly inhibited by clarithromycin and erythromycin but not by azithromycin.[72] The use of clarithromycin and erythromycin will increase serum levels of amlodipine, resulting in an increase of the hypotensive effect. Therefore, it would be prudent to avoid macrolide antibiotics in patients on CCB, although if one is required, azithromycin is the preferred drug.[74]

METFORMIN
Background

Metformin is an oral antihyperglycemic drug marketed as Glumetza (Salix Inc, Raleigh, NC), Fortamet (Watson, Ft. Lauderdale, FL) Glucophage (Bristol-Myers Squibb, Princeton, NJ), and Riomet (Ranbaxy, Jacksonville, FL). It is the seventh most commonly prescribed drug in the United States with 76.9 million prescriptions dispensed in 2014. Metformin is a first-line drug of choice for the treatment of type 2 diabetes mellitus, in particular, in overweight and obese people and those with normal kidney function.

Pharmacology

Metformin lowers blood glucose via several mechanisms. Metformin belongs to the class of oral antihyperglycemic agents referred to as biguanides, which reduce blood glucose synthesis by activating adenosine monophosphate kinase.[75] Metformin acts by countering insulin resistance, particularly in liver and skeletal muscle. It suppresses hepatic gluconeogenesis, increases peripheral insulin sensitivity in insulin sensitive tissues such as muscle and adipose tissue, and enhances the peripheral use of glucose.[76]

Interaction with Dental Treatment

Metallic taste is associated with the use of metformin. This is referred to as dysgeusia. Dysgeusia can interfere with the enjoyment of food and intake of adequate nutrition. This side effect typically will resolve with continued use of the medication.

Long-term use of metformin may result in vitamin B_{12} deficiency. Vitamin B_{12} deficiency may manifest as altered taste, "burning," or "sore" tongue, and/or enlarged or altered tongue appearance.

Patients on metformin can very rarely develop angioedema, which would present as a facial or tongue swelling. The skin of the face, particularly the perioral region, the oral and pharyngeal mucosa, and the tongue, may swell over the period of minutes to hours. This is considered a medical emergency, and if a patient presents as such to a dental office, where angioedema is suspected, the patient should be sent to the emergency department.

OMEPRAZOLE
Background

Omeprazole an antacid marketed as Prilosec (AstraZeneca, Wilmington, DE) is a proton pump inhibitor used in the treatment of dyspepsia, peptic ulcer disease, gastroesophageal reflux disease, laryngopharyngeal reflux, and Zollinger–Ellison syndrome. Omeprazole recently became available over the counter owing to its proven safety and efficacy, so patients may fail to report the use of this drug in their medical history.

Pharmacology

Omeprazole is a selective and irreversible proton pump inhibitor. It suppresses stomach acid secretion by specific inhibition of the H^+/K^+ adenosine triphosphatase system found at the secretory surface of gastric parietal cells. Because this enzyme system is regarded as the acid (proton, or H^+) pump within the gastric mucosa, omeprazole inhibits the final step of acid production.[77]

Interaction with Dental Treatment

Coadministration of omeprazole with warfarin should be avoided. A recent systematic overview of warfarin and its drug and food interactions advised against combining omeprazole with warfarin because it may increase the effects of warfarin.[78] Thus, dental patients on warfarin who may be self-prescribing omeprazole should be monitored before treatment.

In 2012, the FDA informed the public that the use of proton pump inhibitors might be associated with an increased risk of *Clostridium difficile*–associated diarrhea (CDAD).[79] FDA reviewed reports from the FDA's Adverse Event Reporting System and the medical literature for cases of CDAD in patients undergoing treatment with proton pump inhibitors. A diagnosis of CDAD should be considered for patients taking proton pump inhibitors who develop diarrhea that does not improve. Additionally, dentists who prescribe antibiotics known to cause CDAD should remind patients of this risk.

Hypomagnesemia has been reported in patients on omeprazole.[80] The dentist should be aware of signs of hypomagnesemia in patients on omeprazole. Magnesium deficiency may cause weakness, muscle cramps, arrhythmias, depression, tetany, and mental status changes.

ALBUTEROL
Background

Albuterol is a bronchodilator marketed as AccuNeb (Mylan, Morgantown, WV), ProAir HFA (Ivax, Waterford, Ireland), Proventil (Merck, Whitehouse Station, NJ), and Ventolin (GlaxoSmithKline, Research Triangle Park, NC) and is the tenth most commonly prescribed drug in the United States with 67.1 million prescriptions dispensed in 2014. Albuterol is a short-acting β2-adrenergic receptor agonist used for the relief of bronchospasm in conditions such as asthma and chronic obstructive pulmonary disease. Albuterol is also prescribed to prevent breathing difficulties—secondary to bronchoconstriction—during exercise.[81]

Pharmacology

Bronchodilators work through their direct relaxation effect on airway smooth muscle cells. There are 3 major classes of bronchodilators, β2-adrenoceptor agonists, muscarinic receptor antagonists, and xanthines. These medications may be used individually or in combination. Albuterol is the only one of the bronchodilators that is, inhaled; this minimizes systemic effects, such as tremor, headache, muscle cramps, palpitations, and tachycardia. Albuterol is a fast-acting and short lasting bronchodilator for rescue of symptoms, as opposed to maintenance.[81]

Interaction with Dental Treatment

A common side effect of albuterol is tremor, but patients can experience tachycardia or palpitations after use. Chronic use of albuterol is known to cause xerostomia in patients, which can lead to an increased caries risk, gingivitis, increased periodontal disease risk, compromised enamel. Additionally, the risk for oral candidiasis increases with the use of albuterol.

SUMMARY

Owing to an increasing number older patients seeing their dentist and presenting with multiple comorbidities and taking multiple medications, it behooves the dentist to familiarize themselves with the possible interactions between dental treatment and these drugs. Medications may alter the perioral and oral environment resulting in a disturbance in normal function or as in the case of ACEi and metformin, a potentially life-threatening form of angioedema. Specific drug–drug interactions may result in profound morbidity. This document reviewed the top 10 medications prescribed in 2014 and their interactions with dental treatment. In addition to understanding the specific interaction of the top 10 prescribed medications, the dentist hopefully enlightened as how to evaluate any medication their patients may be taking, and how to logically consider the interactions that medication may have with the patient's dental treatment.

REFERENCES

1. United Nations Population Division. World population prospects: the 2002 revision. New York: United Nations; 2003.
2. World Health Organization. The world health report 2003. Shaping the future. Geneva (Switzerland): WHO; 2003.
3. Schou L. Oral health, oral health care, and oral health promotion among older adults: social and behavioral dimensions. In: Cohen LK, Gift HC, editors. Disease prevention and oral health promotion. Copenhagen (Denmark): Munksgaard; 1995. p. 213–70.
4. National Center for Health Statistics. Health, United States, 2013: With Special Feature on Prescription Drugs. Hyattsville, MD. 2014. Available at: http://www.cdc.gov/nchs/data/hus/hus13.pdf.
5. Pinto A, Glick M. Management of patients with thyroid disease: oral health considerations. J Am Dent Assoc 2002;133(7):849–58.
6. Synthroid [package insert]. North Chicago, IL: AbbVie Inc; 2012.
7. Sandler N. Perioperative considerations. In: Miloro M, Peterson LJ, editors. Peterson's principles of oral and maxillofacial surgery. Lewistown (NY): BC Decker; 2004. p. 61–2.
8. Klein I, Danzi S. Thyroid disease and the heart. Circulation 2007;116:1725–35.
9. Substance Abuse and Mental Health Services Administration. Highlights of the 2011 Drug Abuse Warning Network (DAWN) Findings on Drug-related Emergency Department Visits. 2013. Available at: http://www.samhsa.gov/data/sites/default/files/DAWN127/DAWN127/sr127-DAWN-highlights.pdf. Accessed July 8, 2015.
10. Drug Enforcement Administration. Schedules of controlled substances: rescheduling of hydrocodone combination products from schedule III to schedule II. Final rule. 21 CFR Part 1308 [Docket No. DEA-389]. Fed Regist 2014;79(163):49661–82.
11. Ferrante FM. Principles of opioid pharmacotherapy: practical implications of basic mechanisms. J Pain Symptom Manage 1996;11:265–73.
12. Botting RM. Mechanism of action of acetaminophen: is there a cyclooxygenase 3? Clin Infect Dis 2000;31(Suppl 5):S202–10.
13. Schug SA, Sidebotham DA, McGuinnety M, et al. Acetaminophen as an adjunct to morphine by patient-controlled analgesia in the management of acute postoperative pain. Anesth Analg 1998;87(2):368–72.
14. Fitzgerald J. Narcotic analgesics in renal failure. Conn Med 1991;55(12):701–4.
15. Durnin C, Hind ID, Wickens MM, et al. Pharmacokinetics of oral immediate-release hydromorphone (Dilaudid IR) in subjects with renal impairment. Proc West Pharmacol Soc 2001;44:81–2.
16. Vicodin [package insert]. North Chicago, IL: AbbVie Inc; 2014.
17. US Food and Drug Administration (FDA). Acetaminophen prescription combination drug products with more than 325 mg: FDA statement - recommendation to discontinue prescribing and dispensing. U.S. Food and Drug Administration. Available at: http://www.fda.gov/Safety/MedWatch/SafetyInformation/SafetyAlertsforHumanMedicalProducts/ucm381650.htm?source=govdelivery&utm_medium=email&utm_source=govdelivery. Accessed July 8, 2015.
18. Swenson JD, Davis JJ, Johnson KB. Postoperative care of the chronic opioid-consuming patient. Anesthesiol Clin North America 2005;23:37–49.
19. Doverty M, White JM, Somogyi AA, et al. Hyperalgesic responses in methadone maintenance patients. Pain 2001;90(1):91–6.
20. Brill S, Ginosar Y, Davidson EM. Perioperative management of chronic pain patients with opioid dependency. Curr Opin Anaesthesiol 2006;19(3):325–31.

21. Dahl JB, Moiniche S. Preemptive analgesia. Br Med Bull 2004;71:13–27.
22. Rapp SE, Ready LB, Nessly ML. Acute pain management in patients with prior opioid consumption: a case-controlled retrospective review. Pain 1995;61: 195–201.
23. FDA advisory committee. Available at: http://www.fda.gov/downloads/Advisory Committees/CommitteesMeetingMaterials/Drugs/DrugSafetyandRiskManagement AdvisoryCommittee/UCM164897.pdf. Accessed July 8, 2015.
24. Chandok N, Watt KDS. Pain management in the cirrhotic patient: the clinical challenge. Mayo Clin Proc 2010;85(5):451–8.
25. Heard K, Green JL, Bailey JE, et al. A randomized trial to determine the change in alanine aminotransferase during 10 days of paracetamol (acetaminophen) administration in subjects who consume moderate amounts of alcohol. Aliment Pharmacol Ther 2007;26(2):283–90.
26. Whitcomb DC, Block GD. Association of acetaminophen hepatotoxicity with fasting and ethanol use. JAMA 1994;272(23):1845–50.
27. Chopra S. Cirrhosis (beyond the basics). In: Runyon B, editor. UpToDate. Waltham (MA): UpToDate. Available at: http://www.uptodate.com/contents/cirrhosis-beyond-the-basics. Accessed July 8, 2015.
28. Haas DA. Adverse drug interactions in the dental practice: interactions associated with analgesics. J Am Dent Assoc 1999;130:397–407.
29. Howard S. Smith opioid metabolism. Mayo Clin Proc 2009;84(7):613–24.
30. Lurcott G. The effects of the genetic absence and inhibition of CYP2D6 on the metabolism of codeine and its derivatives, hydrocodone and oxycodone. Anesth Prog 1998;45:154–6.
31. Chobanian AV, Bakris GL, Black HR, et al. The seventh report of the joint national committee on prevention, detection, evaluation, and treatment of high blood pressure: the JNC 7 report. JAMA 2003;289(19):2560–72.
32. Sealey JE, Laragh JH. The renin-angiotensin-aldosterone system for normal regulation of blood pressure and sodium and potassium homeostasis. In: Laragh JH, Brenner BM, editors. Hypertension: pathophysiology, diagnosis, and management. New York, NY: Raven Press Ltd; 1990. p. 1287–317.
33. Erdos EG. The angiotensin I converting enzyme. Fed Proc 1977;36:1760–5.
34. Immerman BG, Sybertz EJ, Wong PC. Interaction between sympathetic and renin-angiotensin system. J Hypertens 1984;2:581–7.
35. Biron P, Koiw E, Nowaczynski W. The effects of intravenous infusions of valine-5 angiotensin II and other pressor agents on urinary electrolytes and corticoids including aldosterone. J Clin Invest 1961;40(2):338–47.
36. Padfield PL, Morton JJ. Effects of angiotensin II on arginine-vasopressin in physiological and pathological situations in man. J Endocrinol 1977;74:251–9.
37. Brown NJ, Vaughn DE. Angiotensin-converting enzyme inhibitors. Circulation 1998;97:1411–20.
38. Wolf A, McGoldrick KE. Cardiovascular pharmacotherapeutic considerations in patients undergoing anesthesia. Cardiol Rev 2011;19(1):12–6.
39. Coriat P, Richer C, Douraki T, et al. Influence of chronic angiotensin-converting enzyme inhibition on anesthetic induction. Anesthesiology 1994;81:299–307.
40. Brabant SM, Bertrand M, Eyraud D, et al. The hemodynamic effects of anesthetic induction in vascular surgical patients chronically treated with angiotensin II receptor antagonists. Anesth Analg 1999;89:1388–92.
41. Pigott DW, Nagle C, Allman K, et al. Effect of omitting regular ACE inhibitor medication before cardiac surgery on haemodynamic variables and vasoactive drug requirements. Br J Anaesth 1999;83:715–20.

42. Becker DE. Cardiovascular drugs: implications for dental practice part 1 — cardiotonics, diuretics, and vasodilators. Anesth Prog 2007;54(4):178–86.
43. Bangalore S, Kumar S, Messerli FH. Angiotensin-converting enzyme inhibitor associated cough: deceptive information from the Physicians' Desk Reference. Am J Med 2010;123(11):1016–30.
44. Dicpinigaitis PV. Angiotensin-converting enzyme induced cough: ACCP evidence- based clinical practice guidelines. Chest 2006;129:169S–73S.
45. Levey BA. Angiotensin-cobanverting enzyme inhibitors and cough. Chest 1990; 98(5):1052–3.
46. Brugts JJ, Arima H, Remme W, et al. The incidence and clinical predictors of ACE-inhibitor induced dry cough by perindopril in 27,492 patients with vascular disease. Int J Cardiol 2014;176(3):718–23.
47. Raval P. A case report looking at ACE inhibitors as the cause of angioedema during dental treatment. Br Dent J 2014;216(2):73–5.
48. Seymour RA, Thomason JM, Nolan A. Angiotensin converting enzyme (ACE) inhibitors and their implications for the dental surgeon. Br Dent J 1997;183: 214–8.
49. Wakefield YS, Theaker ED, Pemberton MN. Angiotensin converting enzyme inhibitors and delayed onset, recurrent angioedema of the head and neck. Br Dent J 2008;205:553–6.
50. Gibbs CR, Lip GY, Beevers DG. Angioedema due to ACE inhibitors: increased risk in patients of African origin. Br J Clin Pharmacol 1999;48:861–5.
51. Olin BR, Hebel SK, Dombek CE, editors. Drug interaction facts. St Louis (MO): Facts and Comparisons Inc; 2007.
52. Wolf G, Ritz E. Combination therapy with ACE inhibitors and angiotensin II receptor blockers to halt progression of chronic renal disease: pathophysiology and indications. Kidney Int 2005;67(3):799–812.
53. Loboz KK, Shenfield GM. Drug combinations and impaired renal function – the 'triple whammy'. Br J Clin Pharmacol 2005;59(2):239–43.
54. Schoolwerth AC, Sica DA, Ballermann BJ, et al. Renal considerations in angiotensin converting enzyme inhibitor therapy: a statement for healthcare professionals from the Council on the Kidney in Cardiovascular Disease and the Council for High Blood Pressure Research of the American Heart Association. Circulation 2001;104(16):1985–91.
55. Lopressor [Package insert]. East Hanover, NJ: Novartis Pharmaceuticals Corp; 2015.
56. Freemantle N, Cleland J, Young P, et al. β Blockade after myocardial infarction: systematic review and meta regression analysis. BMJ 1999;318:1730.
57. Holmer SR, Hengstenberg C, Mayer B, et al. Marked suppression of renin levels by beta-receptor blocker in patients treated with standard heart failure therapy: a potential mechanism of benefit from beta-blockade. J Intern Med 2001;249(2): 167–72.
58. Dixit D, Kimborowicz K. Pharmacologic management of chronic stable angina. JAAPA 2015;28(6):1–8.
59. Becker DE, Reed KL. Essentials of local anesthetic pharmacology. Anesth Prog 2006;53(3):98–108.
60. Lipitor [package insert]. New York, NY: Pfizer; Parke-Davis; 2012.
61. Zocor [package insert]. Whitehouse Station, NJ: Merck & Co Inc; 2015.
62. Bakker-Arkema RG, Davidson MH, Goldstein RJ, et al. Efficacy and safety of a new HMG-CoA reductase inhibitor, atorvastatin, in patients with hypertriglyceridemia. JAMA 1996;275:128–33.

63. Goldstein LJ, Brown SM. The low-density lipoprotein pathway and its relation to atherosclerosis. Annu Rev Biochem 1977;46.1:897–930.

64. Assmann G, Gotto AM. HDL cholesterol and protective factors in atherosclerosis. Circulation 2004;109(23 Suppl 1):III8.

65. Westergren T, Johansson P, Molden E. Probable warfarin-simvastatin interaction. Ann Pharmacother 2007;41(7):1292–5.

66. Williams D, Feely J. Pharmacokinetic-pharmacodynamic drug interactions with HMG-CoA reductase inhibitors. Clin Pharmacokinet 2002;41:343–70.

67. Abernethy DR. The pharmacokinetic profile of amlodipine. Am Heart J 1989; 118(5 Pt 2):1100–3.

68. Kimball OP. The treatment of epilepsy with sodium diphenyl hydantoinate. JAMA 1939;112:1244–5.

69. Ellis JS, Seymour RA, Thomason JM, et al. Gingival sequestration of amlodipine induced gingival overgrowth. Lancet 1993;341:1102–3.

70. Sharma S, Sharma A. Amlodipine-induced gingival enlargement–a clinical report. Compendium of continuing education in dentistry (Jamesburg, N.J: 1995). Compend Contin Educ Dent 2012 May;33(5):e78–82.

71. Tripathi AK, Mukherjee S, Saimbi CS, et al. Low dose amlodipine-induced gingival enlargement: A clinical case series. Contemp Clin Dent 2015;6:107–9.

72. Joshi S, Bansal S. A rare case report of amlodipine-induced gingival enlargement and review of its pathogenesis. Case Rep Dent 2013;2013:138248.

73. Ellis JS, Seymour RA, Steele JG, et al. Prevalence of gingival overgrowth induced by calcium channel blockers: a community-based study. J Periodontol 1999; 70(1):63–7.

74. Henneman A, Thornby K-A. Risk of hypotension with concomitant use of calcium-channel blockers and macrolide antibiotics. Am J Health Syst Pharm 2012; 69(12):1038–43.

75. Bridges HR, Jones AJ, Pollak MN, et al. Effects of metformin and other biguanides on oxidative phosphorylation in mitochondria. Biochem J 2014;462(3): 475–87.

76. US Food and Drug Administration. Glucophage (metformin hydrochloride tablets)/Glucophage XR (metformin hydrochloride extended release tablets) (NDA 20-357/S-031 and NDA 21-202/S-016). Princeton (NJ): Bristol-Myers Squibb; 2008. p. 3–32.

77. Prilosec [package insert]. Wilmington, DE: AstraZeneca; 2014.

78. Holbrook AM, Pereira JA, Labiris R, et al. Systematic overview of warfarin and its drug and food interactions. Arch Intern Med 2005;165(10):1095–106.

79. Food and drug administration, Safety announcement on proton pump inhibitors and the risk for CDAD. 2012. Available at: http://www.fda.gov/Drugs/DrugSafety/ucm290510.htm. Accessed August 5, 2015.

80. Epstein M, McGrath S, Law F. Proton-pump inhibitors and hypomagnesemic hypoparathyroidism. N Engl J Med 2006;355(17):1834–6.

81. Cazzola M, Page CP, Calzetta L, et al. Pharmacology and therapeutics of bronchodilators. Pharmacol Rev 2012;64(3):450–504.

Hyposalivation and Xerostomia

Etiology, Complications, and Medical Management

Michael D. Turner, DDS, MD, FACS

KEYWORDS

- Xerostomia • Hyposalivation • Saliva • Dry mouth • Polypharmacy
- Sjögren syndrome • Salivary substitutes

KEY POINTS

- Hyposalivation is the objective, measured decrease in saliva.
- Xerostomia is the subjective feeling of a dry mouth.
- Hyposalivation is mostly caused by the anticholinergic effect of medications.
- Saliva physically protects the hard and soft tissues, lubricates, buffers the oral pH, and is a component of the immune system.
- Complications of hyposalivation are demineralization of teeth, oral candida infections, and mucositis.

INTRODUCTION

Saliva is one of the most versatile, multifunctional substances produced by the body and has a critical role in the preservation of oropharyngeal health. When dysfunction occurs, the effects on the oral environment can lead to severe consequences in the overall patient's health and in their quality of life. This article reviews the role of saliva, the hyposalivation and xerostomia, various disease processes, and their management.

HYPOSALIVATION AND XEROSTOMIA

Although the terms hyposalivation and xerostomia have been and are used interchangeably, they are actually 2 different entities. Hyposalivation is an objective finding of a decreased salivary production. The term xerostomia is the subjective feeling of having dry mouth.[1] Normal, unstimulated salivary secretory rates vary between 800 and 1500 mL per day or 0.3 to 0.4 mL per minute. A flow rate less than 0.1 mL per

Mount Sinai Beth Israel/Jacobi/Einstein Oral and Maxillofacial Surgery, Institute of Head and Neck and Thyroid Cancer, 10 Union Square East, Suite 5B New York, NY 10003, USA
E-mail address: mturner@chpnet.org

Dent Clin N Am 60 (2016) 435–443
http://dx.doi.org/10.1016/j.cden.2015.11.003
0011-8532/16/$ – see front matter © 2016 Elsevier Inc. All rights reserved.

dental.theclinics.com

minute has been determined to be significantly abnormal.[2] A decrease in saliva production by 50% generally will result in the feeling of dry mouth, but xerostomia may occur in patients with a normal salivary flow.[3] For the most part, this article mostly covers the management of hyposalivation, but it will touch on the treatment modalities for xerostomia patients with normal salivary flow rates.

NORMAL SALIVARY FUNCTION

Saliva can be empirically divided into 2 components, mucinous and serous. These 2 components combine to form whole saliva. Whole saliva is secreted by the paired major salivary glands and the thousands of minor salivary glands. There are 3 types of major salivary glands: the parotid, the submandibular, and the lingual (sometimes called the sublingual) glands. The parotid glands mostly secrete serous saliva. The submandibular glands secrete both mucinous and serous saliva. The lingual glands and the minor salivary glands secrete only mucinous saliva.

Saliva also contains hundreds of other substances, such as desquamated cells, glycoproteins, bacteria, debris, complex mixtures of proteins, lipids, ions, and other substances. Although the purpose of many of these components is understood, there are others whose function still remains unknown.[4]

The salivary glands are innervated along the parasympathetic cholinergic pathway. When the gustatory centers are stimulated, acetylcholine is released from the nerve endings and binds to the muscarinic receptors on the salivary gland cells, particularly the muscarinic 3 receptor (M3R), triggering the release of intracellular calcium from the endoplasmic reticulum. These calcium ions activate the transmembrane sodium potassium pump, which increases the intraductal concentration of sodium ions. An ionic gradient then pulls the chloride ions from the ductules, which in turn creates an osmotic gradient that results in the secretion of fluid from the cells.

SALIVARY MUCINS

Salivary mucins serve the important function of sequestering water in the oral mucosa, acting as a lubricating agent, and as a protective layer for the hard and soft tissues of the mouth.[5] Molecularly, they comprise oligosaccharide side chains attached to a central protein strut. The major viscoelastic mucins are the gel-forming MUC5B mucin and the nonpolymeric MUC7 mucin.[6–8] These specific mucins lubricate the mucosa, protecting it from frictional and chemical damage. They also coat ingested food, allowing it to be smoothly swallowed. Mucins also surround the teeth, further protecting the teeth from demineralization and mechanical damage. It has been hypothesized that a loss or a change in concentrations of these molecules is the main etiologic factor in the development xerostomia.[9]

SALIVARY MINERALS

Saliva is rich in minerals, specifically sodium, potassium, calcium, hydrogen, bicarbonate, phosphate, zinc, magnesium, and others. These minerals, along with the salivary proteins, create an osmotic gradient between the intracellular fluid in the salivary cells and the extracellular fluid in the glandular ductules. This osmotic gradient is the driving force that brings the intracellular fluid through the transmembranous channels into the glandular ductules.

The oral pH normally stays in the range of 6.0 to 7.0 and is maintained by the different ions found within the saliva. These ions, particularly bicarbonate and phosphate, stabilize the pH and thereby limit the demineralization of the teeth from bacterial acid and acidic food and drinks. As well as buffering the oral pH, the calcium, phosphate, and fluoride ions that are present in the saliva also remineralize the teeth.[10] The pH range is also necessary for the activation of salivary amylase, the enzyme that begins the hydrolysis of starch into sugars. Finally, by keeping the pH stable, the equilibrium of the oral microbiota is maintained, preventing the overgrowth of Candida and other organisms. The zinc ions that are found in the saliva are crucial for the activation of the taste buds, and for this reason, patients with hyposalivation manifest a decrease or loss in their taste sensation.

IMMUNE SYSTEM FUNCTION

There are immune system components found in the saliva. The salivary glands, particularly the parotid glands, contain B cells and plasma cells that excrete salivary Immunoglobulin A (IgA), which binds to the mucins covering the mucosa. In turn, the IgA binds to bacteria, fungi, and viruses, blocking microbial attachment to the mucosa.[8,11] Other substances that are part of the oral immune system are histatins, lactoperoxidase, lactoferrin, and secretory leukocyte protease inhibitor. These substances also serve to limit the concentration of the oral microbes, helping to further prevent bacterial and fungal overgrowth.

DISEASE ENTITIES

The exact number of patients who have hyposalivation and/or subjective xerostomia is unclear. Meta-analysis of different studies shows a prevalence that ranges from 5% to 47%.[12] This large range is due to a variation in methodology and definitions in the different studies. Regardless of the disparity of the prevalence range, when evaluating the data based on age, it is clear that 20% of the patients 65 years or older have some type of salivary gland abnormality.[13] Ship and colleagues[14] reported that medication-induced hyposalivation is the most common cause of dry mouth in this age category because most older adults take at least one xerogenic medication. The other major diseases that cause hyposalivation are advanced Sjögren syndrome (SS) and head and neck radiation. In these entities, the prevalence of salivary dysfunction is nearly 100%.[15,16]

MEDICATION-INDUCED SALIVARY GLAND DYSFUNCTION

More than 400 medications can cause salivary gland dysfunction, and 80% of the most commonly prescribed medications have been reported to cause hyposalivation.[13,17,18]

It has been found that the incidence and severity of the hyposalivation are directly proportional to the number of medications that the patient is taking.[19] Of the patients over the age of 65, 88% took 1 prescription medication; 76% took 2 prescription medications, and 37% took 5 or more prescription medications.[20]

Medications that have an anticholinergic effect cause the most hyposalivation. The mechanism of this action is at the M3R. Anticholinergic medications decrease the amount of acetylcholine released by the parasympathetic nerves, disabling cell function. The most common xerogenic drug categories are sedative agents, antihistamines, anti-Parkinson, antihypertensive, and antidepressants medications (**Table 1**).

RADIATION-INDUCED HYPOSALIVATION

Radiation therapy is commonly used in the treatment of head and neck malignancies. It causes apoptosis (cell death) of the tumor cells. Unfortunately, when the salivary glands are within the field of radiation, it also damages the salivary acinar and stem

Table 1
Xerogenic medications

Classification	Category	Medication
Sedative agents	Benzodiazepams	Alprazolam, Diazepam, Lorazepam, Oxazepam, Triazolam
Antihistamines	First generation	Carbinoxamine, Clemastine Dexchlorpheniramine, Dimenhydranate Diphenhydramine, Hydroxyzine Meclizine, Promethazine
	Second generation	Cetirizine, Desloratadine Fexofenadine, Levocetirizine, Loratadine
Anti-Parkinsonian	Various	Amantadine, Benztropine Bromocriptine, Carbidopa Entcapone, Levodopa, Pramipexole, Rasagiline, Ropinirole, Selegiline, Trihexyphenidyl
Antihypertensives	α-agonists	Clonidine, Guanabenz, Guanfacine, Methldopa
	β-blockers	Acebutolol, Atenolol, Bebivolol, Betaxolol, Bisoprolol, Carvedilol, Esmolol, Labetalol, Metoprolol, Nadolol, Penbutolol, Pindolol, Propranolol, Stalol, Timolol
	Diuretics	Bumetanide, Furosemide, Torsemide
	Calcium channel blockers	Amlodipine, Diltiazem, Felodipine, Isradipine, Nifedipine, Nimodipine, Verapamil
	ACE inhibitors	Benazepril, Captopril, Enalapril, Fosinopril, Lisinopril, Moexipril, Perindopril, Quinapril, Ramipril, Trandolapril
Antidepressants	Selective serotonin reuptake inhibitors	Fluoxetine, Escitalopram, Fluvoxamine, Sertraline, Paroxetine, Citalopram
	Atypical antidepressants	Bupropion, Duloxetine, Venlafaxine, Mirtazapine, Trazodone
	Tricyclic antidepressants	Amitriptyline, Clomipramine, Desipramine, Doxepin, Imipramine, Nortriptyline, Protriptyline, Trimipramine

cells population, causing a permanent degeneration of the salivary glands. Following radiation, the glands atrophy and become nonfunctional and fibrotic.[21] This damage typically occurs when the exposure dose is 60 Gy or more, although the exact mechanism that leads to gland damage is not clearly understood.

SJÖGREN SYNDROME

SS is an autoimmune disease whereby the salivary gland tissues are targeted by the body's immune system and are either damaged or inactivated. When SS is present as an independent disease, it is called primary SS. When it occurs in conjunction with another autoimmune disease, it is called secondary SS. The reported prevalence of SS varies from 0.05% to 4.8%.[22] Onset is typically between the ages of 40 and 50 with a female-to-male ratio of 9 to 1. The etiologic trigger still remains unknown. Microscopically, the salivary gland cells are infiltrated by plasma cells, B cells, T cells, macrophages, and mast cells.[23] The plasma cells begin to proliferate and produce the autoantibodies anti-Ro and anti-La, also called SSA and SSB, respectively. These autoantibodies are thought to target the M3R and cause cellular dysfunction and glandular atrophy.[23–25] Clinically, enlarged parotid glands are typically found with hyposalivation, ductal inflammation, and acinar destruction.[14]

ORAL EFFECTS OF SALIVARY GLAND HYPOFUNCTION
Dental Caries

Patients with hyposalivation have an increased caries rate as compared with the normal patient population.[26] An increased rate of caries occurs because of the increase of the microbiota, particularly *Strep mutans*, the decreased protection by the mucinous saliva, the decreased efficiency of the salivary debridement of the teeth, and most importantly, the loss of the buffering capacity.[27] When the buffering capacity is impaired, and the pH decreases, demineralization of the teeth occurs.

In the presence of fluoride, calcium, and phosphate, enamel is remineralized, although frequent acid exposures create an irreversible demineralization, resulting in erosion, attrition, and caries.[9] In the elderly, there is an additive effect because of the loss of dexterity and the worsening of oral hygiene.[28] In these patients, the treatment of choice is a neutral sodium fluoride application, which creates a short-term increase in the oral pH and sustains the remineralization of the teeth.[29]

Candidiasis

Saliva prevents Candida overgrowth by mechanical debridement of the mucosa as well as prevents adhesion of the yeast to the tissue (see Immune System Function).[11] Once the volume of the whole saliva decreases and with it the concentration of lactoferrin, IgA, salivary proteins, and peptides, susceptibility to Candida infections increases. These infections can be and should be treated with various topical, oral, and intravenous antifungal agents[30] (**Table 2**).

Mucositis

Inflammation of the mucosa, that is, mucositis, occurs when the oral soft tissues lose their protective mucous layer. The mucosa becomes susceptible to friction and laceration from the teeth, restorations, prosthesis, and food. The keratinized tissue of the tongue also becomes desiccated and forms fissures that trap food and bacteria, leading to an increase in susceptibility to oral candidiasis, glossodynia, and loss or change of the taste sensation. Various agents that coat the mucosa and prevent desiccation can be used (see Salivary Substitutes).[31–33]

Management of Xerostomia and Salivary Hypofunction

Because hyposalivation and xerostomia can be present at the same time as well as be independent of each other, treatment should focus on both the subjective and the objective conditions. Patients with medication-induced hyposalivation can be managed with xylitol, salivary substitutes, peripheral sialagogues, and central sialagogues.

Xylitol

A widespread oral agent is xylitol, a nonfermentable carbohydrate. Xylitol creates an osmotic gradient between the mucosa and the mouth, which draws fluid from the cells to the surface of the tissue, replenishing the outer coating of the tissue, and by extension, the teeth.[34] By increasing the pH of the mouth and coating the teeth, the rate of caries has been found to decrease by 10%.[35]

Salivary Substitutes

The primary functions of the salivary substitutes are to lubricate the oral soft tissue, to relieve the subjective xerostomia, and to protect the teeth from demineralization. There are many combinations and substances that are used to formulate these agents. Currently, the most common substances for oral moisturizers/salivary substitutes are

Table 2
Antifungal agents and dosing

Agent	Dosing
Oral Agents	
Clotrimazole 10 mg troche	Let troche dissolve in mouth 5 times a day for 14 d
Fluconazole 100 mg and 200 mg tablet	200 mg tablet on the first day, then 100–200 mg daily 14 d
Flucytosine capsule 250 mg, 500 mg	Capsule: 50–100 mg/kg/d divided over every 6 h for 7–14 d Suspension: 10 mg/mL dose, rinse with 10 mL and swallow bid for 7–14 d
Ketoconazole 200 mg tablet	1–2 tablets daily until resolution
Miconazole 50 mg buccal tablet	Place in a mucosal vestibule once daily in morning for 14 d
Nystatin oral suspension 100,000 IU/mL	4–6 mL; swish in mouth and then swallow; continue treatment for 48 h after symptoms resolve
Posaconazole	Start 100 mg orally (PO) twice a day, then 100 mg PO once a day for 13 d
Voriconazole	200 mg PO every 12 h treat 14 d minimum and 7 d for following resolution of symptoms
Intravenous Agents	
Anidulafungin	50 mg intravenously (IV) every 24 h for 14 d minimum and 7 d following resolution
Caspofungin	50 mg IV every 24 h and continue for 7–14 d following resolution
Micafungin	150 mg IV every day

Adapted from Muzyka BC, Epifanio RN. Update on oral fungal infections. Dent Clin North Am 2013;57(4):563; with permission.

carboxymethyl cellulose, mucin, hydroxyethyl cellulose, water-glycerin, and glycerate polymer.

In 2009, Hahnel and colleagues[36] reviewed the current in vitro and in vivo evidence of the current salivary substitutes. They found that the viscosity of the agent was one of the most important physical properties for the subjective relief of the patients. Viscosity is how the substance covers the underlying tissues. Unfamiliar and unpleasant sensations were evoked when the viscosity was either too high or too low as compared with natural saliva. It was determined that mucin-based substitutes had viscosities that were more similar to natural saliva than substitutes based on carboxymethyl cellulose, glycerol, or polyethylene oxide. In multiple studies, mucin-based agents were preferred to the carboxymethyl cellulose agents because higher viscosity created a longer duration of action.[37,38]

The second most important physical property was lubrication, which interestingly does not correlate with viscosity. Lubrication is the ability of the substance to reduce friction. Although the data are somewhat inconclusive due to the differences in methods and materials of the various studies, it seems that mucin- and glycerin-based substitutes had a higher reduction in friction than carboxymethyl cellulose substitutes.[36]

Substitutes with the immunologic components of lysozyme, lactoferrin, and lactoperoxidase did reduce microbial count, including Candida, significantly in vitro.

Table 3	
Centrally mediated secretagogues	
Pilocarpine	Head and neck radiation: start 5 mg PO three times a day, maximum 10 mg/dose
	SS: 5 mg PO 4 times a day
Cevimeline	SS: 30 mg PO 3 times a day

Although the results were suggestive in vivo, they were not found to be statistically significant.[36,39]

Peripheral Sialagogues

Peripheral sialagogues function by stimulating a gustatory response. The 2 most common stimulants are ascorbic and malic acids. These peripheral sialagogues are ineffective when there is a complete intrinsic damage to the salivary gland cells because the glands cannot manufacture saliva. Because both of these agents are acidic, and the teeth have a decreased mucous barrier, the rate of the demineralization of the teeth can increase.

Mechanical Stimulation

Mechanical stimulation can increase salivary flow from the parotid glands. Typically, this consists of chewing gum (which should be sugar free). Chewing causes stretching of the parotid capsule and creates compression of the parotid gland and functionally increases salivary flow.[1]

Centrally Mediated Sialagogues

The 2 US Food and Drug Administration–approved centrally mediated secretagogues are pilocarpine and cevimeline (**Table 3**). Both can increase secretions and diminish xerostomic complaints in patients, although they must have functional salivary gland cells. This tissue is not always present in advanced SS and patients with head and neck radiation. Pilocarpine is a nonselective muscarinic agonist that affects all muscarinic receptors in the body. Cevimeline reportedly has a higher affinity for the M3R muscarinic receptor, the receptor associated with salivary gland cell secretion (see Normal Salivary Function). Because of this specificity, there is a reported decrease in the incidence of cholinergic side effects, like sweating and gastrointestinal upset.[40–42]

SUMMARY

The management of patients with hyposalivation and xerostomia can be challenging. There is no ideal agent currently available to treat these specific conditions effectively. The most important aspect that the practitioner must focus on is the prevention and the treatment of the complications that the lack of saliva can cause, specifically, the increase in erosion and caries of the teeth, vulnerability to Candida infections, mucositis, and the sensation of xerostomia.

REFERENCES

1. Furness S, Worthington HV, Bryan G, et al. Interventions for the management of dry mouth: topical therapies. Cochrane Database Syst Rev 2011;(12):CD008934.
2. Madsen V, Lind A, Rasmussen M, et al. Determination of tobramycin in saliva is not suitable for therapeutic drug monitoring of patients with cystic fibrosis. J Cyst Fibros 2004;3(4):249–51.

3. de Almeida Pdel V, Gregio AM, Machado MA, et al. Saliva composition and functions: a comprehensive review. J Contemp Dent Pract 2008;9(3):72–80.

4. Helmerhorst EJ, Oppenheim FG. Saliva: a dynamic proteome. J Dent Res 2007; 86(8):680–93.

5. Tabak LA. Structure and function of human salivary mucins. Crit Rev Oral Biol Med 1990;1(4):229–34.

6. Bobek LA, Tsai H, Biesbrock AR, et al. Molecular cloning, sequence, and specificity of expression of the gene encoding the low molecular weight human salivary mucin (MUC7). J Biol Chem 1993;268(27):20563–9.

7. Thornton DJ, Khan N, Mehrotra R, et al. Salivary mucin MG1 is comprised almost entirely of different glycosylated forms of the MUC5B gene product. Glycobiology 1999;9(3):293–302.

8. Shugars DC, Wahl SM. The role of the oral environment in HIV-1 transmission. J Am Dent Assoc 1998;129(7):851–8.

9. Singh ML, Papas A. Oral implications of polypharmacy in the elderly. Dent Clin North Am 2014;58(4):783–96.

10. Stookey GK. The effect of saliva on dental caries. J Am Dent Assoc 2008; 139(Suppl):11S–7S.

11. Marcotte H, Lavoie MC. Oral microbial ecology and the role of salivary immunoglobulin A. Microbiol Mol Biol Rev 1998;62(1):71–109.

12. Thomson WM. Issues in the epidemiological investigation of dry mouth. Gerodontology 2005;22(2):65–76.

13. Thomson WM. Dry mouth and older people. Aust Dent J 2015;60:54–63.

14. Ship JA, Pillemer SR, Baum BJ. Xerostomia and the geriatric patient. J Am Geriatr Soc 2002;50(3):535–43.

15. Fox PC. Autoimmune diseases and Sjogren's syndrome: an autoimmune exocrinopathy. Ann N Y Acad Sci 2007;1098:15–21.

16. Shiboski CH, Hodgson TA, Ship JA, et al. Management of salivary hypofunction during and after radiotherapy. Oral Surg Oral Med Oral Pathol Oral Radiol Endod 2007;103(Suppl):S66.e1–19.

17. Sreebny LM, Schwartz SS. A reference guide to drugs and dry mouth–2nd edition. Gerodontology 1997;14:33–47.

18. Smith RG, Burtner AP. Oral side-effects of the most frequently prescribed drugs. Spec Care Dentist 1994;14(3):96–102.

19. Sreebny LM. Salivary flow in health and disease. Compend Suppl 1989;(13): S461–9.

20. Gu Q, Dillon CF, Burt VL. Prescription drug use continues to increase: U.S. prescription drug data for 2007-2008. NCHS Data Brief 2010;(42):1–8.

21. Savage NW, Kruger BJ, Adkins KF. The effects of fractionated megavoltage X-irradiation on rat submandibular gland: an assessment by electron microscopy. Aust Dent J 1985;30(3):188–93.

22. Ship JA, Nolan NE, Puckett SA. Longitudinal analysis of parotid and submandibular salivary flow rates in healthy, different-aged adults. J Gerontol A Biol Sci Med Sci 1995;50(5):M285–9.

23. Anaya JM, Talal N. Sjogren's syndrome comes of age. Semin Arthritis Rheum 1999;28(6):355–9.

24. Fox RI, Stern M, Michelson P. Update in Sjogren syndrome. Curr Opin Rheumatol 2000;12(5):391–8.

25. Dawson LJ, Stanbury J, Venn N, et al. Antimuscarinic antibodies in primary Sjogren's syndrome reversibly inhibit the mechanism of fluid secretion by human submandibular salivary acinar cells. Arthritis Rheum 2006;54(4):1165–73.

26. Johnston LL. Caries experience and overall health status. Oral Health Prev Dent 2014;12(2):163–70.
27. Avsar A, Elli M, Darka O, et al. Long-term effects of chemotherapy on caries formation, dental development, and salivary factors in childhood cancer survivors. Oral Surg Oral Med Oral Pathol Oral Radiol Endod 2007;104(6):781–9.
28. Rothen M, Cunha-Cruz J, Zhou L, et al. Oral hygiene behaviors and caries experience in Northwest PRECEDENT patients. Community Dent Oral Epidemiol 2014; 42(6):526–35.
29. Epstein JB, Chin EA, Jacobson JJ, et al. The relationships among fluoride, cariogenic oral flora, and salivary flow rate during radiation therapy. Oral Surg Oral Med Oral Pathol Oral Radiol Endod 1998;86(3):286–92.
30. Muzyka BC, Epifanio RN. Update on oral fungal infections. Dent Clin North Am 2013;57(4):561–81.
31. Pretty IA, Gallagher MJ, Martin MV, et al. A study to assess the effects of a new detergent-free, olive oil formulation dentifrice in vitro and in vivo. J Dent 2003; 31(5):327–32.
32. Ship JA, McCutcheon JA, Spivakovsky S, et al. Safety and effectiveness of topical dry mouth products containing olive oil, betaine, and xylitol in reducing xerostomia for polypharmacy-induced dry mouth. J Oral Rehabil 2007;34(10): 724–32.
33. Lapiedra R, Gómez GE, Sanchez BP, et al. The effect of a combination saliva substitute for the management of xerostomia and hyposalivation. J Maxillofac Oral Surg 2015;14(3):653–8.
34. Ritter AV, Bader JD, Leo MC, et al. Tooth-surface-specific effects of xylitol: randomized trial results. J Dent Res 2013;92(6):512–7.
35. Bader JD, Vollmer WM, Shugars DA, et al. Results from the xylitol for adult caries trial (X-ACT). J Am Dent Assoc 2013;144(1):21–30.
36. Hahnel S, Behr M, Handel G, et al. Saliva substitutes for the treatment of radiation-induced xerostomia–a review. Support Care Cancer 2009;17(11): 1331–43.
37. Dirix P, Nuyts S, Vander Poorten V, et al. Efficacy of the BioXtra dry mouth care system in the treatment of radiotherapy-induced xerostomia. Support Care Cancer 2007;15(12):1429–36.
38. Shahdad SA, Taylor C, Barclay SC, et al. A double-blind, crossover study of Biotene Oralbalance and BioXtra systems as salivary substitutes in patients with post-radiotherapy xerostomia. Eur J Cancer Care 2005;14(4): 319–26.
39. Sugiura Y, Soga Y, Tanimoto I, et al. Antimicrobial effects of the saliva substitute, Oralbalance, against microorganisms from oral mucosa in the hematopoietic cell transplantation period. Support Care Cancer 2008;16(4):421–4.
40. Vivino FB, Al-Hashimi I, Khan Z, et al. Pilocarpine tablets for the treatment of dry mouth and dry eye symptoms in patients with Sjogren syndrome: a randomized, placebo-controlled, fixed-dose, multicenter trial. P92-01 Study Group. Arch Intern Med 1999;159(2):174–81.
41. Johnson JT, Ferretti GA, Nethery WJ, et al. Oral pilocarpine for post-irradiation xerostomia in patients with head and neck cancer. N Engl J Med 1993;329(6): 390–5.
42. Lovelace TL, Fox NF, Sood AJ. Management of radiotherapy-induced salivary hypofunction and consequent xerostomia in patients with oral or head and neck cancer: meta-analysis and literature review. Oral Surg Oral Med Oral Pathol Oral Radiol 2014;117(5):595–607.

Updates of Topical and Local Anesthesia Agents

Ricardo A. Boyce, DDS, FICD*, Tarun Kirpalani, DMD, Naveen Mohan, DDS

KEYWORDS

- Topical and local anesthetics • Local anesthetic overdose • Adverse drug response
- Potency/toxicity • Auxiliary techniques • Periodontal anesthetics
- Trigger point injections • Intraosseous injections • Intrasulcular infusion

KEY POINTS

- Fear and anxiety are the main reasons patients do not go to or follow up with the dentist.
- The modern-day dentist has the responsibility of educating fearful patients on the many advances to minimize pain.
- Educating patients of the advances in anesthesia practiced in dentistry can alleviate psychogenic pain.
- Depending on the procedure, it is imperative that the clinician choose the best anesthesia for the job at hand.
- Clinicians who provide care to toddlers should be aware of the low safety margin in children that can lead to local anesthetic overdose.

Topical and local anesthetics (LAs) are the unsung heroes in modern-day dentistry. There are times when older patients sit in a dental chair and share the experiences they endured as a child or stories they heard of dentistry being performed with not enough or without any LA. The experiences are often described as torturous or barbaric. These stories of bad experiences over time have allowed fear to set into the minds of many patients. Fear and anxiety (usually involving the needle or the injection) are the main reasons patients do not go to or follow up with a dentist. Although in contrast, pain is the reason a fearful patient will present to the dental office.

Dentistry has evolved to a point where we can now focus on preventive treatment to avoid dental caries, which oftentimes contribute to a host of painful experiences (ie, injections, abscess, and so forth). This will involve the Dentist educating the "fearful" patients of the many advances in dentistry to minimize pain and to improve the overall oral hygiene, which will lessen the likelihood of discomfort in future visits. Educating patients of the advances in anesthesia practiced in dentistry can oftentimes

---

Department of Dentistry/Oral and Maxillofacial Surgery, The Brooklyn Hospital Center, 121 DeKalb Avenue, Box 187, Brooklyn, NY 11201, USA
* Corresponding author.
E-mail address: raboycedds@yahoo.com

Dent Clin N Am 60 (2016) 445–471
http://dx.doi.org/10.1016/j.cden.2015.12.001
0011-8532/16/$ – see front matter © 2016 Elsevier Inc. All rights reserved.

alleviate psychogenic anxiety. Trust is also an important factor; if patients trust their doctor, they may be more willing to try procedures with multiple visits in order to save as opposed to extracting a tooth or a group of teeth. The experienced clinician will more likely have a variety of techniques learned over the years that can help build a trusting relationship with patients.

Pain is defined as an "unpleasant sensory and emotional experience associated with actual or potential tissue damage"[1] by the International Association for the Study of Pain. Acute pain is caused by a noxious stimulation (trauma, abnormal function of a muscle, or a disease) that lasts less than or cured within 6 months' duration. Chronic pain often lasts longer than 6 months and can be associated with a disease and possibly have psychological effects. "Pain initiated or caused by a primary lesion or dysfunction in the nervous system" is known as Neuropathic pain.[2] Nasri-Heir and colleagues[3] went further to state "chronic pain disorders, such as neuralgias, chronic musculoskelatal disorders, and various forms of neurovascular pain, may produce equivalent pain but usually are not secondary to tissue damaging events."[3]

There are 2 common methods to evaluate pain management: the visual analog scale (VAS) and the McGill Pain Questionnaire (MPQ). The latter (MPQ) involves a checklist of words describing symptoms and a scoring system related to the quality of pain from head to toe. This tool is quite lengthy (not recommended for private practice or high-volume dental clinics) and is used in the management of pain syndromes. Now the VAS is basic, simple, and can be used to determine the intensity of pain from children to the elderly (**Fig. 1**). Essentially it is a horizontal line numbered from 0 to 10, with 0 representing no pain and 10 as the worst possible pain. Gomella and Haist[4] state that it is called the "fifth vital sign" and is commonly used in the hospital setting.

An experienced and oftentimes skilled clinician will give serious thought to the type of topical anesthesia and LA administered before, during (if needed), and after the procedure (if needed). Depending on the procedure (minimally invasive, invasive, minor, or major surgery), it is imperative that the clinician choose the best anesthesia for the job at hand. Malamed[5] offers a rational approach to selecting an appropriate LA:

1. The length of time for which pain control is necessary
2. The requirement for pain control after treatment (postoperative pain control)
3. The requirement for hemostasis during the procedure
4. Any contraindications involving a selected or specific group of anesthetics (ie, true documented reproducible allergy)

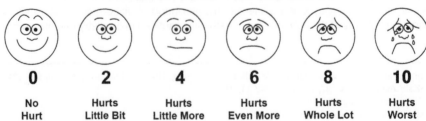

Wong-Baker FACES® Pain Rating Scale

0	2	4	6	8	10
No Hurt	Hurts Little Bit	Hurts Little More	Hurts Even More	Hurts Whole Lot	Hurts Worst

Fig. 1. Pain scale used to determine the intensity of pain from children to the elderly. (Copyright 1983, Wong-Baker FACES® Foundation, www.WongBakerFACES.org. Used with permission. Originally published in Whaley & Wong's Nursing Care of Infants and Children. © Elsevier Inc.)

Clinician's who provide care to toddlers and children should be aware of the *low safety margin* in children that can lead to LA overdose. Hersh and colleagues[6] mention that "the cardiovascular effects of local anesthetic overdosage include vasodilation, which in turn can lead to a drop in systemic blood pressure... Death can occur due to either respiratory depression or cardiac arrest." The modern-day dentist should be knowledgeable of the number of LA–induced toxicities involving children and the administration of 2% plain lidocaine and 3% mepivacaine (ie, Carbocaine, Polocaine, Scandonest). Yagiella[7] stated "it is advisable to use a preparation containing a vasoconstrictor, if not doing so would result in more total drug being administered."[7]

Isolated systolic hypertension is commonly seen in middle-aged and elderly patients, with blood pressure (BP) greater than 160 mm Hg/less than 90 mm Hg; dental care is commonly treated under appropriate LA and compliance of medications (along with follow-up visits by their primary care physician). Any patient with a systolic BP of 180/100 should *not* be seen or treated with elective dental care (ie, LA with or without epinephrine) but should be given a medical consult, only to return after the BP is controlled and patients have written clearance from their physician and/or cardiologist. In cases with a BP >180/120 is Malignant Hypertension, is considered a medical emergency.

Today, the most popular treatment in dentistry involves the planning, placement, and restoration of implants. Steinberg and Kelly[8] state that "when placing mandibular implants, it is not necessary to administer an inferior alveolar block injection for adequate local anesthesia... Local infiltration provides sufficient anesthesia to place an implant with either flap or flapless techniques."[8] They explained further that the primary advantage of not giving a block injection for implant placement in the mandible "is so the patient has some awareness and perception around the inferior alveolar nerve (IAN)."[8] Paresthesia is defined as persistent anesthesia or altered sensation well beyond the expected duration of anesthesia, which involves sensations of numbness, swelling, tingling, and itching.[5] Malamed[5] went further to state that "...paresthesia is one of the most frequent causes of dental malpractice litigation." The dentist must be well aware of this term as it relates to

1. The administration of certain LAs and the various techniques
2. Extraction of third molars (wisdom teeth)
3. Surgical incisions/flaps injuring the lingual or mental nerve (neurotmesis)
4. Drilling an osteotomy and/or implant placement in which the regional nerve is crushed (neuropraxia, axonotmesis) and so forth

Hillerup and Jensen[9] recommended in 2006 that "articaine should *not* be used by inferior alveolar nerve block... it had a greater propensity for paresthesia."[9]

A complete Blood Count (CBC) and differential, if needed, should be obtained on medically compromised patients suspected of bleeding and thrombotic disorders. It is imperative for the dentist to avoid the administration of local anesthesia to a patient with < 50,000 Platelets. Any invasive treatment without platelet replacement therapy will lead to excess bleeding.

One advancement in modern-day dentistry is the use of LAs as diagnostic nerve blocks when trying to *rule out* a local versus a central cause of pain.

It is each clinician's responsibility to know about the classification, potency, toxicity, metabolism, excretion, pregnancy classification, contraindications, and manufacturer's recommended dosage (MRD) for the use of LAs according to the patients' body weight (children, elderly, or adults).

Multiple sources of reference (especially evidenced-based studies) should be used to eliminate biased opinions related to LAs.

TOPICAL ANESTHETICS

Topical anesthetics are used in dentistry and medicine to minimize painful stimuli or manage chronic pain. Studies have shown the benefits of decreased pain when performing an ultrasound with the use of topical anesthetics.[10,11] It can be prepared and compounded as gels, creams, ointments, liquids, lotions, sprays, and powders.

- *Benzocaine* is an ester derivative topical anesthetic. Common US brand names include *Anbesol* (over the counter [OTC]), *Babee Teething* (OTC), *HurriCaine*, *Orajel* (OTC), *Orabase* (OTC), *Brace-Aid Oral Anesthetic* (OTC), and *Vick's Chloraseptic* Sore Throat (OTC). There are other brand names in many local pharmacies including topical benzocaine. It binds selectively to the intracellular surface of sodium channels to block the influx of sodium into the axon.[12] In dentistry, it is used on the oral mucosa to provide surface anesthesia before needle penetration of LA. As mentioned earlier, it lessens the often-described painful experiences associated when getting a shot or injection of the LA. It is also used in OTC products to provide temporary relief of pain from toothaches, canker sores, and sore throats.
- The combination preparation of *benzocaine, butyl aminobenzoate, tetracaine, and benzalkonium chloride* is a topical spray LA used for pain control and gagging. *Cetacaine* is the brand name for this combination (*see later, Cetacaine spray*).
- The combination preparation of *benzocaine, gelatin, pectin, and sodium carboxy-methylcellulose* is a topical anesthetic used for oral lesions. The brand name for this combination is *Orabase*.
- *Dibucaine* is an amide derivative topical LA used for the temporary relief of pain and itching. Examples for the use of dibucaine include minor burns and hemorrhoids. The brand name is *Nupercainal*.
- The combination preparation of *dichlorodifluoromethane and trichloromonofluoromethane* is a topical spray LA used in the management of myofascial pain in patients with temporomandibular dysfunction (TMD). This spray technique is often used with trigger-point therapy and should be used by the clinician trained in the treatment and management of orofacial pain and TMD. It is extremely important to first cover patients' eyes. The inverted bottle should be at least 12 in away from the muscle, at a rate of 10 cm/s.[12] The *spray and stretch therapy* is performed by cooling the skin with a refrigerant spray and then gently stretching the involved muscle.[13] The brand name is *Fluori-Methane*.
- *Dyclonine hydrochloride* (HCL) is a topical preparation (0.5% and 1.0% solution) that can be used in patients who are allergic to esters or amides. The duration of the anesthesia is 60 minutes. Nonetheless, in the past, dyclonine has been used as an active ingredient in *Sucrets* (an OTC throat lozenge) and *Cepacol* (sore throat spray). The Dyclone brand is no longer on the North American market.[5] It is widely marketed outside of the United States (in sex pills and sex sprays) known as a Stiff Delay Cream.
- *Ethyl chloride* is a topical spray anesthetic used in minor operative procedures, insect stings, and burns. It is also used for discomfort from

myofascial and visceral pain syndromes (see *spray and stretch therapy* mentioned earlier).

- *Ethyl chloride and dichlorotetrafluoroethane* is a topical spray anesthetic used in minor surgical procedures, contusions, dermabrasion, injections, and strains (see *spray and stretch therapy* mentioned earlier).
- *Eutectic Mixture of Local Anesthetic (EMLA cream)* is an amide-type topical anesthetic used as an adjunct for phlebotomy (ie, intravenous cannulation or venipuncture) for patients with a phobia of needles. The composition consists of 2.5% of lidocaine and 2.5% of prilocaine. It must be applied 1 hour before the procedure to provide surface anesthesia on the skin and lasts 2 to 3 hours. It is *not* recommended on mucous membranes (according to the manufacturer), even though studies have shown its effectiveness in dental procedures.[5,14] It is contraindicated in patients with congenital or methemoglobinemia.
- *Lidocaine* is an amide, which is available as a topical (base 5% and 2% water soluble) and 2% injectable solution (2% plain is no longer available in dental cartridges in North America[5]); 2% lidocaine HCL with epinephrine (1:50,000 and 1:100,000) is discussed later in this article. Two-percent lidocaine is still readily stocked in hospitals by physicians (especially obstetricians and gynecologists) and oral medicine techniques (*see Auxiliary Techniques*). Lidocaine is also available by prescription in the United States in a viscous (0.5%, 1.0%, and 2.0%) form. In the viscous state, lidocaine can be used as a rinse to help patients experiencing severe pain from mucositis secondary to radiation and chemotherapy. In oral medicine, it is one of the active ingredients in Magic Mouth Wash rinse. It is *important to note* that, although local applications of topical anesthetics are useful for pain relief, there should be *caution* with the use of potent topical anesthetics. Potent topical anesthetics have the ability to cause decreased gag reflex, central nervous system (CNS) depression or excitation, or cardiovascular effects, which may follow excessive absorption.[15] Brand names include Xylocaine, Dilocaine, Solarcaine, Lidoderm, L.M.X.4, Denti Patch, Duo-Trach, Nervocaine, Octocaine, and Zilactin-L. When it comes to pregnant and lactating patients, plain lidocaine is the drug of choice by most obstetricians and gynecologists. One main advantage of using plain lidocaine is the low incidence of allergic reactions. In pediatrics and pedodontics, the disadvantage of plain lidocaine includes the history of LA overdose in children. Thus, 2% plain lidocaine is no longer available in carpules/cartridges. Malamed[5] states as a rule the pediatric dentist administers a plain LA only "when treatment is limited to one quadrant... If treatment extends to two or more quadrants in one visit, a vasopressor-containing LA is selected."[5] There are times (poor behavior by the child or the parents inability to take off from work for multiple visits) when children may need to be treated in the operating room for oral rehabilitation under general anesthesia. If this is the case, the clinician should avoid the use of 2% plain lidocaine while providing treatment of all 4 quadrants. In the operating room, the dentist should use 1% lidocaine with 1:100,000 epinephrine calculated according to the child's weight in kilograms (see **Fig. 10**).
- *Tetracaine HCL* is an ester-type LA (2.0% topically and 0.15% as an injection). It is metabolized in plasma and in the liver by plasma pseudocholinesterase. It is contraindicated in patients with known liver disease. Tetracaine is used in medicine for spinal anesthesia and as LA to the eye and nose for diagnostic purposes and examinations. In dentistry it can be applied as a spray to the

soft palate region (see later, Cetacaine spray) for gaggers and for diagnostic purposes and also for pain relief associated with cancer sores and fever blisters. Note: When applied topically, it is 5 to 8 times more potent than cocaine.[5]

LOCAL ANESTHETICS

Local anesthesia is a loss of sensation in a circumscribed area of the body caused by a depression of excitation in nerve endings or an inhibition of the conduction process in peripheral nerves.[5] All LAs' main mechanism of action is to decrease the rate of depolarization by decreasing the permeability of the ion channels to sodium. The depolarization is not sufficient to reduce the membrane of a nerve fiber to its firing potential.[16] They are either esters or amides; all of them have an aromatic ring that gives them lipid solubility in order for them to work.[16]

Ester LAs include propoxycaine, benzocaine, procaine, and tetracaine (**Table 1**). Para aminobenzoic acid (PABA) is formed from the metabolism, which can cause allergic reactions, including dermatitis and sloughing of tissues. For this reason, injectable esters are no longer used in dentistry. They are also more potent vasodilators.[18] Vasodilation increases the rate of absorption of the LAs, which decreases its duration of action and increases the potential for overdose. They are hydrolyzed in the plasma by pseudocholinesterase.[16]

Amide LAs include lidocaine, mepivacaine, prilocaine, articaine, bupivacaine, and etidocaine (**Tables 2** and **3**). They are metabolized in the liver, and no PABA is formed. They have an amine terminus end that gives the LA some water solubility.

Kidneys are the primary excretory organ for both the LAs and the metabolites.[18] The maximum calculated drug dose should always be decreased in medically compromised, debilitated, or elderly persons. However, the dose should not be altered if nitrous oxide or oxygen anxiolysis is administered.

Drugs that have the same mechanism of action usually have additive effects when used together. It has been suggested that the dose of LA be adjusted down when sedating children with opioids. The use of LA has also been found to reduce the dose of inhalation anesthetics for patients undergoing general anesthesia (GA). Local anesthetic with epinephrine can cause dysrhythmias when used with halogenated hydrocarbons (ie, halothane).[23]

1. **Factors that affect LA biotransformation and distribution in the body**[5]
   a. Liver function (for amide LA): half-lives of amide LA increased with decreased liver function
   b. Plasma protein binding
   c. Blood volume

   • **When administering two LAs, the total dose of both should not exceed the lower of the two maximum doses for the individual agents**.

2. **Desirable properties of LAs**[5]
   a. They are not irritants.
   b. They do not cause permanent alteration of nerve structure.
   c. There is low systemic toxicity.
   d. They are effective both when injected into tissue and in mucous membranes.
   e. There is a short duration of onset.
   f. Duration of action must be long enough to permit completion of procedure but not so long as to require extended recovery.
   g. There is potency for anesthesia without the use of harmful concentrations.

Table 1 Ester LAs		
Drug	**Facts[17]**	**Comments**
1. Procaine	• Classification = ester • Potency = 1 • Toxicity = 1 • Metabolism = hydrolyzed in plasma by plasma pseudocholinesterase • Excretion = 90% as PABA, 8% as diethylaminoethanol, 2% unchanged in the urine • pKa = 9.1 • pH (with epi) = 3.5–5.5 • Onset = 6–10 min (slow) • Half-life = 30 min	• It is the first injectable LA synthesized. • It has the greatest vasodilation properties: increased bleeding at surgical site. • It is not available as a topical. • It has a slow onset. • Use it when there is an allergy to PABA. • Toxicity may present initial mild sedation instead of excitatory symptoms.[18]
2. Propoxycaine	• Classification = ester • Potency = 7–8 • Toxicity = 7–8 • Metabolism = hydrolyzed in plasma and liver • Excretion = kidneys • pH/pKa = not available • Onset = 2–3 min • Half-life = not available	• It is combined with procaine for a more rapid onset and longer duration. • It is not available because of high toxicity. • It is not available as a topical.
3. Cocaine HCL	• Metabolism = liver • Excretion: urine • Onset (topical) = 1 min	• It is the first LA to be widely used in dentistry. • It is highly soluble in water. • It is the only anesthetic that consistently produces vasoconstriction.[18] • It is absorbed rapidly but eliminated slowly. • It blocks reuptake and enhances release of NE; there is increased accumulation of NE.[16] • It readily crosses the BBB and elevates mood.[16] • It should not be administered to patients who have taken cocaine in previous 48 h. The beta receptors in the heart and the dopamine receptors in the brain have been sensitized, and the epinephrine can cause cardiac arrhythmias and a hypertensive crises.[16] • Because of its abuse potential, it is not recommended to be used as a topical. • It has a short duration of action, which means more of the drugs need to be injected, which increases the potential for systemic toxicity.

Abbreviations: BBB, blood-brain barrier; PABA, para-aminobenzoic acid.
   Data from Refs.[16–18]; and *Courtesy of* Kirpalani T, DMD, Brooklyn, NY.

Table 2
Amide LAs

Drug	LA (%)	Vasoconstrictor	Duration	MRD
1. Lidocaine	2	None *short acting*	Pulpal = 5–10 min Soft tissue = 1–2 h	4.4/kg 2.0/lb Max = 300
		Epi (1:50,000) for *hemostasis*	Pulpal 1.0–1.5 h Soft tissue = 3–5 h	4.4/kg 2.0/lb Max = 300
		Epi (1:100,000)	Pulpal = 1.0–1.5 h Soft tissue = 3–5 h	4.4/kg 2.0/lb Max = 300
2. Mepivacaine (Carbocaine)	3	None	Pulpal = 20–40 min Soft tissue = 2–3 h	4.4/kg 2.0/lb Max = 300
	2	Levonordefrin (1:20,000)	Pulpal = 1.0–1.5 h Soft tissue = 3–5 h	4.4/kg 2.0/lb Max = 300
		Epi (1:200,000)	Pulpal = 45–60 min Soft tissue = 2–4 h	4.4/kg 2.0/lb Max = 300
		Epi (1:100,000)	Pulpal = 60–85 min Soft tissue = 2–5 h	4.4/kg 2.0/lb Max = 300
3. Prilocaine	4	None	Pulpal = 10–60 min Soft tissue = 1.5–4.0 h	6.0/kg 2.7/lb Max = 400
		Epi (1:200,000)	Pulpal = 1.0–1.5 h Soft tissue = 3–8 h	6.0/kg 2.7/lb Max = 400
4. Articaine (Septocaine)	4	Epi (1:100,000)	Pulpal = 60–75 min Soft tissue = 3–6 h	• Adult = 7/kg, 3.2/lb • Child = 5/kg, 2.3/lb • Max = 500
		Epi (1:200,000)	Pulpal = 45–60 min Soft tissue = 2–5 h	• Adult = 7/kg, 3.2/lb • Child = 5/kg, 2.3/lb • Max = 500
5. Bupivacaine (Marcaine)	0.5	Epi (1:200,000) *long acting*	Pulpal = 1.5–3.0 h Soft tissue = 4–9 h	1.3/kg 0.6/lb Max = 90
6. Etidocaine	1.5	Epi (1:200,000)	Pulpal = 1.5–3.0 h Soft tissue = 4–9 h	8.0/kg 3.6/lb Max = 400

Abbreviation: Max, maximum.
From Malamed SF. Clinical actions of specific agents. Handbook of local anesthesia by Malamed. 6th edition. Philadelphia: Elsevier; 2013. p. 52–75; with permission.

    h. They do not cause allergic reactions.
    i. They are available in solution and undergo biotransformation in the body.
    j. They are sterile/capable of being sterilized.
3. Duration varies depending on[17]
    a. Individual variation to the drug, depicted by a normal distribution
    b. Accuracy of administration. Deposition close to nerve will provide greater depth and duration of anesthesia compared with an anesthetic deposited a greater distance from the nerve.

Table 3
Amide LAs in detail

Drug	Facts[17]	Comments
1. Lidocaine	• Classification: amide • Potency = 2 • Toxicity = 2 • Metabolism = liver • Excretion = kidneys (>80% metabolites, <10% unchanged) • pH (with epi) = 7.9 • pKa = 5.0–5.5 • Onset = 2–3 min (rapid) • Half-life = 1.6 h	• It was introduced in 1948. • It is most commonly used is the 2% solution with (1:100,000 epi).[16] • There are several generics on the market.[16] • Toxicity may present initial mild sedation instead of excitatory symptoms.[18] • It has less vasodilation than procaine but more than prilocaine or mepivacaine. • It produces a greater depth of anesthesia with a longer duration over a larger area than a comparable volume of procaine. • Topical anesthetic is available. • It is the first amide anesthetic to be marketed. • Relative to procaine, it has a more rapid onset of action, longer duration of action, and greater potency. • Epi-sensitive patients are limited to 1 carpule of 1:50,000 epi and 2 carpules of 1:100,000 epi. • Use 1:50,000 epi for hemostasis.
2. Mepivacaine	• Classification: amide • Potency = 2 • Toxicity = 2 • Metabolism = liver • Excretion = kidneys (<16% excreted unchanged) • pKa = 7.6 • pH (plain solution) = 4.5 • Onset = 1.5–2.0 min • Half-life = 1.9 h	• It was introduced in 1960. • It produces only slight vasodilation, so it produces a longer duration of anesthesia relative to other anesthetics without vasoconstrictor. • Use 3% without epi in patients in whom a vasoconstrictor is not indicated and for dental procedures of short duration. • It is common in pediatric and geriatric dentistry.
3. Prilocaine	• Classification = amide • Potency = 2 • Toxicity = 1 • Metabolism = in the liver, kidney, and lung • Excretion = via kidneys	• It was introduced in 1960. • Topical is not available. • Renal clearance is faster than other amides.

(continued on next page)

Table 3
(continued)

Drug	Facts[17]	Comments
	• pKa = 7.9 • pH (with epi) = 3.0–4.0 • Onset = 2–4 min • Half-life = 1.6 h	• Metabolism in the liver produces carbon dioxide, orthotoluidine, and N-propylalanine. In large doses, orthotoluidine can lead to methemoglobinemia, which reduces the blood's oxygen-carrying capacity. • Plasma levels decrease more rapidly than lidocaine, so it is less toxic. • It has less tissue vasodilation than lidocaine and can be used in plain solution for short-duration procedures. • CNS toxicity signs are briefer and less severe than the same doses of lidocaine. • Cardiac patients can receive a maximum of 4 carpules of prilocaine with 1:200,000 epi. • It is indicated for epi-sensitive patients who require prolonged anesthesia. • It has a relative contraindication in patients with methemoglobinemia, sickle cell anemia, or symptoms of hypoxia. • There are reports of paresthesia, particularly alveolar and lingual nerve blocks. The hypothesis is that it is the chemical toxicity that is the cause of these paresthesias.[19] This hypothesis has been supported by reports of neurologic defects with 4% lidocaine in animal studies[20] and in human studies using 5% lidocaine for spinal anesthesia.[21]
4. Articaine	• Classification: amide • Potency = 3.5 • Toxicity = 2 • Metabolism = plasma and liver producing free carboxylic acid • Excretion = via kidneys (<10% unchanged, >90% metabolites) • pKa = 7.8 • pH (with epi) = 4.4–5.4 • Onset = 1–3 min • Half-life = 1.25 h	• It was introduced in 1976. • It is claimed to have enhanced tissue penetration.[16] • It has a slightly faster onset of action relative to other amides. • There are anecdotal claims that clinicians get better anesthesia compared with other locals, especially with patients who are difficult to get numb.[16] • It is an analogue of prilocaine in which the benzene ring found in all other amide LAs has been replaced with a thiophene ring. • Paresthesia unrelated to surgery most often involves the tongue, followed by the lip, and is most common with 4% solutions of articaine (as with prilocaine).[22] Most cases resolve in 8 wk.[21] • It has vasodilatory properties similar to lidocaine. • Methemoglobinemia is a potential side effect. • It is no longer contraindicated in patients with idiopathic/congenital methemoglobinemia.[23] • It is contraindicated in patients with sulfur allergies because it contains methylparaben. • For a hot tooth, consider intrapulpal or intraosseous articaine.

| 5. Bupivacaine | • Classification = amide
• Potency = 4 times that of lidocaine
• Toxicity = 4 times less than lidocaine
• Metabolism = liver
• Excretion = kidneys
• pKa = 8.1 (high)
• pH (with epi) = 3.0–4.5
• Onset = 6–10 min
• Half-life = 2.7 h | • It was introduced in 1983.
• It has added carbons to the mepivacaine molecule that increases potency and duration of action.[16]
• It has greater vasodilation than lidocaine but less than procaine.
• It is not available as a topical.
• It is indicated when lengthy pulpal anesthesia is required and for management of postoperative pain.
• It has a longer onset relative to lidocaine or mepivacaine.
• It is not recommended for pediatrics or physically/mentally disabled patients because of prolonged effects, which increase the risk of soft tissue injury.[17] |
| 6. Etidocaine | • Classification = amide
• Potency = 4 times that of lidocaine
• Toxicity = 2–4 times that of lidocaine
• Metabolism = N-dealkylation in the liver
• Excretion = kidneys
• pKa = 7.7
• pH (with epi) = 3.0–3.5
• Onset = 1.5–3.0 min
• Half-life = 2.6 h | • It has added carbons to the lidocaine molecule that increases potency and duration of action.[16]
• It is no longer on the market.[16]
• It has greater vasodilation than lidocaine but less than procaine.
• No topical is available.
• It is long acting and has similar indications to bupivacaine. |

All potencies/toxicities are relative to procaine of 1.
Data from Refs. [16-23]; and *Courtesy of* Kirpalani T, DMD, Brooklyn, NY.

    c. Vascularity/pH of the tissues. Inflammation and infection usually decrease the duration of action. Increased vascularity leads to more rapid absorption of the anesthetic reducing the duration.

    d. Anatomic variation

    e. Type of injection administered; nerve block or supraperiosteal

4. Factors in selection of LA[23]

    a. Anticipated duration of dental procedure

    b. Potential for discomfort in the posttreatment period

    c. Possibility of self-mutilation in the postoperative period

    d. Requirement for hemostasis during treatment

    e. Medical/developmental status of patients

    f. The planned administration of other agents, such as nitrous oxide, sedative agents and general anesthesia

    g. Allergies

5. Toxicity of LAs[18]

Systemic Effects of LAs

Systemic actions of LAs are related to the plasma levels. The central nervous system (CNS) and the cardiovascular system (CVS) are the most susceptible to their actions, and the blood level of the anesthetic depends on its rate of uptake and on the rate of distribution/biotransformation. Overdose can result from high blood levels caused by a single inadvertent intravascular injection or repeated injections.

    a. CNS: LAs can cross the blood-brain barrier (BBB) and cause CNS depression. At toxic levels, they can cause seizures and a biphasic reaction (excitation followed by depression).

    b. CVS: LAs' action decreases electrical excitability of the myocardium, conduction rate, and force of contraction. It is also a biphasic reaction: As plasma levels of anesthetic increase, vasodilation occurs followed by depression of the myocardium and subsequent decrease in BP. The depressive effects on the CVS are at significantly elevated levels.

    c. Respiratory system: It can lead to respiratory arrest due to CNS depression. At lower levels, LAs can also have a direct relaxant action on bronchial smooth muscle.

    d. Symptoms of overdose include headaches, light-headedness, dizziness, blurred vision, ringing in ears, numbness of tongue and perioral tissues, flushed feeling, drowsiness, disorientation, and loss of consciousness.

Terminology/Synonyms of Common Amide Drugs Used

1. *Lidocaine HCL/Alpha-Caine HCL/Xylocaine HCL/Octocaine HCL/Lignospan[17]*
2. *Mepivacaine HCL/Arestocaine HCL/Carbocaine HCL/Isocaine HCL/Polocaine HCL/Scandonest HCL*
3. *Prilocaine/Citanest*
4. *Articaine/Septocaine/Septanest/Ultracaine D-S*
5. *Bupivacaine/Marcaine HCL*
6. *Etidocaine/Duranest*

Vasoconstrictors in Local Anesthetics

- It is added to constrict blood vessels in the area of injection, which lowers the rate of absorption of the LA into the blood stream, thereby lowering the risk of toxicity and prolonging the anesthetic action in the area.[23]

- Norepinephrine causes hypertensive problems.
- Dosages should be kept to a minimum in patients receiving tricyclic antidepressants (TCAs) because dysrhythmias may occur. Levonordefrin and norepinephrine (NE) are contraindicated in patients receiving TCAs.[23]
- When halogenated gases (eg, halothane) are used for GA, the myocardium is sensitized to epinephrine. Such situations dictate caution with use of epinephrine, which also includes patients with cardiovascular disease, thyroid dysfunction, diabetes, or sulfite sensitivity.
- It is added to anesthetics to oppose vasodilatory properties.
- *Levonordefrin* is purely synthetic but is an isomer of epinephrine. It does not provide the intensity of hemostasis noted with epinephrine. It is less likely to produce more cardiac side effects than epinephrine, but it is more likely to increase BP and does have a higher potential of interaction with TCAs.
- These catecholamines do not cross the BBB; all side effects are peripheral.
- *Ephedrine* and *tyramine* are noncatecholamines. Hence, they can cross the BBB and act as stimulants. Instead of directly stimulating alpha and beta receptors, they enhance the release of neurotransmitters. Do not administer to patients on monoamine oxidase inhibitors because they can cause hypertensive crises.
- Advantages of epinephrine include reduced blood levels of locals, longer pulpal anesthesia, and reduced blood loss which gives you a clearer surgical field.
- Epinephrine overdose signs are elevated systolic BP, increased heart rate, abnormal rhythm, cardiac conduction abnormalities, cardiac dysrhythmias, and cardiac arrest.[18]
- A bisulfite preservative is used in LAs containing epinephrine. For patients having an allergy to bisulfites, use of an LA without vasoconstrictor is indicated.
- Epinephrine overdose symptoms are anxiety, restlessness, headache, tremor, dizziness, sweating, pallor, palpitations, and respiratory difficulty.
- Maximum doses of vasoconstrictor (based on a 70-kg individual) are 0.2 mg for healthy patients and 0.04 mg for cardiac patients.[18]

Dose Calculations

- The maximum dose of LAs is limited by either the maximum dose of the LA or the maximum dose of the vasoconstrictor. One must calculate the maximum number of carpules of LA and that of the vasoconstrictor that can be given to patients, and the smaller number will be the maximum number of carpules of LA that one can administer to a given patient.

(i) Maximum doses of local anesthetic

- $X\% = (1000X)$ mg/100 mL
- MRD $= Y$ mg/kg
- Weight of individual $= Z$ kg
- Volume of one carpule $= 1.8$ mL/carpule
- Total amount of anesthetic that can be given to patients $= (Z * Y)$ mg
- Total amount of anesthetic in one carpule $= [(1.8/100)*(1000X)]$ mg/carpule $= (18X)$ mg/carpule

Maximum number of carpules that can be given to patients $= [(Z*Y)/18X]$ carpules

(ii) Maximum doses of vasoconstrictor

- Dosage equivalence of epinephrine (epi) = A mg/mL (from **Table 4**)
- Amount of epi in one carpule = (A mg/mL)*(1.8 mL/carpule) = 1.8 A mg/carpule
- Maximum dose of epinephrine for patients = B mg

Maximum number of carpules that can be given to patients = [(B/1.8 A)] carpules

Determining Factors for Effect of Anesthetic

The role of pKa and pH

LAs are typically manufactured with a pH from 3.5 to 6.0.[24] When injected into body tissue at physiologic pH, the anesthetic will dissociate. An equilibrium between the uncharged basic form and the cationic form is established:

Base/H+ ↔ Base + H+

The uncharged basic form is the active form of LAs. This property of LAs allows for the anesthetic to diffuse through the membrane of the neuronal tissue. The pKa of the anesthetic describes the amount of uncharged form versus cationic form is present at a given pH. When the pKa equals the pH of surrounding tissue, an equilibrium will be established with 50% basic form and 50% cationic form. This point is illustrated by the Henderson-Hasselbalch equation:

pKa = pH − log [base]/[acid]

LAs have pKas typically ranging from 7.7 to 8.9 (**Table 5**).[25] As the pH of the surrounding tissue decreases, the equilibrium will shift left, which results in less availability of the uncharged base form. The pKa determines the onset time, as LAs with a higher pKa will have slower onset times.

Lipid solubility

The lipid solubility of an LA is another characteristic that effects the ability to penetrate the neuronal tissue. Lipid solubility determines the potency of an LA. Potency describes the amount of the drug required to have a similar effect compared with another anesthetic.[25] The higher the lipid solubility, the more potent the anesthetic will be. In turn, a lesser dosage is required to achieve the same effect compared with an anesthetic that is not as lipid soluble (**Table 6**).

In addition to potency, the anesthetics with higher lipid solubility will also have a longer duration of action. Furthermore, the degree of protein binding will also effect the duration.

Table 4
Maximum doses of vasoconstrictor[24]

Concentration	Dose Equivalence (mg/mL)
1:1000	1.0
1:10,000	0.1
1:100,000	0.01
1:200,000	0.005

Courtesy of Naveen Mohan, DMD, Brooklyn, NY.

Table 5 Characteristics of commonly used LAs at physiologic pH[24]		
Medication	**pKa**	**Free Base (%)**
Mepivacaine	7.7	33
Lidocaine	7.8	29
Articaine	7.8	29
Bupivacaine	8.1	17
Procaine	8.9	3

Auxiliary Techniques (Topicals and Injections)

When it comes to the use of LAs in dentistry, the delivery can be in the form of infiltration (anterior superior alveolar [ASA], middle superior alveolar [MSA], posterior superior alveolar [PSA], buccal/facial), palatal (incisive foramen, greater palatine), regional block (IAN, buccal, mental, incisive), periodontal ligament (PDL), and intrapulpal. Although the Gow-Gates technique and the Vazirani-Akinosi closed-mouth mandibular block are proven ways of administering LAs, they should be used by oral and maxillofacial surgeons or other experienced specialist in medicine and dentistry. When it comes to routine dental procedures, the 2 aforementioned techniques are not needed because of *increased risks* of (1) temporary or transient paralysis, (2) hematoma, and (3) being in arbitrary space (ie, vessels or accidental needle breakage). It is imperative to make contact with bone while using the Gow-Gates technique; otherwise, do not inject the LA into arbitrary space. As mentioned earlier, local infiltration is sufficient anesthesia for implant placement instead of IAN block.

There are other techniques that are being introduced to the dental profession or that are selectively practiced by specialist that are discussed in this section. Trigger-point injections are usually not taught on the undergraduate dental school level; therefore, patients in need of this treatment should be referred to a pain specialist in dentistry (ie, oral medicine specialist, orofacial pain specialist, oral and maxillofacial surgeon, and so forth). Referral to any of the specialist mentioned earlier should be indicated when

1. The disability greatly exceeds what is expected from physical findings.
2. Patients make excessive demands for tests and treatments that are not indicated.
3. Patients display significant psychological distress (ie, depression).
4. Patients display aberrant behavior, such as continual nonadherence to treatments.[26]

Patients who are suspected of having or diagnosed with TMD or orofacial pain usually respond well to treatment managed by the specialists mentioned

Table 6 Lipid solubility of commonly used anesthetics[24]	
Medication	**Lipid Solubility**
Articaine	40
Mepivacaine	42
Lidocaine	110
Bupivacaine	560

earlier; but there are times when these patients may need to be referred to a physiotherapist, psychiatrists, neurologist, anesthesiologist, or other health care professionals when considering a central (as opposed to peripheral) cause of pain.[27] Diagnostic nerve blocks can be used by the dentist to rule out an odontogenic/peripheral versus centralized pain source before referral. This topic of discussion is of extreme importance to the general dentist because a proper diagnosis should be established before they feel the pressure to initiate invasive treatment (ie, root canal, extraction) that is considered ineffective and inappropriate.[28]

Finally, soft tissue injury (lip biting or cheek biting) is a fairly common complication that occurs in pediatric, physically disabled, or mentally disabled patients after dental treatment with the use of LAs. The best way to prevent this occurring in pediatric patients is educating children and parents before dismissal. This instruction may present a challenge with the special needs patients mentioned earlier. It also should be noted that PDL injection is not recommended in deciduous teeth because of the high risk of enamel hypoplasia.[29] Today some pedodontists, dentists, and dental hygienists are equipped with phentolamine mesylate (Ora-Verse) (**Figs. 2** and **3**). Phentolamine mesylate is used as an option to decrease prolonged anesthesia in patients who are at risk for soft tissue injury (mentioned earlier) or patients that may need to return to work or may have a speaking engagement.[30] Phentolamine mesylate is *not* recommended in children younger than 6 years or weighing less than 15 kg (33 lb), and its dosage depends on the number of cartridges administered.[5]

PERIODONTAL ANESTHETICS

- *HurriPAK*, which contains 20% benzocaine (in multiple flavors), is an anesthetic liquid. It is marketed as a needle-free periodontal anesthetic kit. This product *must* be used with a plastic syringe (3 mL) and disposable periodontal irrigation tips (**Figs. 4–6**). The plastic tip is injected deep into the gingival sulcus. The onset is 30 seconds and the duration is 15 minutes. Realistically, 15 minutes duration *will not* provide adequate anesthesia for a routine dental visit on adult patients, so multiple administration of the liquid anesthetic or the need for needle infiltrations or PDL injections on adult patients would be needed.
- *Cetacaine*, which contains 14% benzocaine, 2% butamben, 2% tetracaine HCL, is indicated for topical pain control of all accessible mucous membranes except the eyes. It is *not* suitable and should *never* be used for injection. It is marketed as an anesthetic liquid clinical kit that includes liquid bottle, delivery syringes, and microcapillary delivery tips for delivery into periodontal

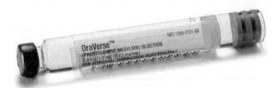

Fig. 2. Phentolamine mesylate (Ora-Verse) is used as an option to decrease prolonged anesthesia in patients who are at risk for soft tissue injury or patients who may need to return to work or may have a speaking engagement. (*Courtesy of* Septodont, Lancaster, PA; with permission.)

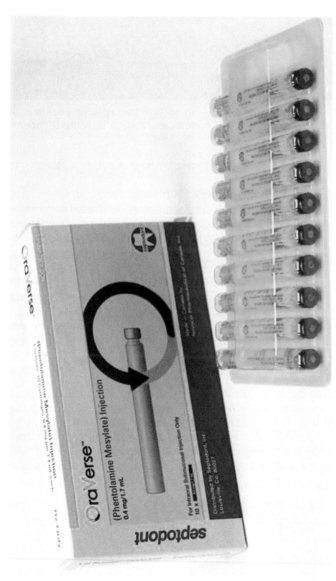

Fig. 3. Phentolamine mesylate (Ora-Verse) is used as an option to decrease prolonged anesthesia in patients who are at risk for soft tissue injury or patients who may need to return to work or may have a speaking engagement. (*Courtesy of Septodont, Lancaster, PA; with permission.*)

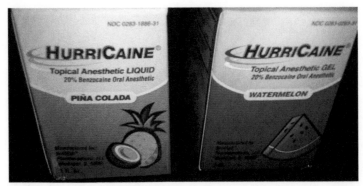

Fig. 4. HurriPAK contains 20% benzocaine (in multiple flavors) as an anesthetic liquid and gel. It is marketed as a needle-free periodontal anesthetic kit. (Beutlich Pharmaceuticals, LLC, Waukegan, IL.)

    pockets. It can also be applied topically using a cotton swab or microbrush (**Fig. 7**).

- *Oraqix* contains 2.5% lidocaine and 2.5% prilocaine and comes with 20 cartridges and blunted tips. Oraqix has a unique dispenser that is favored by dental hygienists and some periodontists for ease of use (**Figs. 8** and **9**). Oraqix is *not* to be injected; instead, it is deposited into periodontal pockets during scaling and root planning. It is imperative that the clinician be cautious when using Oraqix in combination with other LAs. It is contraindicated in patients with a known allergy or hypersensitivity to amide-type LAs. Oraqix should *not* be used in patients with known deficiency of glucose-6-phosphate dehydrogenase or methemoglobinemia (congenital, idiopathic) or children younger than 12 months who are receiving treatments with methemoglobin-inducing agents. It is the clinician's responsibility to consult, interpret patients' medical condition, and determine if it is safe to administer this product (based on their dental/medical training).

Trigger-Point Injections

This technique involves the injection of an LA into the muscle causing the pain. A trigger point has been defined as any cutaneous or muscular areas that, when stimulated, bring about an acute neuralgic or referred musculoskeletal pain, respectively.[31] *The choice of LA for this treatment is 2% lidocaine (without vasoconstrictor) because of the low toxicity into the muscle.* As mentioned earlier, 2% plain lidocaine is no longer

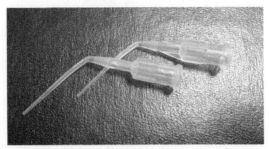

Fig. 5. The HurriPAK must be used with a plastic syringe (3 mL). (*Courtesy of* Beutlich Pharmaceuticals, LLC, Waukegan, IL; with permission.)

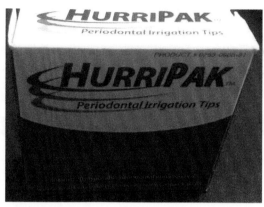

Fig. 6. Disposable periodontal irrigation tips. (*Courtesy of* Beutlich Pharmaceuticals, LLC, Waukegan, IL; with permission.)

available in dental cartridges (since August 2011) in North America; however, it is readily available for the dentist working in a hospital environment (**Fig. 10**). Phero and colleagues[32] describe it as "injections given to a muscle group in a series of weekly treatments for 3 to 5 weeks... may be continued with intervals between injections, depending on the response." If properly administered, the injections will decrease or eliminate the pain associated with the trigger point area as well as any referred pain.[33]

Intraosseous Injection

This technique is excellent for patients presenting to the dental office with the classic "hot tooth" and want to save the tooth via root canal therapy. LA properly delivered will decrease if not eliminate acute pain, but a high-speed handpiece with bur introducing air and water on an inflamed and/or infected tooth will set off pain that will have patients either crying or literally jumping out of the chair. Even

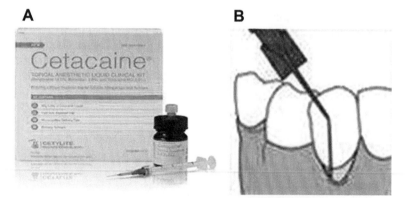

Fig. 7. Cetacaine contains 14% benzocaine, 2% butamben, and 2% tetracaine hydrochloride and is indicated for topical pain control of all accessible mucous membranes except the eyes. (*A*) It is marketed as an anesthetic liquid clinical kit that includes liquid bottle, delivery syringes, and microcapillary delivery tips for delivery into periodontal pockets. (*B*) It can also be applied topically using a cotton swab or microbrush. (*Courtesy of* Cetylite Industries, Inc, Pennsauken, NJ; with permission.)

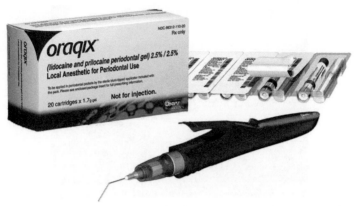

Fig. 8. Oraqix contains 2.5% lidocaine and 2.5% prilocaine and comes with 20 cartridges and blunted tips. (*Courtesy of* DENTSPLY Pharmaceutical, York, PA; with permission.)

a patient experiencing all the signs of profound anesthesia can become symptomatic when a bur (in combination with air and water) is applied to exposed dentinal tubules. Hargreaves and Keiser[34] reported an 8-fold increase in LA failure after an IAN block injection.

Intraosseous injection involves an LA to be deposited in bone between 2 teeth.[35] The brand names popular to use in North America are Stabident and X-Tip, which have guide sleeves that allow a short 27-gauge needle (**Figs. 11–15** show the X-Tip). It is *important* for the clinician to be trained by a dentist or specialist in the dental profession with experience. The clinician should have a good bitewing and periapical radiograph in order to prevent perforation on any root structure. Selection of the injection site is 2 to 4 mm apical to the crest of bone. The site chosen should be distal to the tooth being worked on. Next, the cortical plate will be perforated with the use of a drill (X-Tip) or perforator (Stabident). Both systems have a guide sleeve for the 27-gauge needle with LA. If LA with epinephrine is chosen, the clinician should alert patients about the high probability of heart palpitations while injecting. After proper administration, all symptoms mentioned earlier are completely alleviated, giving the skilled clinician the opportunity to perform the pulpectomy. It is *imperative* that the clinician remove the guide sleeve before dismissal of patients. The guide sleeve has a metal component that if left accidentally can be dislodged and be swallowed by patients. It is the clinician's responsibility to check

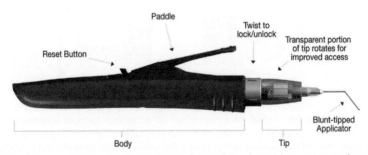

Fig. 9. Oraqix has a unique dispenser that is favored by dental hygienists and some periodontists for ease of use. (*Courtesy of* DENTSPLY Pharmaceutical, York, PA; with permission.)

A   B

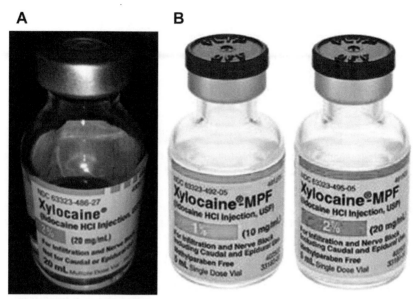

Fig. 10. The choice of LA for trigger-point injections is 2% lidocaine (without vasocon-strictor) because of the low toxicity into the muscle. Two-percent plain lidocaine is no longer available in dental cartridges (since August 2011) in North America; however, it is readily available for the dentist working in a hospital environment for (*A*) multiple doses and (*B*) single doses. (App Pharmaceuticals, Schaumburg, IL.)

and count all sharps used before discharging any patient. Accidental aspiration will involve immediate attention in the emergency department to chest radiograph to *rule out* lung *verses* gastrointestinal involvement. Each system has specific manufacturer instructions and should be reviewed before each use if not used on

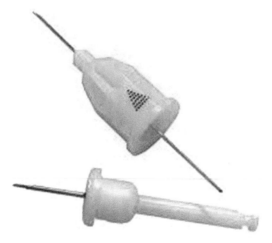

Fig. 11. The 27-gauge ultrashort needle (in *yellow*) and the drill, which latches to the slow speed and guide sleeve (in *white*). (*Courtesy of* DENTSPLY Maillefer, Ballaigues, Switzerland; with permission.)

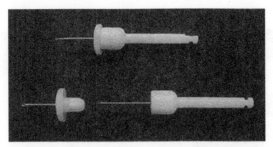

Fig. 12. There is separation between the drill and guide sleeve. (*Courtesy of* DENTSPLY Maillefer, Ballaigues, Switzerland; with permission.)

a daily/weekly basis. This technique is not for every dentist; only those who have been trained, feel confident in the delivery system, and do not have a problem owning up to responsibilities should use the product.

Intrasulcular Infusion

The last but certainly not least to mention is a new product on the market called The NumBee (Novoject USA LLC, Austin, TX), a plastic hub that attaches to all standard dental syringes. The blade is plastic, thinner than most toothpicks, and only needs to be placed under the gum and into the sulcus as deep as the bristles on a toothbrush would penetrate. Most importantly, there is no piercing of any tissue. The plastic blade encases a rounded-tip steel cannula that carries the anesthetic through the blade. At the tip of the NumBee, a small tip encircles the end of the cannula. This tip achieves a superior seal between the device and the ligament, which, in turn, makes it easier to deliver the anesthetic under pressure. There is

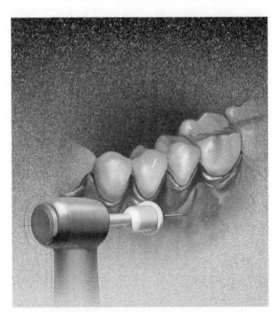

Fig. 13. Step 1: Note the separation shows the drill and hand piece in place. (*Courtesy of* DENTSPLY Maillefer, Ballaigues, Switzerland; with permission.)

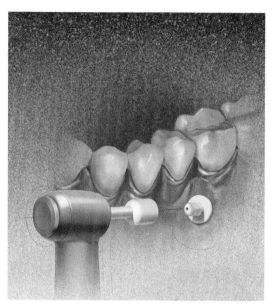

Fig. 14. Step 2: Note the separation of the drill and guide sleeve. (*Courtesy of* DENTSPLY Maillefer, Ballaigues, Switzerland; with permission.)

no sharp tip, which can be demonstrated on the hand of fearful patients prior to administration. This product eliminates the hypodermic needle, which, in turn, would be great on pediatric patients and those adults who have a phobia of the needle (**Figs. 16–18**).

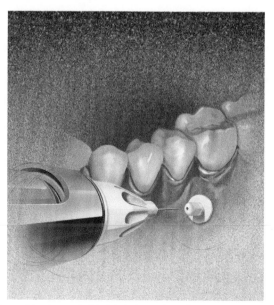

Fig. 15. Step 3: The guide sleeve (*white*) is left in place for insertion and administration of the LA. (*Courtesy of* DENTSPLY Maillefer, Ballaigues, Switzerland; with permission.)

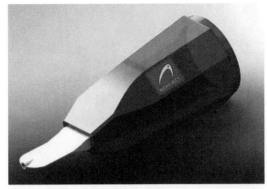

Fig. 16. The Numbee by Novoject. (*Courtesy of* Novoject USA LLC, Austin, TX; with permission.)

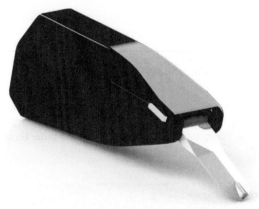

Fig. 17. This image shows the ability to move the plastic blade to maneuver difficult areas. (*Courtesy of* Novoject USA LLC, Austin, TX; with permission.)

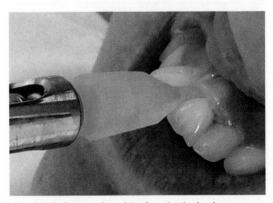

Fig. 18. Numbee plastic blade being placed in the gingival sulcus on a patient. (*Courtesy of* Novoject USA LLC, Austin, TX; with permission.)

SUMMARY

As described in this article, there are many advances in the area of topical anesthetics and LAs. If it were not for these advances, several procedures in medicine and dentistry would be considered barbaric. Topical anesthetics and LAs have played a great role in dentistry in alleviating the fears of patients, eliminating pain, and providing pain control. LAs with epinephrine are beneficial to pediatric dental patients because of the high risks involved with 2% plain lidocaine and 3% mepivacaine. When vasoconstrictors (ie, epinephrine) are used, caution is a *must* in patients with hyperthyroidism; it is discouraged for use by many obstetricians and gynecologists in pregnant patients. It is imperative for each clinician to screen patients before treatment (eg, health history, obtain a base line BP), definitely before any invasive surgical procedure. Isolated systolic hypertension is commonly seen in middle-aged and elderly patients, with BP greater than 160 mm Hg/less than 90 mm Hg; dental care is commonly treated under appropriate LA and compliance of medications. Any patient with a systolic BP of 180/100 should *not* be seen or treated with elective dental care (ie, LA with or without epinephrine) but should be given a medical consult, only to return after the BP is controlled and patients have written clearance. Malignant hypertension (>180/120 mm Hg) is a medical emergency; symptomatic patients should be sent directly to the emergency department. Liu and colleagues[36] summed it up best: "Clinicians should enhance their awareness of dosage, concentration, and combination of drugs of LAs to decrease the incidence of adverse drug reactions (ADR)… also should know clearly about the local anatomic structures and practice skillfully to avoid wrong administration, such as intravascular injection." They went further by stating, "It is important to evaluate the patients' health condition, psychological condition, and allergic history before using local anesthetics."[36]

LA still remains the unsung hero in modern-day dentistry. Many invasive procedures simply would not be performed without the use and advances of topical anesthetics and LAs.

Each clinician should have a good foundation about the classification, potency, toxicity, metabolism, excretion, pregnancy classification, contraindications, and MDR for the use of LAs according to patients' body weight (children, elderly, or adults). The modern-day dentist has the responsibility of knowing the variety of the products on the market and should have *at least 3 (updated)* references to access before, during, and after treatment. This practice will ensure proper care with topical anesthetics and LAs for the masses of patients entering dental offices worldwide.

REFERENCES

1. Melzack R, Wall PD. Pain mechanisms: a new theory. Science 1965;150(3699): 971–9.
2. Merskey H, Bogduk N. Classification of chronic pain: descriptions of chronic pain syndromes and definition of pain terms. 2nd Edition. Seattle (WA): IASP; 1994.
3. Nasri-Heir C, Khan J, Heir GM. Topical medications as treatment of neuropathic orofacial pain. Dent Clin North Am 2013;57:541.
4. Gomella LG, Haist SA. Clinician's pocket reference: pain management. 9th Edition. Blacklick (OH): McGraw-Hill Medical Publishing Division; 2002. p. 315–23.
5. Malamed SF. Handbook of local anesthesia by Malamed. 6th Edition. St. Louis (MO): Elsevier; 2013.
6. Hersh EV, Helpin ML, Evans OB. Local anesthetic mortality: report of case. J Dent Child 1991;58(6):489–91.
7. Yagiella JA. Local anesthetics. Pharmacology and therapeutics for dentistry by Neidle and Yagiella. 3rd edition. St. Louis (MO): C.V. Mosby Co; 1989. p. 230–48.

8. Stienberg MJ, Kelly PD. Implant-related nerve injuries. Dent Clin North Am 2015; 59(2):357–73.

9. Hillerup S, Jensen R. Nerve injury caused by mandibular block analgesia. Int J Oral Maxillofac Surg 2006;35:437–43.

10. Becker BM, Helrich S, Baker E, et al. Ultrasound with topical anesthetic rapidly decreases pain of intravenous cannulation. Acad Emerg Med 2005;12(4):289–95.

11. Stowell CP, Trieu MQ, Chuang H, et al. Ultrasound-enabled topical anesthesia for pain reduction of phlebotomy for whole blood donation. Transfusion 2009;49(1): 146–53.

12. Wynn RL, Meiller TF, Crossley HL. Drug information handbook for dentistry: oral medicine for medically-compromised patients & specific oral conditions. 7th edition. Hudson (OH): Lexi-Comp Inc; 2002. p. 352.

13. Blasberg B, Greenberg MS. Temporomandibular disorders: Burket's oral medicine by Greenberg and Glick. 10th edition. Hamilton (Ontario): BC Decker; 2003. p. 271–306.

14. Bernardi M, Secco F, Benech A. Anesthetic efficacy of a eutectic mixture of lidocaine and prilocaine (EMLA) on the oral mucosa: prospective double-blind study with a placebo. Minerva Stomatol 1999;48:9–43.

15. Greenberg MS, Glick M. Burket's oral medicine. Oral cancer. 10th edition. Hamilton (Canada): BC Decker; 2008. p. 220.

16. Hersh, EV. "Local anesthetics" lecture. U Penn SDM 8/28/2010.

17. Malamed SF. Clinical actions of specific agents. Handbook of local anesthesia by Malamed. 6th edition. St. Louis (MO): Elsevier; 2013. p. 52–75.

18. Hersh, EV. "Local anesthetics" lecture. U Penn SDM 9/10/2010.

19. Miller PA, Haas DA. Incidence of Local Anesthetic-Induced Neuropathies in Ontario from 1994–1998 (Abstract 3869). J Dent Res 2000;79(special issue):627.

20. Fink BR, Kish SJ. Reversible inhibition of rapid axonal transport in-vivo by lidocaine hydrochloride. Anesthesiology 1976;44:139–46.

21. Kane RE. Neurologic deficits following epidural or spinal anesthesia. Anesthesiol 1981;60(3):150–61.

22. Haas DA, Lennon D. A 21 year retrospective study of reports of paresthesia following local anesthesia administration. J Can Dent Assoc 1995;61(4):319–30.

23. Turk DC. Assess the person, not just the pain. Pain: Clinical updates 2013;1:1–4.

24. Massoomi N. Local anesthetics. In: Fonseca RJ, editor. Oral and maxillofacial surgery, vol. I, 2nd edition. St Louis (MO): Saunders Elsevier; 2009. p. 35–56.

25. Drasner K. Local anesthetics. In: Miller R, Pardo M, editors. Basics of anesthesia. 6th edition. Philadelphia: Elsevier Saunders; 2011. p. 130–42.

26. Turk D. Assess the person, not just the pain. Pain Clin Updates 1993;1(3):1–4.

27. Greenberg MS, Glick M. Burkett's oral medicine. Temporomandibular disorders. 10th edition. Hamilton (Canada): BC Decker; 2008. p. 288.

28. Greenberg MS, Glick M. Burkett's oral medicine. Orofacial Pain. 10th Edition. Hamilton (Canada): BC Decker; 2008. p. 324.

29. Brannstrom M, Lindskog S, Nordenvall KJ. Enamel hypoplasia in permanent teeth induced by periodontal ligament anesthesia of primary teeth. J Am Dent Assoc 1984;109:535–736.

30. Ora-Verse prescribing information. San Diego (CA): Novalar Pharmaceuticals; 2015.

31. Okeson JP. Orofacial pain: guidelines for assessment, diagnosis, and management. Carol Stream (IL): Quintessence Publishing Co; 1996. p. 266.

32. Phero J, Raj P, McDonald J. Transcutaneous electrical nerve stimulation and myoneural injection therapy for management of chronic myofascial pain. Dent Clin North Am 1987;31:703–23.

33. Travell JG, Simons DG. Myofascial pain and dysfunction: the trigger point manual. Baltimore (MD): Williams and Wilkins; 1983. p. 63–158.
34. Hargreaves K, Kaiser K. Local anesthetic failure in endodontics: mechanisms and management. Endod Top 2002;1:26–39.
35. Cassamani F. Une Nouvelle Technique d" Anesthesia Intraligamentarie: la seringue. [PhD thesis]. Paris: PERI Press; 1924.
36. Liu W, Yang X, Li C, et al. Adverse drug reactions to local anesthetics: a systemic review. Oral Surg Oral Med Oral Pathol Oral Radiol Endod 2013;115(3):319–27.

Current Concepts of Prophylactic Antibiotics for Dental Patients

Mehran Hossaini-zadeh, DMD

KEYWORDS

• Antibiotic prophylaxis • Infective endocarditis • Prosthetic joint infection

KEY POINTS

- There is no evidence to support the routine use of antibiotic prophylaxis before dental procedures to prevent infective endocarditis.
- There is no evidence to support the routine use of antibiotic prophylaxis before dental procedures to prevent prosthetic joint infection.
- There is no evidence to support an association between the bacteremia after dental procedures and incidence of IE or PJI.

INTRODUCTION

The theoretic need for the use of antibiotic prophylaxis is summarized in the context of bacteremia, presumably from the oral cavity. Oral organisms entering the bloodstream, via invasive dental procedures, can potentially colonize vulnerable areas, such as defective heart valves, prosthetic joints, and implanted devices, such as cardiac stents or hemodialysis shunts. The colonization of these vulnerable sites can result in various sequlae, such as valvular damage, infective endocarditis (IE), and failure of prosthesis or implanted devices. Despite the theoretic context, there are multitudes of variables that often are not included into the equation. These variables include, but are not limited to, the extent of bacteremia, species of bacteria, host susceptibility, presence of comorbidities, type of implanted devices, type of antibiotics used, bacteria response to the antibiotics, and the nature of dental procedures. Practitioners often balance these variables with the perceived benign nature of antibiotics, and elect to use antibiotics rather than considering the risks and benefits of not using them. This is further complicated by an unrealistic fear of legal reprisal and whether a practitioner can justify their decision to an unrelenting legal team.

Oral and Maxillofacial Surgery, Temple University Kornberg School of Dentistry, 3223 North Broad Street, Philadelphia, PA 19140, USA
E-mail address: Mehran.Hossaini@temple.edu

Dent Clin N Am 60 (2016) 473–482
http://dx.doi.org/10.1016/j.cden.2015.12.002
0011-8532/16/$ – see front matter © 2016 Elsevier Inc. All rights reserved.

dental.theclinics.com

HISTORY OF ANTIBIOTIC PROPHYLAXIS GUIDELINES FOR INFECTIVE ENDOCARDITIS

In 1955, the American Heart Associations (AHA) published its first recommendations for prevention of infective endocarditis.[1] These guidelines have evolved over the past decades by work of the AHA and American College of Cardiology Task Force groups. International societies have also published their own recommendations and guidelines, further contributing to the evolution of most recent guidelines.

The updates in the available guidelines, from 1955 through 2007, have taken several factors into consideration. Such factors as drug resistance bacteria, risk stratification of the patient population, etiology of bacteremia, and the complexity of the prophylaxis regiment have been included in development of these guidelines. The 1997 guidelines were the first to acknowledge that IE is often not associated with invasive procedures, and more frequently caused by random bacteremia from routine activities. The rational for these guidelines was largely based on expert opinion and what seemed prudent practice to prevent a life-threatening infection.[2] The evidence used to develop these guidelines could be scored as class IIB, and level of evidence C.

In 2007, the most recent guidelines were developed based on the publications and data questioning the efficacy of antibiotics therapy in prevention of IE, and in an attempt to reduce the complexity of the previous guidelines. These new guidelines have significantly reduced the use of antibiotic prophylaxis to prevent IE.

Justification for Antibiotic Prophylaxis in Prevention of Infective Endocarditis

Despite advances in diagnosis and treatment of IE, it continues to be a dangerous disease. Morbidity and mortality are 50% in high-risk patients, such as those with prosthetic valves, congenital heart disease, and previous history of IE.[3]

Development of IE is the net result of a complex set of circumstances involving bloodstream pathogens interacting with the tissue matrix and platelets at the site of endothelial cell damage. This process is summarized in the stages noted next. It is also important to note that the clinical manifestations of IE are further affected by the host immune system.[4]

1. Formation of nonbacterial thrombotic endocarditis (NBTE): Some cardiac anomalies, congenital or acquired, can result in turbulent blood flow, which can cause endothelial injury. Adhesion of platelets and fibrin to the site of trauma can potentially lead into NBTE.
2. Transient bacteremia: Trauma to oral mucosal surfaces can result in transient bacteremia from the site of injury, populating the bloodstream with viridans group streptococci and other common oral microflora
3. Bacterial adhesion: The bacteria within the bloodstream can adhere to the site of endothelial injury and NBTE. Some microorganisms, such as viridans group streptococci, have surface components that allow their adhesions to various surfaces. This surface characteristic can serve as a virulence factor in development of IE.[5] The adhesion of other organisms, such as staphylococci, is facilitated either by surface components or formation of a biofilm, particularly on the surface of implanted devices. There has been some work on vaccines directed to the adhesion characteristics of viridian group streptococci and staphylococci resulting in some protection against IE in experimental models.[6,7]
4. Proliferation of bacteria: On adherence to NBTE, microorganisms rapidly proliferate forming bacterial vegetation within the damaged endothelial surface. These isolated foci can be potentially unaffected by the host immune system, allowing their further growth and invasion. More than 90% of these vegetations are metabolically inactive rendering them less responsive to antibiotics.[8] The bacterial vegetation

within the injured endothelial surfaces can ultimately result in further damage to the cardiac tissue and development of IE.

Gene sequencing, such as 16S rRNA, has identified more than 6 billion bacteria representing more than 700 species.[9] These bacteria and their colonies commonly exist in the form of biofilm in oral environment, including but not limited to soft tissue, teeth, and prostheses. A unique feature of oral bacterial and plaque biofilm is their close proximity to the highly vascularized tissue bed, particularly in the periodontal pockets.[10]

These organisms can gain access into the bloodstream via multitude of mechanisms and portals. Perhaps the most obvious and common route is via trauma-induced procedures, such as periodontal probing, dental extractions, scaling, and other instrumentation resulting in exposure of vascular bed to spillage of bacteria from the plaque biofilm. Although this trauma is often attributed to invasive dental procedures, other activities, such as chewing, brushing, and flossing, fall under this category and induce bacteremia.

For example, it has been shown that 20% of patients demonstrated bacteremia after chewing.[11–13] Bacteremia has been detected in 75% of patients with periodontitis and 20% of patient experiencing gingivitis.[12,14] In one study, bacteremia was noted after tooth brushing in 23% of patients compared with 60% after single tooth extraction. However, the authors suggested that the frequency of tooth brushing may potentially expose patients to a higher cumulative risk from bacteremia compared with single tooth extraction.[15]

In summary, bacteremia can be quantified based on two general parameters. First is the degree of inflammation present at the site, which demonstrates the type and microbial load of the biofilm. Second is the extent of trauma or tissue damage that has occurred exposing the bloodstream to the biofilm.

The guidelines recommending antibiotic prophylaxis for prevention of IE are primarily based on three main observations: (1) bacteremia has been recognized as a cause of IE, (2) viridans group streptococci can result in a critical bacteremia, and (3) these organisms are susceptible to common antibiotics.

The role of dental procedures as a source of bacteremia and the efficacy of antibiotics to prevent IE from such bacteremia continues to be nebulous. Several case-controlled studies have questioned the proposed relationship between invasive dental procedures and IE. A study of 275 patients in the Netherlands demonstrated that IE was caused by random bacteremia rather than invasive dental procedures.[16] Studies in France and the United States demonstrated no correlation between dental treatment and IE compared with control subjects.[17,18]

However, these studies have not addressed the ineffectiveness of antibiotics use in prevention of IE. The incidence of IE from dental procedure without the use of antibiotics has been estimated at 1 in 46,000. In comparison, the incidence of IE in patients with antibiotic use before dental procedures is estimated at 1 in 150,000.[19] The authors of this study have therefore concluded that a huge number of prophylaxis doses of antibiotics would be needed to prevent a very small number of potential IE cases. In light of this high number needed to treat, there is a greater concern for the adverse effects and complications associated with the antibiotics use.

Generally speaking, the risk of adverse effects from a single dose of antibiotics is minor. Risk of fatal anaphylaxis reaction has been reported at 15 to 25 people per million.[20] Antibiotic resistance is less likely to occur for a single dose of antibiotics. However, with continued use, resistance becomes a more concerning factor. Spillage of antibiotics and other pharmaceuticals in the drinking water has captured the attention of the world community and resulted in several health-related concerns.[21]

PATIENT EVALUATION AND MANAGEMENT

Limitations of the available evidence and continuous changes in the clinical profile of IE have led to revision of antibiotic prophylaxis guidelines by various organizations worldwide.[22] In general, all these guidelines aim to reduce the ambiguity, complexity, and requirements for antibiotic prophylaxis use toward prevention of IE. In the United States, the AHA established the most recent guidelines in 2007 gaining endorsement from the American Dental Association (ADA). These guidelines recommend antibiotic prophylaxis use only for patients with highest risk of developing IE. Such guidelines have been received with mixed reactions, and some cardiologists consider them quite alarming and a deviation from the previously accepted clinical practices. Dental providers equally have been confused by the new guidelines, and unable to navigate between the AHA recommendations and medical providers discomfort with changing their established practice.

These debates behoove dental providers to take a more active role in the decision-making process for the use of antibiotic prophylaxis. In general, patients in good health, with healthy dentition and peridontium should not be prescribed antibiotics prophylaxis for prevention of IE, unless they meet the specific criteria for the highest risk groups outlined by the AHA guidelines.[2] The review of various guidelines and their revisions point out to three general domains for consideration: (1) the patient's medical risk factors and state of oral health, (2) invasiveness of the dental procedures, and (3) stratification of the risks for IE.

The relevance of the patient's medical risk factors and state of oral health has been well supported by the literature (all articles). Patients with compromised immune system, such as those with uncontrolled diabetes or recent history of chemotherapy, may be at great risk for adverse event from bacteremia regardless of their compliance with the AHA antibiotic prophylaxis guidelines. If invasive dental treatment is indicated, the dental provider should consider the use of antibiotics before such procedures even though patients may not be considered high risk for IE. Defining the immune competence of patients and determining their potential risk for postprocedure adverse events is an important step in evaluation and caring for all patients. In the context of IE, it becomes an important factor in determining the justification for use of antibiotic prophylaxis.

Another common denominator in the discussion surrounding IE has been the patient's overall oral health status. Characteristics of oral biofilm, presence of advance periodontal disease, the extent of dental carries, and homecare habits have been the centerpiece for concerns associated with bacteremia from oral origin. Identification of viridian group streptococci and *Staphylococcus* spp in patients with IE, in absence of dental procedures, has been linked to the occurrence of random bacteremia.

Although the maintenance of oral health should be a routine aspect of a dental practice, clinical outcomes are not always favorable. Dental providers should consider identifying patients with higher risk of IE and consider implementation of more rigorous oral hygiene care plan. Even patients with moderate risk for IE may benefit from antibiotic prophylaxis in preparation for provision of invasive dental procedures in highly inflamed areas or sites with extensive presence of biofilm.

Compared with cardiologists or other medical providers, dental providers can most appropriately estimate the invasiveness of the planned procedure, extent of local inflammation, and potential for bacteremia secondary to their treatment. Based on this information, dental providers can more objectively support the value of antibiotic prophylaxis for prevention of IE, given the patient's risk factor. Similarly, despite empiric recommendations, dental providers should resist the unnecessary use of antibiotic prophylaxis when not justified by the invasiveness of the procedure and health of local soft tissue.

The risk assessment for IE at times requires a collaboration with the patient's health care team. There is no evidence to support the benefit of antibiotics prophylaxis in patients with low or moderate risk for IE. Therefore, in absence of any other relevant health history or clinical findings patients in these categories do not require antibiotic prophylaxis. The dental providers should evaluate medical consultations or other recommendations by medical providers very critically. In absence of the four high-risk categories defined by the AHA, any medical opinion recommending antibiotic prophylaxis should contain supporting information to support deviation from the proposed guidelines.

From the quality of care perspective, exposure of patients to unnecessary antibiotics, regardless of the safety margin, is inappropriate. From the medical-legal perspective, medical consultations or recommendations are simply one health care provider's opinion. The dental provider is withheld to the standard of analyzing those opinions and formulating a logical decision based on the established treatment guidelines. In such circumstances, and in the event of an adverse antibiotic-related incident, the dental provider may be placed in a position to defend the unnecessary use of antibiotic prophylaxis. This defense may be challenging given guidelines set forth by the AHA, ADA, and other organizations.

HISTORY OF ANTIBIOTIC PROPHYLAXIS TO PREVENT PROSTHETIC JOINT INFECTION

According to the Centers for Disease Control and Prevention, every year approximately 719,000 total knee and 332,00 total hip replacement surgeries are performed in the United States. It is estimated that 7% of these procedures are revision surgeries.[23] Prosthetic joint infection (PJI) often results in failure and significant morbidity for patients. The use of antibiotics and other improvements have resulted in significant reduction of PJI in the past decades.

It has been noted that bacteremia from various sources, including oral cavity, can result in bacterial seeding of joint implants and ultimately cause infection in the early postoperative period and potentially many years after the surgery.[24] The most vulnerable period for damage to joint implants caused by bacteremia is the first 2 years after insertion.[25] PJI can occur in three time periods[26,27]:

1. Early: usually occurs within the first 3 months after the placement of joint implant. This is often caused by bacterial seeding during the perioperative period.
2. Delayed: occurs between 3 and 24 months after the placement of the joint implant. This is caused by less virulent organisms seeded during the perioperative period, partially treated previous infection, or bacteremia initiated from an infected distant site.
3. Late: occurs after the first 24 months of the joint implant placement. These are often to hematogenous bacterial seeding of the prosthesis.

The rate of PJI during the first year after the placement of joint implant has been reported to range between 0.58% and 1.6% for knee arthroplasty, and 0.67% and 2.4% for hip arthroplasty.[28–31]

The most common bacterial causes of PJI include coagulase-negative staphylococcus, *Staphylococcus aureus*, mixed bacteria, *Streptococcus* spp, gram-negative rods, *Enterococcus* spp, and anaerobes. Bacteria present in the oral cavity account for 6% to 13% of PJI, and approximately 11% of PJI are culture-negative.[32]

Similar to its relationship with IE, dental procedures have long been considered a source of bacteremia potentially resulting in PJI. However, the analogy between these two conditions is anatomically invalid because of differences between their anatomy, blood supply, microorganisms, and mechanism of infection.[33,34] Although maintenance of good oral health prior, during, and after joint replacement is critical, there has been significant controversy about the impact of bacteremia from dental procedures on PJI in the past few years.

In 2003, the ADA and American Academy of Orthopaedic Surgeons (AAOS) published a set of guidelines in management of patients with joint implants.[35] The 2003 guidelines categorized the use of antibiotic prophylaxis for prevention of PJI based on patients' risk factors and the expected incidence of bacteremia from dental procedures. Based on these guidelines, patients were candidates for antibiotic prophylaxis only within the first 2 years after their joint replacement, and only in the context of invasive dental procedures with higher incidence of bacteremia, such as dental extractions and periodontal procedures.

There is limited available evidence to demonstrate any correlation between immune-compromised patients or those with comorbidities, such as human immunodeficiency virus infection, and increased risk of PJI after dental procedures. However, the 2003 guidelines recommended empirical antibiotic prophylaxis regiment for this patient population when receiving dental procedures with highest risks for bacteremia.

In 2009, AAOS released an information statement recommending the use of antibiotic prophylaxis for any patient at potential increased risk for hematogenous total joint infections.[33] In this document, effectively all patients with prosthetic joint replacement were defined as lifelong candidates for antibiotic prophylaxis before dental procedures. There is little evidence to support the recommendation of this information statement, particularly in the context that no consideration was given to stratify the risk for bacteremia among various dental procedures. Also, the risk of nonprocedural bacteremia, such as during function, was not considered.

In 2012, the AAOS in collaboration with the ADA published a document to define clinical practice guidelines based on the available evidence.[36] This group considered 222 questions in regards to the relationship between dental procedures, bacteremia, and risk of developing PJI. In this report, bacteremia was considered an intermediate outcome and PJI defined as a clinical end point.

The 2012 panel identified significantly variable evidence regarding the correlation between dental procedures and bacteremia. The panel was unable to identify a mean value; however, it reported a median incident rate of bacteremia ranging from 5% for chewing up to 65% for single tooth extraction and gingivectomy. Despite the incidence of bacteremia, this panel was unable to identify any direct evidence to support the association between bacteremia and PJI. The quality of these recommendations ranges from limited, to inconclusive, to consensus.

In 2014 an ADA panel further investigated the available evidence to continue the development of an evidence-based clinical practice guideline on the use of antibiotic prophylaxis in patients with prosthetic joints undergoing dental procedures.[37] This panel elected to focus only on the link between the clinical end point of PJI and dental procedure. The 2012 panel identified only one study providing direct evidence to identify dental procedure as potential risk factor for PJI.[38] The panel identified three additional studies exploring this link.[39–41] These three additional studies failed to show an association between dental procedures and PJI. Based on this and other reviews, the 2014 ADA panel concluded that the evidence has failed to demonstrate the association between dental procedures and PJI or the effectiveness of antibiotic prophylaxis. Therefore, this panel did not recommended antibiotic prophylaxis before dental procedures to prevent PJI. Both the 2012 and 2014 panels identified the need for additional case-controlled studies to provide higher level of certainty of evidence.

ANTIBIOTIC REGIMENT RECOMMENDATION

The choice of the appropriate antibiotics for the purpose of prophylaxis has been not been without its own controversies. Several studies have demonstrated the effectiveness of antibiotics against bacteremia. However, there is no evidence to support the impact of antibiotics on clinical end points, such as IE and PJI. The recommendations for the specific antibiotic regiments have been further complicated by the increasing incidence of bacterial resistance to common antibiotics, such as amoxicillin. In otherwise healthy patients, the viridians group streptococci have shown 32% resistance to penicillin and 41% resistance to erythromycin.[42] Streptococci resistance to azithromycin and clindamycin has been noted in 82% and 71% of the strains, respectively.[43]

The effect of viridans group streptococci resistance on antibiotic prevention of IE is unknown. If resistance is predictive for the lack of clinical efficacy, then the high resistance of the viridans group streptococci further supports the assertion that antibiotic prophylaxis before dental procedures is of little to no value.[2] There are highly active antibiotics against viridans group streptococci, such as vancomycin and fluoroquinolone. However, recommending these antibiotics for routine prophylaxis before dental treatment is impractical, and their impact on prevention of IE or JPE is questionable.

Amoxicillin continues to be the preferred antibiotic in patients with no penicillin allergy because of its superior absorption through the gastrointestinal tract and sustained serum concentration. Cephalosporins have been suggested for patients who are unable to tolerate penicillins or amoxicillin. However, there is no evidence to support the improved effectiveness, therefore preference, of one cephalosporin versus another.

The AAOS/ADA recommendations for antibiotic prophylaxis regimen for prevention of JPI are essentially parallel to those recommended by the AHA. Similarly, the effectiveness of one antibiotic versus another against occurrence of the clinical end point of JPI is not well supported by the available evidence.

SUMMARY

There have been great improvements in patient quality of life over the past decades, in part because of innovations in surgical and medical care. Antibiotics have served a critical role, and arguably revolutionized many aspects of health care. However, their use and overuse have resulted in several public health issues. Also, their risks and side effects have inadvertently and negatively impacted patients' quality of life. Oral microflora and health continues to be an important focus and concern toward the overall health of patients. This relationship cannot be ignored, and meticulous maintenance of good oral health should remain an important path toward good overall health. However, it is important to examine this relationship carefully and objectively when considering clinical end points, such as the incidence of IE and JPI. Based on the current review of evidence by several groups of experts including, but not limited to, the AAOS, ADA, AHA, and National Institute for Health and Care Excellence, the use of antibiotics prophylaxis for the purpose of prevention of IE and JPI is not supported. Although some cohorts of patients may benefit from this practice, there is no need for antibiotic prophylaxis for all patients with a perceived potential risk for IE and JPI. Dental providers should consider more engagement in this dialogue and take an active role in improvement of their patients' quality of life by educating their colleagues and other health care professionals regarding the impact of oral health in relationship to IE, JPI, and other health-related clinical outcomes.

REFERENCES

1. Jones TD, Baumgartner L, Bellows MT, et al, Committee on Prevention of Rheumatic Fever and Bacterial Endocarditis, American Heart Association. Prevention of rheumatic fever and bacterial endocarditis through control of streptococcal infections. Circulation 1955;11:317–20.
2. American College of Cardiology and American Heart Association Task Force on Practice Guidelines. Manual for ACC/AHA guideline writing committees: methodologies and policies from the ACC/AHA Task Force on Practice Guidelines. Available at: http://circ.ahajour-nals.org/manual/. Accessed May 2, 2007.
3. Prendergast BD. The changing face of infective endocarditis. Heart 2006;92: 879–85.
4. Wilson W, Taubert KA, Gewitz M, et al. Prevention of infective endocarditis: guidelines from the American Heart Association. J Am Dent Assoc 2008;139:S11–24.
5. Burnette-Curley D, Wells V, Viscount H, et al. FimA, a major virulence factor associated with *Streptococcus parasanguis* endocarditis. Infect Immun 1995;63: 4669–74.
6. Viscount HB, Munro CL, Burnette-Curley D, et al. Immunization with FimA protects against *Streptococcus parasanguis* endocarditis in rats. Infect Immun 1997;65:994–1002.
7. Kitten T, Munro CL, Wang A, et al. Vaccination with FimA from *Streptococcus parasanguis* protects rats from endocarditis caused by other viridans streptococci. Infect Immun 2002;70:422–5.
8. Durack DT, Beeson PB. Experimental bacterial endocarditis, II: survival of a bacteria in endocardial vegetations. Br J Exp Pathol 1972;53:50–3.
9. Parahitiyawa NB, Jin LJ, Leung WK, et al. Microbiology of odontogenic bacteremia: beyond endocarditis. Clin Microbiol Rev 2009;22(1):46–64.
10. Nanci A, Bosshardt DD. Structure of periodontal tissues in health and disease. Periodontol 2000 2006;40:11–28.
11. Cobe HM. Transitory bacteremia. Oral Surg Oral Med Oral Pathol 1954;7: 609–15.
12. Forner L, Larsen T, Kilian M, et al. Incidence of bacteremia after chewing, tooth brushing and scaling in individuals with periodontal inflammation. J Clin Periodontol 2006;33:401–7.
13. Geerts SO, Nys M, De MP, et al. Systemic release of endotoxins induced by gentle mastication: association with periodontitis severity. J Periodontol 2002; 73:73–8.
14. Daly C, Mitchell D, Grossberg D, et al. Bacteremia caused by periodontal probing. Aust Dent J 1997;42:77–80.
15. Lockhart PB, Brennan MT, Sasser HC, et al. Bacteremia associated with tooth brushing and dental extraction. Circulation 2008;117(24):3118–25.
16. Van der Meer JT, Van Wijk W, Thompson J, et al. Efficacy of antibiotic prophylaxis for prevention of native-valve endocarditis. Lancet 1992;339:135–9.
17. Lacassin F, Hoen B, Leport C, et al. Procedures associated with infective endocarditis in adults. A case control study. Eur Heart J 1995;16:1968–74.
18. Strom BL, Abrutyn E, Berlin JA, et al. Dental and cardiac risk factors for infective endocarditis. A population-based, case-control study. Ann Intern Med 1998;129: 761–9.

19. Duval X, Alla F, Hoen B, et al. Estimated risk of endocarditis in adults with predisposing cardiac conditions undergoing dental procedures with or without antibiotic prophylaxis. Clin Infect Dis 2006;42:e102–7.

20. Ahlstedt S. Penicillin allergy: can the incidence be reduced? Allergy 1984;39: 151–64.

21. Pharmaceuticals in Drinking Water. World Health Organization Report. 2011.

22. Harrison JL, Hoen B, Prendergast BD. Antibiotic prophylaxis for infective endocarditis. Lancet 2008;371:1317–9. Available at: www.thelancet.com.

23. Number of Patients, Number of Procedures, Average Patient Age, Average Length of Stay - National Hospital Discharge Survey 1998-2005. U.S. Department of Health and Human Services; Centers for Disease Control and Prevention; National Center for Health Statistics.

24. Rubin R, Salvati EA, Lewis R. Infected total hip replacement after dental procedures. Oral Surg 1976;41:13–23.

25. Hansen AD, Osmon DR, Nelson CL. Prevention of deep prosthetic joint infection. J Bone Joint Surg Am 1996;78-A(3):458–71.

26. Young H, Hirsh J, Hammerberg EM, et al. Dental disease and periprosthetic joint infection. J Bone Joint Surg Am 2014;96(2):162–8.

27. Zimmerli W. Infection and musculoskeletal conditions: prosthetic-joint associated infections. Best Pract Res Clin Rheumatol 2006;20(6):1045–63.

28. Suleiman LI, Ortega G, Ong'uti SK, et al. Does BMI affect perioperative complications following total knee and hip arthroplasty? J Surg Res 2012;174(1):7–11.

29. Edwards JR, Peterson KD, Mu Y, et al. National Healthcare Safety Network (NHSN) report; data summary for 2006 through 2008, issued December 2009. Am J Infect Control 2009;37(10):783–805.

30. Kurtz SM, Ong KL, Lau E, et al. Prosthetic joint infection risk after TKA in the Medicare population. Clin Orthop Relat Res 2010;468(1):52–6.

31. Ong KL, Kurtz SM, Lau E, et al. Prosthetic joint infection risk after total hip arthroplasty in the Medicare population. J Arthroplasty 2009;24(6 Suppl):105–9.

32. Zimmerli W, Trampuz A, Ochsner PE. Prosthetic-joint infections. N Engl J Med 2004;351(16):1645–54.

33. Antibiotic Prophylaxis for Patients after Total Joint Replacement. Information Statement from the American Academy of Orthopapedic Surgeons. 2009.

34. McGowan DA. Dentistry and endocarditis. Br Dent J 1990;169:69.

35. American Dental Association, American Academy of Orthopedic Surgeons. Antibiotic prophylaxis for dental patients with total joint replacements. J Am Dent Assoc 2003;134(7):895–9.

36. Prevention of orthopaedic implant infection in patients undergoing dental procedures-evidence based guideline and evidence report. American Academy of Orthopedic Surgeons/American Dental Association. 2012.

37. Sollecito TP, Abt E, Lockhart PB, et al. The use of prophylactic antibiotics prior to dental procedures in patients with prosthetic joints: evidence-based clinical practice guideline for dental practitioners. A report of the American Dental Association Council on Scientific Affairs. J Am Dent Assoc 2015;146: 11–6.

38. Berbari EF, Osmon DR, Carr A, et al. Dental procedures as risk factors for prosthetic hip or knee infection: a hospital-based prospective case control study. Clin Infect Dis 2010;50(1):816 [erratum appears in Clin Infect Dis 2010;50(6): 944].

39. Jacobson JJ, Millard HD, Plezia R, et al. Dental treatment and late prosthetic joint infections. Oral Surg Oral Med Oral Pathol 1986;61(4):413–7.

40. Skaar DD, O'Connor H, Hodges JS, et al. Dental procedures and subsequent prosthetic joint infections: findings from the Medicare Current Beneficiary Survey. JADA 2011;142(12):1343–51.

41. Swan J, Dowsey M, Babazadeh S, et al. Significance of sentinel infective events in haematogenous prosthetic knee infections. ANZ J Surg 2011;81(1–2):40–5.

42. Diekema DJ, Beach ML, Pfaller MA, et al, SENTRY Participants Group. Antimicrobial resistance in viridans group streptococci among patients with and without the diagnosis of cancer in the USA, Canada and Latin America. Clin Microbiol Infect 2001;7:152–7.

43. King A, Bathgate T, Phillips I. Erythromycin susceptibility of viridans streptococci from the normal throat flora of patients treated with azithromycin or clarithromycin. Clin Microbiol Infect 2002;8:85–92.

Medication Management of Jaw Lesions for Dental Patients

Orrett E. Ogle, DDS[a,b,*], Arvind Babu Rajendra Santosh, MDS[c]

KEYWORDS

- Inralesional injections • Jaw lesions • Sclerosing agent • Giant cell lesion

KEY POINTS

- Most pathologic lesions of the jaws or of oral mucosa are treated successfully by surgical interventions.
- For treatment of the central giant cell lesion, aneurysmal bone cysts (ABC), histiocytosis of the mandible, hemangioma, odontogenic keratocyst, Paget disease, oral submucous fibrosis (OSF), and oral lichen planus (OLP), medical management consisting of intralesional injections, sclerosing agents, and systemic bisphosphonates is as successful as surgical procedures with fewer complications.
- Medication management of jaw lesions involves the use of pharmacologic agents to modify, slow, or eradicate a pathologic process that is affecting the jaw.

Medication management of jaw lesions involves the use of pharmacologic agents to modify, slow, or eradicate a pathologic process that is affecting the jaw. For a majority of pathologic lesions seen in the jaws, surgical procedures are indicated and are curative. For large lesions, however, surgical procedures may have poor neurologic, functional, or esthetic results. Several alternative nonsurgical therapies, such as intralesional injections, the use of sclerosing agents, and bisphosphonates, have been described for the management of certain intrabony or mucosal diseases. This article discusses the treatment of jaw lesions that are amenable to localized drug treatment and the pharmacology of the agents used most frequently used (**Table 1**). Drugs that require systemic administration are only briefly presented. For completion, a few soft tissue lesions are also discussed.

The authors have nothing to disclose.

[a] Mona Dental Program, Faculty of Medical Sciences, University of the West Indies, Kingston, Jamaica; [b] Oral and Maxillofacial Surgery, Woodhull Medical Center, Brooklyn, NY, USA; [c] Mona Dental Program, Faculty of Medical Sciences, University of the West Indies, Mona, Kingston 7, Jamaica
* Corresponding author. 4974 Golf Valley Court, Douglasville, GA 30135.
E-mail address: oeogle@aol.com

Table 1
Diseases amenable to treatment by intralesional injection and agents used

Disease	Agents Used
Central giant cell lesion	Corticosteroids, calcitonin, interferon alfa, bisphosphonates
ABCs	Ethibloc, calcitonin, aqueous calcium sulfate.
Histiocytosis of the mandible	Corticosteroids
Low-flow VM	Absolute ethanol, sodium morrhuate, sodium tetradecyl sulfate, ethanolamine oleate
Hemangioma	Corticosteroids, bleomycin, sodium morrhuate
Odontogenic keratocyst	Carnoy solution
Paget disease	Calcitonin, bisphosphonates
OLP	Corticosteroids
OSF	Corticosteroids, interferon gamma

The methods used to treat jaw lesions by pharmaceutical or chemical agents involve

- Intralesional injection
- Topical application
- Systemic administration

INTRALESIONAL INJECTION

Intralesional injection is the direct delivery of medication into the body of the lesion. The purpose is to obtain a high concentration of the drug at the diseased site, with minimal systemic absorption. Intralesional injections are easily performed and are relatively safe. The operator must take into consideration, however, the anatomy of the area. Adjacent nerves should not be compromised and intravascular injections should be avoided.

CENTRAL GIANT CELL LESION

The central giant cell granuloma (CGCG) was classified by the World Health Organization in 2005 as an aggressive idiopathic benign intraosseous lesion that occurs almost exclusively in the jaws. It is most frequently seen in young women (women:-men ratio = 2:1) and typically presents in the second and third decades.[1,2] The lesion is osteolytic and histologically consists of multinucleated giant cells throughout a fibroblastic stroma that are often clustered around areas of hemorrhage.[3] Surgery (ranging from aggressive curettage to peripheral ostectomy to en bloc resection) is the most common treatment, but because of a high recurrence rate, alternative medical treatments have been introduced. The most widely used agents are corticosteroids, calcitonin, and interferon alfa. Both steroids and calcitonin affect the giant cells rather than the stromal cells, even though it may be the stromal cells (fibroblasts) that are the etiologic cells of CGCG and the giant cells only secondary or reactive. Glucocorticoid receptors and calcitonin receptors have been identified on both multinucleated giant cells and mononuclear spindle-shaped cells.[4]

Steroids

The rationale for using corticosteroids to treat CGCC was based on its histologic resemblance to sarcoid. Because corticosteroids have been effective in the treatment of sarcoid, it was thought that they may have a similar therapeutic effect on the CGCC.

In addition, corticosteroids may act by suppressing the angiogenic component of the lesion.[5] Steroids seem to inhibit the extracellular production of bone resorption mediating lysosomal proteases in multinucleated giant cells and by inducing apoptosis of osteoclastic cells.[6]

The drugs used are triamcinolone acetonide (10 mg/mL or 40 mg/mL) or triamcinolone hexacetonide (20 mg/mL). The injections are administered weekly or biweekly.

Triamcinolone acetonide

Triamcinolone acetonide is a more potent derivative of triamcinolone. It is a synthetic glucocorticoid corticosteroid with marked anti-inflammatory action and no mineralocorticoid action. Its potency is 5 times that of cortisol. It is packaged as a sterile aqueous suspension suitable for intralesional injection, in doses of 10 mg/mL or 40 mg/mL. It should be injected directly into the jaw lesion.

The general protocol is to start with triamcinolone acetonide, 10 mg/mL, and inject 2 mL of the drug for every 2 cm of radiolucency noted on the standard panoramic jaw radiograph (panorex). The drug is mixed 50/50 with 2% lidocaine, with 1:100,000 epinephrine and injected into the body of the lesion. The site of injection is determined by clinically selecting the site where cortical bone is most expanded and is thinnest and, once inside the lesion, small amounts are injected into different areas. At times, several spots may have to be selected. The injections are repeated weekly for 6 weeks.

Allergic reactions are rare and dose independent. Systemic side effects are not likely to follow these intralesional injections because the doses are confined locally and the actual systemic absorbed dose is small. Intralesional steroids should not be injected at the site of active infection – including the presence of herpes labialis – nor where there is previous history of triamcinolone hypersensitivity. Side effects include pain at the injection site, bleeding, bruising, infection, and impaired wound healing.

Triamcinolone hexacetonide

Triamcinolone hexacetonide (Aristospan [Sandoz Inc., Princeton, NJ]) is the hexacetonide (containing 6 acetonide groups) ester of triamcinolone and is practically insoluble. When injected intralesionally, it is absorbed slowly from the injection site. The pharmacologic action of triamcinolone hexacetonide is less intense but more prolonged. Its activity is due to the slow release of triamcinolone acetonide through hydrolysis. After this reaction, the pharmacology is identical to triamcinolone acetonide. Its use in CGCC is that using triamcinolone hexacetonide, 20 mg/mL, allows for a biweekly interval of injections.[7]

Calcitonin

Similar to the use of steroids, the rationale for using calcitonin to treat CGCC was that its histology appears similar to brown tumor of hyperparathyroidism and only blood calcium levels can distinguish between the two. For this reason, calcitonin— the antagonist for parathormone—was introduced, although parathyroid hormone has never been identified in the CGCG. Calcitonin receptors, however, have been identified on the giant cells of the lesion, antagonizing osteoclastic bone resorption.[8]

Calcitonin takes longer than steroids to affect CGCGs and is, therefore, not suitable for treating patients with aggressive lesions (especially in a younger age group) or those with associated pain or paraesthesia where a quick result would be beneficial.

Calcitonin is commercially available as human calcitonin and salmon calcitonin but salmon calcitonin is the one most widely used. Salmon calcitonin is approximately

50 times more potent than human calcitonin.[9] Its high potency in human is due to its high affinity (40 times that of human calcitonin) for the human calcitonin receptor and its slow rate of clearance.[10] It inhibits osteoclastic bone resorption, altering both the number and/or resorptive activity of osteoclasts, and decreases the rate of bone turnover in conditions with an increased rate of bone resorption and formation, such as active Paget disease and CGCG. The bioavailability of salmon calcitonin is approximately 70% after injection.[11] It is supplied as ready-for-injection ampules of 100 IU, where each ampule of 1 mL contains 100 IU, and as 50 IU, where each ampule of 1 mL contains 50 IU.

Being a polypeptide, calcitonin may give rise in rare cases to localized or generalized hypersensitivity reactions. Antibody formation can limit its effectiveness. Allergic-type reactions, including single cases of anaphylactic shock, have been reported.[11] Side effects are rare and generally mild.

A suggested treatment regimen is 100 IU of calcitonin per day, until it is ascertained radiographically that there is no further resolution of the disease. Radiographically, resolution does not normally commence until 6 to 9 months of treatment, and treatment is continued for up to 24 months to see the maximum resolution.[12]

Interferon

The use of interferon alfa derives its rationale from the hypothesis that the central giant cell lesion is an angiogenic tumor that is characterized by vascular proliferation and bone resorption. Antiangiogenic activity is a known property of interferon alfa. It directly interferes with the ability of endothelial cells to form new capillary blood vessels.[13] Interferon also seems to encourage bone formation, through stimulation of osteoblasts and preosteoblasts, and to inhibit bone resorption.[14]

Interferon alfa is a *biologic response modifier* and is classified as a pleiotropic cytokine. This drug has multiple serious side effects and patients need to be followed closely. Hematocrit, hemoglobin, white blood cell and platelet counts, and liver function tests should be performed every 6 weeks. Side effects include headache, fatigue, diarrhea, upset stomach, loss of appetite, dizziness, xerostomia, dysgeusia, nausea/vomiting, anemia, neutropenia, and thrombocytopenia. Tooth and gum problems may sometimes occur during treatment. Having a dry mouth can worsen the periodontal side effects. Contraindications are hypersensitivity to interferon alfa, autoimmune hepatitis, decompensated liver disease, and pregnancy.

The protocol for using interferon to treat the CGCG is a combination of surgery and medical treatment. After enucleation, interferon alfa-2a or interferon alfa-2b is started on postoperative day 3 at a once-daily dose of 2,000,000 units to 3,000,000 units subcutaneously. The daily doses are continued until the defect seems to be filled in with bone on a panoramic radiograph or on a confirmatory CT scan. The mean duration of treatment was reported to be 7.3 ± 0.8 months.[15]

ANEURYSMAL BONE CYSTS

The ABC is a benign cystic type lesion of bone, composed of blood-filled spaces separated by connective tissue septa containing fibroblasts, osteoclast-type giant cells, and reactive woven bone.[16,17] The lesion, however, is neither an aneurysm nor a cyst. It is characterized by a rapid growth pattern with resultant bony expansion and facial asymmetry. It affects young individuals under 20 years of age, with no gender predilection, and is seen more frequently in the mandible than the maxilla (3:1) with preponderance for the body, ramus, and angle region.[18] ABC can be classified into 3 types: vascular cystic type (95%), a solid noncystic type (5%), and a rare mixed variant that demonstrates features of both the vascular and solid types.

Treatment of ABC is usually the complete surgical removal of the lesion. This may prove difficult at times because the lesions are often multilocular and may be divided by multiple bony septae. In addition to curettage or block resection, pharmaceutical management includes intralesional injection of calcitonin in combination with methyl-prednisolone, intralesional fibrosing Ethibloc (Ethicon), and aqueous calcium sulfate.

Intralesional injection of calcitonin in combination with methylprednisolone requires long-term repeated multiple injections and the response is unpredictable and has not been consistent. Methylprednisolone has an antiangiogenesis and fibroblastic effect whereas calcitonin has an osteoclastic inhibitory effect and promotes trabecular bone formation.

Methylprednisolone

Methylprednisolone sodium succinate (Medrol and Solu-Medrol [Pfizer Inc., NY]) is a synthetic glucocorticoid that is typically used for its anti-inflammatory effects. It is an intermediate-acting steroid that can stay active for 12 to 36 hours. Methylprednisolone at very low doses can inhibited angiogenesis. For the treatment of ABC, 125 mg of methylprednisolone is injected with 200 IU of calcitonin into the center of the lesion. Side effects are rare.

Ethibloc (Ethicon, Norderstedt, Germany) is an emulsion of zein, alcohol, oleum papaveris, propylene glycol, and a contrast medium, which thickens immediately when in contact with aqueous solution. As the alcohol dissolves in blood, zein precip-itates and forms a filler with chewing gum–like consistency. The gelatinous material that is formed is biodegradable. Ethibloc injection is a simple, minimally invasive alter-native procedure for the treatment of ABC and makes open operation unnecessary by stopping the expansion of the cyst and inducing endosteal new bone formation.[19] It is not currently available in the United States but it has been used successfully in Europe and Canada. It is applied as a single injection and basically acts as a fibrosing agent.

Aqueous Calcium Sulfate

Aqueous calcium sulfate (BonePlast [Biomet, Warsaw, Indiana]) is another agent sug-gested for the treatment of ABC. The contents of the lesion is first aspirated. It may take a few attempts to aspirate the cavity, but the aspiration should be done until there is no return of aspirant from the cavity. After aspiration is completed, aqueous calcium sulfate is injected into the cavity. The aqueous calcium sulfate completely fills the cystic cavity and solidifies, thus preventing refill. The material is osteoconductive and has been used as a bone graft substitute in bony cavities. The calcium sulfate cement is reportedly absorbed completely within 8 weeks and replaced with new bone.[20] Limited data exist, however, regarding the use of calcium sulfate for the treat-ment of ABC in the jaw.

HISTIOCYTOSIS

Histiocytosis refers to a group of rare disorders of the reticuloendothelial system. Specifically, Langerhans cell disease (LCD), formerly known as histiocytosis X or idio-pathic histiocytosis, is a rare disorder characterized by a proliferation of cells exhibit-ing phenotypic characteristics of Langerhans cells. The term, *Langerhans cell histiocytosis*, comprises 3 morphologically similar lesions: eosinophilic granuloma, Hand-Schüller-Christian syndrome, and Abt-Letterer-Siwe syndrome. The localized

LCH (monostatic or multifocal eosinophilic granuloma) refers to a form of the disease typified by solitary or multiple skeletal lesions without extraskeletal involvement; it commonly affects children and young adults. The disseminated, chronic form, named Hand-Schüller-Christian syndrome, consists of skeletal and extraskeletal lesions with a progressive chronic course and usually affects children older than 3 years. The disseminated, acute, or subacute form, named Abt-Letterer-Siwe syndrome, refers to the form of the disease that is most often fatal because of the extensive skeletal and extraskeletal lesions; this form usually affects infants and children younger than 3 years.[21] The skull, mandible, ribs, vertebrae, and long bones are often involved.[22] Typically, Langerhans cell histiocytosis that affects many body systems occurs in children younger than 2, whereas single-site disease occur in people of any age and is the type dentists encounter. The disease peaks in the first 3 decades and boys and men are affected twice as often as girls and women.

The most common oral findings are localized pain and swelling, mucosal ulceration, gingival necrosis, and destruction of alveolar bone with tooth mobility and exfoliation. Many lesions, however, remain asymptomatic and are discovered accidentally during routine dental radiological examination. Radiologically, the lesions are localized radiolucencies with no sclerosis or reactive borders. With severe alveolar bone resorption there is an appearance of teeth floating in space.

Treatment options for LCD of the jaws are surgery (curettage), radiotherapy, chemotherapy, and intralesional injection of corticosteroids. Surgical curettage is the principal treatment modality, but its success is dependent on the extent and accessibility of the lesion. Extensive or radical surgery leading to loss of function and disfigurement is contraindicated. Local injection of corticosteroids is an effective treatment in localized disease. In children with mandibular LCD, 1 dose of methylprednisolone succinate injection has proved adequate.[23] Prednisone and triamcinolone acetonide have also been used.

Steroids

It is postulated that a transient immune dysfunction stimulates the cytokine-mediated proliferation of pathologic Langerhans cells within the hematopoietic marrow of the bone. Stimulated histiocytes (monocytes/macrophages) are a source of mediators, such as tumor necrosis factor α, interleukin 1, and prostaglandin E2, which can cause osteolysis.[24,25] Corticosteroids have the ability to inhibit the production of such mediators.[24,25] Glucocorticoids inhibit monocyte/macrophage tumor necrosis factor α and interleukin 1p production at the transcriptional and post-transcriptional levels[26] whereas the suppression of the production of prostanoids occurs by blocking phospholipase A2 activity.[27] The injected steroid also serves to inhibit additional inflammatory cells and impede fibrosis, which produces better bone formation.

Methylprednisolone

Intralesional injections of 165 mg[28] to 200 mg[29] of methylprednisolone to mandibular lesion in which complete resolution was achieved have been reported. Complete resolution of the lesion reportedly occurs in 8 to 17 months after a single injection of methylprednisolone.[30]

LOW-FLOW VASCULAR MALFORMATION

A vascular malformation (VM) is congenital abnormal links between blood vessels, which tends to grow as a child grows. (VM should not be confused with hemangioma, which is a tumor. The hemangioma is not present at birth.) Low-flow VMs are abnormal connections between veins and exhibit a low flow rate because they are postcapillary lesions and have no arteriovenous shunts. These venous anomalies usually expand because of hormonal changes such as puberty and, therefore, are often not noted until a child reaches adolescence.

In the oral cavity, VM can present at any site but most commonly on the anterior two-thirds of tongue, leading to macroglossia and difficulty in mastication, speech, and deglutition. Other sites that may be involved are palate, gingiva, and buccal mucosa.[31] Oral vascular lesions are of clinical importance to the dentist because they pose serious bleeding risk, which may be induced during normal dental procedures, such as orthodontics, periodontics, or oral surgery.[32] Arteriovenous malformations of the jaws are high-flow lesions and are rare. Their importance lies in their potential to result in extensive life-threatening blood loss, most often after tooth extraction, with the dentist unaware of the existence of the arteriovenous malformations.

The most frequently used treatment of a VM is the injection of an agent to induce inflammation and obliteration of the veins. For small mucosal lesions, local injection is often effective. Intralesional sclerotherapy using liquid sclerosing agents produces good outcomes in smaller lesions.

Agents used are

- Alcohol
- Sodium morrhuate
- Sodium tetradecyl sulfate
- Ethanolamine oleate
- Polidocanol
- Corticosteroid

The agents are injected directly into the middle of the affected area.

HEMANGIOMA

Hemangiomas are benign tumors of infancy that display a rapid growth phase with endothelial cell proliferation and involution phases. They are not present at birth but manifest within the first few months of life. Oral hemangiomas are rare but have been reported to occur in regions of the gingiva, palatal mucosa, lips, jawbone (usually maxilla), and salivary gland.[33]

Treatment options includes surgical excision, intralesional injections, interferon α-2b, radiation, electrocoagulation, cryosurgery, laser therapy, and embolization.[33] The choice of treatment depends on the age of the patient, the size and extent of the lesion, and its clinical characteristics. Superficial lesions that are not an esthetic problem and are not subject to masticatory trauma should be left alone. Most oral lesions tend to be small and can be easily treated by surgical excision. Deeper lesions may pose a risk of severe bleeding, whereas lesions of the lip, if excised, may result in unfavorable esthetics. Intralesional pharmaceutical management includes corticosteroids, bleomycin, hypertonic saline, sodium morrhuate, or psylliate.

Triamcinolone Acetonide

The intralesional injection of triamcinolone is accompanied by a significant increase in mast cell density, reduced transcription of cytokines, and an enhanced expression of the mitochondrial cytochrome b gene, resulting in vasoconstriction and inhibition of angiogenic signals.[34] For the treatment of proliferative hemangioma (<3 cm in diameter) intralesional injection of triamcinolone in 1 mg/kg to 3 mg/kg of body weight is administered and followed every 4 to 6 weeks. Side effects are rare and generally mild.[35]

Bleomycin

Bleomycin is a glycopeptide antitumor antibiotic and antiviral drug, and whose mechanism of action is (1) DNA cleavage via oxidative damage caused by free radicals, which form when its metal binding core is oxidized; (2) induces apoptosis in cells that exhibit rapid growth; and (3) a sclerosing effect on vascular endothelium.[36] The rationale for using bleomycin is based specifically on its high sclerosing effect on vascular endothelium.

A dose of 1 mg to 15 mg (based on the size of the lesion) of bleomycin is injected intralesionally per session.[37] The interval between each session should fall between 3 and 4 weeks.

Sodium Morrhuate

Sodium morrhuate is a mixture of the sodium salts of the saturated and unsaturated fatty acids of cod liver oil. Sodium morrhuate stimulates thrombus formation in the injected area by triggering inflammatory events at the tunica intima layer of a vessel. The newly formed thrombus obliterates the vessel and subsequent fibrosis is the result. The endothelial cells within the hemangioma undergo apoptotic death initiated through mitochondrial apoptotic pathway after exposure to sodium morrhuate. The 5% sodium morrhuate solution contains morrhuate sodium, 50 mg; benzyl alcohol 2%; and pH adjusted to approximately 9.5 with hydrochloric acid and/or sodium hydroxide. It is used primarily for cavernous hemangioma.

ORAL LICHEN PLANUS

Lichen planus is chronic mucocutaneous disease that predominantly affects skin and is often observed in oral mucosa. Treatment of lichen planus varies with the clinical form, but the primary goal is to eliminate painful, erythematous, erosive, or bullous lesions. No treatment is indicated in the absence of pain or other subjective symptoms.

Systemic corticosteroids have been the mainstay of management of oral lichen planus (OLP). Topical corticosteroid is reported to be an acceptable approach of localized symptomatic treatment of OLP. This includes 0.05% fluocinonide, 0.05% clobetasol, 0.05% betamethasone, or 0.1% triamcinolone. Topical application of 0.1% triamcinolone in treatment of OLP is reported as an effective drug in managing the symptomatic patients.[38] The greatest disadvantage in using topical corticosteroids is their lack of adherence to the mucosa for a sufficient length of time.

Intralesional injections of corticosteroid in OLP is reported to diminish the oral lesions. The intralesional injection of 5 mg per mL to 10 mg per mL of triamcinolone acetonide (Kenalog [Bristol-Myers Squibb Company, Princeton, NJ]) has been shown an acceptable treatment.[39]

ODONTOGENIC KERATOCYST

Odontogenic keratocyst has been reclassified as a neoplastic condition, designated as keratocystic odontogenic tumor by the World Health Organization in 2005 and defined as a benign unicystic or multicystic intraosseous tumor of odontogenic origin, with a characteristic lining of parakeratinized stratified squamous epithelium and potential for aggressive infiltrative behavior.[40] It is frequently seen in young men and typically presents in the second and third decades. The lesion is exceedingly rare in individuals under age 10 years with gradual decline in incidence above 30 years.[41,42]

Surgical procedures, such as marsupialization, enucleation, and curettage, had been the most traditional methods of treatment; however, due to high recurrence and neoplastic potential of the condition peripheral ostectomy or chemical fixation with Carnoy solution have been used. Intralesional management of keratocystic odontogenic tumor include Carnoy solution and cryotherapy as adjunctive therapy.[43]

Carnoy Solution

Carnoy solution is a nuclear fixative chemical agent that is used in histologic technique. The Carnoy solution is prepared by the mixture of 24 mL ethanol (60%), 12 mL chloroform (30%), 4 mL glacial acetic acid (10%), and 1 g ferric chloride. Theoretically, this solution helps in nuclear fixation of remnants of the dental lamina, cystic epithelium, and daughter or satellite cystic epithelial structures and favors in reduction of recurrence potential.[44] Five minutes' application of Carnoy solution penetrates the bone to a depth of 1.5 mm without injuring the neurovascular structures. Precaution must be taken, however, with lesions that extend near the inferior alveolar canal or to the inferior border of the mandible. Direct contact of the solution over the nerve is not recommended. The presence of daughter cyst, satellite cyst, and remnants of cystic epithelium is usually adjacent to the main lesion and they are reported to be the 3 most common causes for recurrence of the lesions. It is likely that fixation of 5 minutes and a depth of 2 mm to 3 mm are adequate for intralesional management. Reports have suggested that the use of Carnoy solution facilitates easier removal of the cystic lining and enhances visual identification of soft tissue cystic remnants.[45,46]

Modified Carnoy solution
  Ferric chloride—1 g
  Glacial acetic acid—1 mL
  Absolute alcohol—6 mL
  Carnoy solution containing chloroform has carcinogenic activities.

Liquid Nitrogen

Liquid nitrogen, not a typically a pharmaceutical agent, is used in the intralesional management of keratocystic odontogenic tumor with the indications similar to those discussed with Carnoy solution. Liquid nitrogen produces osseous necrosis while maintaining the inorganic framework. The cellular lysis is promoted by intracellular and extracellular damage by osmotic disturbance and electrolyte imbalance and it usually occurs at temperatures below −20°C. For the intralesional management of keratocystic odontogenic tumor, a single minute of liquid nitrogen (below −20°C) penetrates 1 mm to 3 mm of osseous tissue and produces bone necrosis of the same depth. Liquid nitrogen use may damage the surrounding structures and immediate osseous grafting is recommended in the surgical defects that are greater than 4 cm, which reduces the complications of wound dehiscence and pathologic fractures.[47,48]

ORAL SUBMUCOUS FIBROSIS

OSF is a chronic, progressive precancerous condition of the oral cavity and oropharynx due to the chronic placement of the betel quid or paan in the mouth and is frequently reported in Indian and Southeast Asian individuals. OSF is characterized by mucosal rigidity, reduced mouth opening, and burning sensation of oral cavity.[49]

Moderate to severe OSF is irreversible. Medical treatment is symptomatic and predominantly aimed at improving jaw opening. The treatment of OSF consists of intralesional injections of corticosteroid or interferon gamma and nutritional supplementation of lycopene, 16 mg daily. For mild cases, 0.5 mL of hyaluronidase, 1500 IU (fibrinolytic and modifies permeability of connective tissue), can be used. The combination of steroids and topical hyaluronidase shows better long-term results than either agent used alone. Hydrocortisone acetate (corticosteroid and relieves inflammation), 25 mg/mL, is injected intralesionally at multiple site once a week. The intralesional injections can be given for 12 weeks. For patients with reduced mouth opening and mucosal burning, intralesional injection of interferon gamma, 0.01 U/mL to 10.0 U/mL, is administrated weekly for a maximum of 12 weeks.[50,51] Interferon gamma is a known antifibrotic cytokine and has an immunoregulatory effect. Interferon gamma, through its effect of altering collagen synthesis, reduces/slows the fibrosis process.

PAGET DISEASE

Paget disease is a condition characterized by abnormal and anarchic resorption and deposition of bone, resulting in distortion and weakening of the affected bone. It usually affects middle-aged individuals older than 45 years with male predilection, and whites are more frequently affected. The disease may be monostotic or polyostotic. Of the jaw bones, the maxilla is most commonly involved.

Treatment is not indicated in patients with limited jaw involvement and who are asymptomatic. Symptomatic patients (bone pain) are usually treated symptomatically with nonsteroidal anti-inflammatory drugs. The pharmaceutical management of antiresorptive therapy is strongly recommended for patients with more severe bone pain. Calcitonin, bisphosphonate, alendronate, and risedronate are the routinely used drugs in the management of Paget disease.[52]

Calcitonin

Calcitonin is one of the traditional drugs in the management of Paget disease individuals. The rationale for using calcitonin is to inhibit the osteolytic mechanism in the disease process. Intralesional administration of calcitonin (dose and delivery) is similar with CGCC management. In the recent treatment modality, however, the calcitonin is replaced greatly by bisphosphonate therapy.[53]

SUMMARY

Most pathologic lesions of the jaws or of oral mucosa are treated successfully by surgical interventions. For certain lesions, several conservative nonsurgical therapies have been shown as successful as surgical procedures, with fewer complications. For the treatment of these select intrabony or mucosal diseases, medical management, consisting of intralesional injections, sclerosing agents, and systemic bisphosphonates, have been successful. The addition of pharmaceutical methods of treating larger lesions for which surgical procedures may have poor neurologic, functional or esthetic outcomes, or where surgical training is deficient, is a valuable tool for dental practitioners.

REFERENCES

1. Nicolai G, Lorè B, Mariani G, et al. Central giant cell granuloma of the jaws. J Craniofac Surg 2010;21(2):383–6.
2. World Health Organization IARC Screening Group: WHO histological classification of odontogenic tumours. Bone-related lesions. Central giant cell lesion

(granuloma). 9262/0. Available at: http://screening.iarc.fr/atlasoralclassifwho2. php. Accessed May, 2015.

3. de Lange J, van den Akker HP, van den Berg H. Central giant cell granuloma of the jaw: a review of the literature with emphasis on therapy options. Oral Surg Oral Med Oral Pathol Oral Radiol Endod 2007;104(5):603–15.

4. Vered M, Buchner A, Dayan D. Immunohistochemical expression of glucocorticoid and calcitonin receptors as a tool for selecting therapeutic approach in central giant cell granuloma of the jawbones. Int J Oral Maxillofac Surg 2006;35:756–60.

5. Ferretti C, Muthray E. Management of central giant cell granuloma of mandible using intralesional corticosteroids: case report and review of literature. J Oral Maxillofac Surg 2011;69(11):2824–9.

6. Vered M, Buchner A, Dayan D. Central giant cell granuloma of the jawbones – new insights into molecular biology with clinical implications on treatment approaches. Histol Histopathol 2008;23(9):1151–60.

7. Nogueira RL, Teixeira RC, Cavalcante RB, et al. Intralesional injection of triamcinolone hexacetonide as an alternative treatment for central giant-cell granuloma in 21cases. Int J Oral Maxillofac Surg 2010;39:1204–10.

8. Penfold CN, Evans BT. Giant cell lesions complicating Paget's disease of bone and their response to calcitonin therapy. Br J Oral Maxillofac Surg 1993;31(4):267.

9. Banga AK. Transdermal delivery of peptides and proteins. Chapter 8.5.5. In: Banga AK, editor. Transdermal and intradermal delivery of therapeutic agents: application of physical technologies. Boca Raton (FL): Taylor and Francis Group; 2011. p. 208.

10. Rosen HN. Calcitonin in the prevention and treatment ot osteoporosis. Up to Date. Available at: http://www.uptodate.com/contents/calcitonin-in-the-prevention-and-treatment-of-osteoporosis. Accessed May, 2015.

11. Miacalcic. Drug information. Sponsored by NOVARTIS Pharmaceuticals.

12. Pogrel MA. The diagnosis and management of giant cell lesions of the jaws. Ann Maxillofac Surg 2012;2(2):102–6.

13. Folkman J, Ingber D. Inhibition of angiogenesis. Semin Cancer Biol 1992;3(2): 89–96.

14. Abukawa H, Kaban LB, Williams WB, et al. Effect of interferon-Alpha-2b on porcine mesenchymal stem cells. J Oral Maxillofac Surg 2006;64(8):1214–20.

15. Chatta MR, Ali K, Aslam A, et al. Curent concepts in central giant cell granuloma. Pakistan Oral & Dent Jr 2006;26(1):71–88.

16. Rosenberg AE, Nielsen GP, Fletcher JA. World Health Organisation classification of tumours. Pathology and genetics of tumours of soft tissues and bone. Lyon (France): IARC Press; 2002. p. 338.

17. Devi P, Thimmarasa VB, Mehrotra V, et al. Aneurysmal bone cyst of the mandible: a case report and review of literature. J Oral Maxillofac Pathol 2011;15(1):105–8.

18. Kiattavorncharoen S, Joos U, Brinkschmidt C, et al. Aneurysmal bone cyst of the mandible: a case report. Int J Oral Maxillofac Surg 2003;32:419–22.

19. George H, Unnikrishnan PN, Garg NK, et al. Long-term follow-up of Ethibloc injection in aneurysmal bone cysts. J Pediatr Orthop B 2009;18(6):375–80.

20. Clayer M. Injectable form of calcium sulphate as treatment of aneurysmal bone cysts. ANZ J Surg 2008;78(5):366–70.

21. Can JH, Kurt A, Özer E, et al. Mandibular manifestation of Langerhans cell histiocytosis in children. Oral Oncol 2005;41(8):174–7.

22. Stewart JCB. Benign nonodontogenic tumors. Chapter 12. In: Regezi JA, Sciubba JJ, Jordan RCK, editors. Oral pathology-clinical pathological correlations. 6th edition. St Louis (MO): Elsevier/Saunders; 2012. p. 307.

23. Esen A, Dolanmaz D, Kalayci A, et al. Treatment of localized Langerhans' cell histiocytosis of the mandible with intralesional steroid injection: report of a case. Oral Surg Oral Med Oral Pathol Oral Radiol Endod 2010;109(2):e53–8.

24. Hart PH, Vitti GF, Burgess DR, et al. Potential antiinflammatory effects of interleukin 4: suppression of human monocyte tumor necrosis factor alpha, interleukin 1, and prostaglandin E2. Proc Natl Acad Sci USA 1989;86:3803–7.

25. Harris GJ, Woo KI. Eosinophilic granuloma of the orbit: a paradox of aggressive destruction responsive to minimal intervention. Trans Am Ophthalmol Soc 2003; 101:93–105.

26. Beutler B, Krochin N, Milsark IW, et al. Control of cachectin (tumor necrosis factor) synthesis: mechanisms of endotoxin resistance. Science 1986;232(4753): 977–80.

27. Flower RJ, Blackwell GJ. Anti-inflammatory steroids induce biosynthesis of a phospholipase A2 inhibitor which prevents prostaglandin generation. Nature 1979;278(5703):456–9.

28. Jones LR, Toth BB, Cangir A. Treatment for solitary eosinophilic granuloma of the mandible by steroid injection: report of a case. J Oral Maxillofac Surg 1989;47: 306–9.

29. Moralis A, Kunkel M, Kleinsasser N, et al. Intralesional corticosteroid therapy for mandibular langerhans cell histiocytosis preserving the intralesional tooth germ. Oral Maxillofac Surg 2008;12:105–11.

30. Esen A, Işık K, Dolanmaz D. Treatment of mouth and jaw diseases with intralesional steroid injection. World J Stomatol 2015;4(2):87–95.

31. Shatty DC, Urs AB, Rai HC, et al. Case series on vascular malformation and their review with regard to terminology and categorization. Contemp Clin Dent 2010; 4(1):259–62.

32. Patel A, Davies SJ, Sandler PJ. The potentially fatal vascular anomaly and orthodontic treatment–a case report. Dent Update 2004;31(4):230–6.

33. Dilsiz A, Aydin T, Gursan N. Capillary hemangioma as a rare benign tumor of the oral cavity: a case report. Cases J 2009;2:8622. Available at: http://www.ncbi.nlm. nih.gov/pmc/articles/PMC2827094/. Accessed June, 2015.

34. Hasan Q, Tan ST, Gush J, et al. Steroid therapy of a proliferating hemangioma: histochemical and molecular changes. Pediatrics 2000;105(1 Pt 1):117–20.

35. Couto JA, Greene AK. Management of problematic infantile hemangioma using intralesional triamcinolone: efficacy and safety in 100 infants. J Plast Reconstr Aesthet Surg 2014;67(11):1469–74.

36. Smit DP, Meyer D. Intralesional bleomycin for the treatment of periocular capillary hemangiomas. Indian J Ophthalmol 2012;60(4):326–8.

37. Hassan Y, Osman AK, Altyeb A. Noninvasive management of hemangioma and vascular malformation using intralesional bleomycin injection. Ann Plast Surg 2013;70(1):70–3.

38. Usatine RP, Tinitigan M. Diagnosis and treatment of lichen planus. Am Fam Physician 2011;84(1):53–60.

39. Lee YC, Shin SY, Kim SW, et al. Intralesional injection versus mouth rinse of triamcinolone acetonide in oral lichen planus: a randomized controlled study. Otolaryngol Head Neck Surg 2013;148(3):443–9.

40. Barnes L, Eveson JW, Reichart P, et al, editors. Pathology and genetics of head and neck tumours. Lyon (France): IARC Press; 2005. WHO classification of tumours series.

41. Brannon RB. The odontogenic keratocyst: a clinicopathological study of 312 cases-Part 1: clinical features. Oral Surg Oral Med Oral Pathol 1976;42:54–71.

42. Meara JG, Shah S, Li KK, et al. The odontogenic keratocyst: a 20-year clinico-pathologic review. Laryngoscope 1998;108(2):280–3.
43. Madras J, Lapointe H. Keratocystic odontogenic tumor: reclassification of the odon-togenic keratocyst from cyst to tumor. J Can Dent Assoc 2008;74(2). 165–165h.
44. Dashow JE, McHugh JB, Braun TM, et al. Significantly decreased recurrence rates in keratocystic odontogenic tumor with simple enucleation and curettage using carnoy's versus modified carnoy's solution. J Oral Maxillofac Surg 2015; 73(11):2132–5. Available at: http://www.unboundmedicine.com/medline/ citation/26044601/Significantly_Decreased_Recurrence_Rates_in_Keratocystic_ Odontogenic_Tumor_With_Simple_Enucleation_and_Curettage_Using_Carnoy's_ Versus_Modified_Carnoy's_Solution_. Accessed June, 2015.
45. Morgan TA, Burton CC, Qian F. A retrospective review of treatment of the odonto-genic keratocyst. J Oral Maxillofac Surg 2005;63(5):635–9.
46. Abdullah WA. Surgical treatment of keratocystic odontogenic tumour: a review article. Saudi Dent J 2011;23(2):61–5.
47. Schmidt BL, Pogrel MA. The use of enucleation and liquid nitrogen cryotherapy in the management of odontogenic keratocysts. J Oral Maxillofac Surg 2001;59(7): 720–5.
48. Schmidt BI. The use of liquid nitrogen cryotherapy in the management of the odontogenic keratocyst. Oral Maxillofac Surg Clin North Am 2003;15(3):393–5.
49. Samuel HB, Renukananda GS. Comparative study between intralesional steroid injection and oral lycopene in the treatment of oral submucous fibrosis. Int J Sci Stud 2015;2(10):20–2.
50. Haque MF, Meghji S, Nazir R, et al. Interferon gamma (IFN-gamma) may reverse oral submucous fibrosis. J Oral Pathol Med 2001;30(1):12–21.
51. Krishnamoorthy B, Khan M. Management of oral submucous fibrosis by two different drug regimens: a comparative study. Dent Res J 2013;10(4):527–32.
52. Singer FR. Clinical efficacy of salmon calcitonin in Paget's disease of bone. Calcif Tissue Int 1991;49(Suppl 2):S7–8.
53. Siris ES, Lyles KW, Singer FR, et al. Medical management of Paget's disease of bone: indications for treatment and review of current therapies. J Bone Miner Res 2006;21(Suppl 2):P94–8.

Antimicrobial Therapy in Management of Odontogenic Infections in General Dentistry

Curtis J. Holmes, DDS[a],*, Robert Pellecchia, DDS[b]

KEYWORDS

- Odontogenic infections • Antimicrobial therapy • Antibiotic therapy • Dental abscess
- Antibiotics • Allergy • Diagnosis and treatment plan

KEY POINTS

- This article focuses on the diagnosis and management of odontogenic infections.
- Current antibiotic regimens are reviewed and discussed including use of alternative antibiotics with patients known to have a penicillin allergy.
- Emphasis is made on proper examination of the patient with use of diagnostic aids to provide the correct treatment of choice.

In the dental office, there are a number of conditions that can be classified as unscheduled dental emergencies ranging from tooth pain, to a fractured or avulsed tooth, to odontogenic infections. For the general dentist management of odontogenic infections can be the most concerning of these office based emergencies owing to the complex microbiology of odontogenic infections and potential for advancement to life-threatening medical emergencies. Odontogenic infections encompass a variety of conditions ranging from localized abscesses to deep space head and neck infections.[1] Deep space infections can carry a high incidence of morbidity and mortality.[2] Because these patients often present to the dental office unexpectedly, it is imperative for the dental professional to have an understanding of treatment and management of such infections. Management of patient with an odontogenic infection is a multifaceted approach involving an examination and assessment of the patient, identifying the source of the infection, anatomic considerations, surgical intervention, administration of the appropriate antimicrobial therapy, and referral to an appropriately trained

[a] Department of Dentistry and Oral and Maxillofacial Surgery, The Brooklyn Hospital Center, Brooklyn, NY, USA; [b] Department of Dentistry and Oral and Maxillofacial Surgery, Geisinger Medical Center, Danville, PA, USA
* Corresponding author. 100 North Academy Avenue, Danville, PA 17821.
E-mail address: dr.cjholmes@gmail.com

Dent Clin N Am 60 (2016) 497–507
http://dx.doi.org/10.1016/j.cden.2015.11.013
0011-8532/16/$ – see front matter © 2016 Elsevier Inc. All rights reserved.

provider if indicated. This article provides a basic understanding of the diagnosis and pharmacologic management of patients with infections that are odontogenic in origin. This article is limited to management in the outpatient setting. It is recommended that providers with desires to manage infections in the inpatient setting to review the literature on therapeutic management of these patients before treatment.

EXAMINATION AND ASSESSMENT

A thorough patient examination is a critical component of treatment of odontogenic infections. Patient evaluation begins with a comprehensive history and physical examination followed by an assessment of the pertinent findings. This is then followed by a diagnosis and development of a treatment plan for patient care. Failure to complete a comprehensive history and examination of the patient can lead to improper treatment and/or delayed treatment of infections, potentially leading to serious complications, including but not limited to airway compromise, mediastinitis, sepsis, and death.[2]

A patient history includes attaining information regarding the symptoms, onset, and duration of the present illness. This information helps to form an understanding of the severity of the patient's infection. Common signs and symptoms that should alert a provider of a developing or established infection include trismus, fever, difficulty swallowing, pain, difficulty breathing, and pain on swallowing.[1–3] The patient's medical history and current medications are key in assessing the patient's ability to fight infection as well as providing insight to potential drug interactions.

The physical examination oftentimes begins before the provider enters the room with the recording of vital signs or on introduction with visual inspection swelling or general appearance and posturing. Airway assessment is a critical component of this examination. It allows for assessment of the necessity for emergent referral. Palpation, percussion, and thorough visual examination of the extraoral and intraoral cavities provide necessary information for identifying the source and location of the infection. Providers should pay close attention size of swelling, tongue position, floor of the mouth swelling or elevation, visual disturbances, voice changes, vestibules, and uvula position. This should be followed by radiographic examination.

After subjective and objective information has been gathered and interpreted an appropriate diagnosis is made, which guides the plan of treatment. This treatment could vary based on the findings present but can involve antibiotic therapy, surgical management, or a combination of both with or without an urgent referral to an oral and maxillofacial surgeon or hospital.

STAGES OF ABSCESS DEVELOPMENT

The source of odontogenic infections is commonly bacteria native to the oral cavity. This bacteria acts on a tooth or the periodontium. In periodontal infections, attachment loss of the gingival fibers and destruction of supportive structures expose the teeth and tissues to bacterial introduction. Periapical infections begin with a carious lesion causing pupal necrosis, which introduces the pulp to microorganisms. This process then proceeds until the bacteria invades the periapical tissues.[1,4] Upon accessing the periapical tissues, the process can remain localized to the bony structures as a cyst, granuloma, or focal osteomyelitis. A second alternate a progressive process may ensue as periapical infection spreads through cortical bone involving cellulitis, and localized and deep space abscess formation.

After inoculation of bacteria into deeper tissues abscess, development progresses through cellulitis to abscess formation without early intervention. Cellulitis is an acute disorder associated with warm, diffuse, painful, indurated swelling of soft tissues that also may present with erythema. Next, the indurated swelling begins to soften as an abscess develops represented by localized area fluctuance. An abscess is collection of purulent material containing necrotic tissue, bacteria, and dead white blood cells. Patients may present at varying stages of the process. Bacteria from a dental infections also has the ability spread hematogenously owing to the high vascularity of head and neck structures, allowing infections to present in distant sites including the orbit, brain, and spine.[1,4]

ANATOMIC CONSIDERATIONS

Odontogenic infections spread from the bony structures through the cortical bone along the path of least resistance, with the affected fascial spaces determined by the structures in proximity to the tooth roots.[5] This necessitates an understanding of fascial spaces and anatomy to effectively diagnose and develop a surgical plan for management of infections. The spaces that are primarily affected by odontogenic infections are located adjacent to the origin. Those spaces are categorized as primary fascial spaces. They include buccal, canine, sublingual, submandibular, submental, and vestibular spaces.

After infection spreads to primary spaces, they can progress to include secondary spaces (**Table 1**). Secondary spaces include pterygomandibular, infratemporal, masseteric, lateral pharyngeal, superficial and deep temporal, masticator, and retropharyngeal.

A basic understanding of the spread of infections into the primary spaces is established by understanding the origin and insertions of the buccinator and mylohyoid muscles in relation to the maxilla and the mandible. The buccinator inserts superiorly into the alveolus of the maxilla and inferiorly in the alveolus of the mandible. An infection that spreads within the constraints of those insertions results in a vestibular abscess and spread of infection above or below these insertions forms a buccal space infection. The mylohyoid muscle's origin is from the mylohyoid line of the mandible. Teeth with root apices below this origin are the mandibular second and third molars. Infectious spread of these teeth through the lingual plate forms submandibular space infections. The roots of the mandibular premolars and first molars lie above the mylohyoid and, therefore, infectious spread lingually associated with these teeth create sublingual space infections. Relations of teeth to primary fascial spaces are provided in **Table 2**. The teeth most frequently identified as the source of an infection are the mandibular molars, followed by the mandibular premolars.[2,3,5]

A special note should be made of an indurated cellulitis involving bilateral submandibular, sublingual, and submental spaces with drooling, tongue displacement, dysphagia, and patient head positioned in the "sniffing" position. This is the classic description of Ludwig's angina. This is a medical emergency in need of definitive

Table 1		
Fascial spaces of odontogenic infections		
Primary	Vestibular	Sublingual
	Buccal	Submandibular
	Canine	Submental
Secondary	Masseteric	Infratemporal
	Masticator	Superficial temporal
	Pterygomandibular	Deep temporal
	Lateral pharyngeal	Retropharyngeal

Table 2		
Relationship of teeth and primary fascial spaces		
Vestibular	Maxillary incisors	Mandibular incisors
	Maxillary canines	Mandibular canines
	Maxillary premolars	Mandibular premolars
	Maxillary molars	Mandibular molars
Buccal	Maxillary premolars	
	Maxillary premolars	
	Maxillary molars	
	Mandibular premolars	
Canine	Maxillary incisors	
	Maxillary canines	
	Maxillary premolars	
Sublingual	Mandibular premolars	
	Mandibular first molars	
Submandibular	Mandibular second	
	Mandibular third molars	
Submental	Mandibular incisors	
	Mandibular canines	

airway management and timely surgical management, and should be referred immediately to the nearest hospital for treatment. Patients with infections associated with maxillary molars may also present with maxillary sinusitis owing to the close proximity of roots apices with the floor of the maxillary sinus. Conversely, patients with maxillary sinusitis may also present with symptoms of an infection, so it is prudent to perform an examination to develop the appropriate diagnosis.

SURGICAL INTERVENTION

Resolution of an odontogenic infection occurs after pharmacotherapy, but it is often studied in combination with surgical treatment.[2,3,6] Surgical invention is believed by many to be the most important aspect of management of odontogenic infection.[1] The goal of surgical intervention is to remove the source of the infection. Eradication of the infection source is performed by tooth extraction, root canal therapy, or incision and drainage with intervention as early in the infectious process as possible. The extent of the general dentists' involvement in treating an odontogenic infection lies in the training and comfort level of the provider. Root canal therapy and tooth extractions are routinely performed by dental professionals; however, these procedures with associated fascial space spread of infection could lead to a decision to refer the patient to a specialist for management of the infection. Many general dentists are trained to manage some primary space infections, but should use their judgment based on subjective and objective findings on examination of the patient to guide the decision to treat or refer immediately. Patients presenting with infections of the secondary fascial spaces should be referred immediately to owing to the sequelae of potential complications of improper treatment, advancement of infection to other fascial spaces, the necessity for extraoral approaches, and potential for surgical or nonsurgical airway management.

Microbiology of an Odontogenic Infection

It has been stated that odontogenic infections arise from bacterial introduction in the deeper tissues of the head and neck. There is vast array of bacterial species all residing contemporaneously in the oral cavity and contribute the normal oral flora. Odontogenic infections are characterized as a combination of aerobic and anaerobic bacteria. This is why they are considered mixed infections. Streptomyces species are often responsible for orofacial cellulitis and abscess. Aerobic bacteria including *Streptococcus viridans*, *Streptococcus milleri* group species, beta-hemolytic strepto-coccus, and coagulase-negative staphylococci have been cultured from odontogenic infections. Within the *S milleri* group, the members *S anginosus*, *S intermedius*, and *S constellatus* are most often associated with cellulitis. Anaerobic bacteria is often isolated from sites with chronic abscess formation. These pathogens include *Peptostreptococcus*, *Prevotella*, *Prophyromonas*, *Fusobacterium*, *Bacteroides*, and *Elkenella*.[1,3,7–10] The most common microorganisms isolated from odontogenic infec-tions has been consistent over the years.[3,8] However, what has changed is the prev-alence, the ability to isolate and the ability to classify them owing to changes in nomenclature.[1,5,11]

Over the years, studies have shown that there has been a change in the antibiotic susceptibility of isolated organisms. Although many strepotococci are still sensitive to penicillin,[1,12] especially those that are prevalent during the first 3 days of clinical symptoms, the gram-negative obligate anaerobes, present abundantly after 3 days, are producing penicillin-resistant strains.[7,13] It has also been found that there is an in-crease in aerobes and anaerobes that are resistant to clindamycin regimens.[1,14] This complicates recommendations for therapeutics for orofacial infections; however, traditionally used empirical antibiotics are excellent options if culture and sensitivity testing are not performed at or before the time of surgery. Nonetheless, providers must not forget about the potential resistant organisms to empirical antibiotics.

ANTIBIOTICS OF CHOICE

Antibiotics are antimicrobials used for the treatment and prevention of infections. They are classified as either bactericidal or bacteriostatic. Bactericidal antibiotics kill bac-teria by inhibiting cell wall synthesis and bacteriostatic antibiotics inhibit bacterial growth and reproductions. **Table 3** lists common antibiotics and their classification. The choice of antimicrobial therapy for patients with an odontogenic infections can be complex owing to numerous variables that must be considered. Factors involved in antibiotic selection include host-specific factors and pharmacologic factors.

Table 3
Bactericidal and bacteriostatic antibiotics

Bactericidal	Bacteriostatic
Beta-lactams	Macrolides
Penicillins	Erythromycin
Cephalosporins	Clarithromycin
Carbapenems	Azithromycin
Monobactams	
Aminoglycosides	Clindamycin
Vancomycin	Tetracyclines
Metronidazole	Sulfa antibiotics
Fluoroquinolones	—

From Flynn TR, Halpern LR. Antibiotic selection in head and neck infections. Oral Maxillofac Surg Clin North Am 2003;15(1):21; with permission.

Host factors include the microbiology of odontogenic infections, history of allergic responses or intolerance, previous antibiotic therapy, age, pregnancy status, and immune system status.[7] Traditional pathogens found to be in association with orofacial infections are mixed in origin and consist of facultative and obligate anaerobic bacteria. The duration of the infectious process aids in deciphering which organisms predominate. Allergy to antibiotics is collected during acquisition of medical history as well as information regarding antibiotic intolerance. Previous antibiotic therapy, especially on a consistent basis, yields a propensity for resistant organisms to an antibiotic. Certain antibiotics should be avoided in children as well as pregnant patients. The immunocompetence of a patient may direct antibiotic therapy toward bactericidal, rather than bacteriostatic, agents.

Pharmacologic factors of interest include spectrum of antibiotics, pharmacokinetics, tissue distribution of antimicrobials, cost of antibiotics, adverse reactions, and potential drug interactions.[7] The antibiotic spectrum is of important consideration, because it is best for the patient to receive therapy to be geared toward antibiotics that are effective against the involved microorganisms. Pharmacokinetically, the effectiveness of such antibiotics depend on serum concentrations needed to kill bacteria or the time necessary to maintain adequate serum levels. Beta-lactams and vancomycin are time dependent, whereas fluoroquinolones are concentration dependent. The ability of an antibiotic to reach the site of an infection should be considered, because abscess cavities are avascular. Thus, antibiotic effectiveness is based on the ability to penetrate an abscess. Adverse reactions and potential drug interactions are discussed elsewhere in this article.

Pathogen-specific antibiotic therapy is driven by results of culture and sensitivity testing. Site cultures are not obtained until surgical intervention has occurred and patients with orofacial infections warrant timely therapeutic management. Empirical antibiotic therapy for odontogenic infections is based on an understanding of common pathogens cultured from infection site. Empiric antibiotics may be difficult to ascertain owing to the complex microbiology of such infections, the timing of antibiotic administration and antibiotic resistance. **Table 4** shows empiric antibiotics of choice for odontogenic infections in the outpatient setting. Penicillin remains the antibiotic of choice in the outpatient setting for the management of odontogenic infections when there is no history of allergy,[1–3,6,7,13] especially in infections of less than 3 days' duration.[3,7] Clindamycin is the antibiotic of choice for patients with an allergy to penicillin.[1–3,6,7,13] This may also be considered for infections of greater than 3 days' duration owing to the increase in penicillin-resistant organisms present at this stage.[7,13] Of the macrolides, azithromycin has fewer drug–drug interactions and is used to treat infections; however, resistance to macrolides has been reported.[13] Cephalosporins have been found to be effective in treatment of orofacial infections,

Table 4	
Empiric antibiotics of choice for odontogenic infections in outpatient setting	
No Penicillin Allergy	**Penicillin Allergy**
Amoxicillin	Clindamycin
Clindamycin	Azithromycin
Azithromycin	Metronidazole
	Moxifloxacin

Adapted from Flynn T. What are the antibiotics of choice for odontogenic infections, and how long should the treatment course last? Oral Maxillofac Surg Clin North Am 2011;23(4):533; with permission.

but there are pathogens that produce cephalosporinases. There also must be consideration for cross-allergy in penicillin-allergic patients. Metronidazole is excellent for obligate anaerobes and studies have shown its effectiveness in the outpatient setting6, however, it is often used in the inpatient setting in combination with other antibiotics.[2,6,7,13] Moxifloxacin, a fourth-generation fluoroquinolone, has a spectrum of coverage including oral aerobes and anaerobes, including *Eikenella corrodens*, which is clindamycin resistant. Moxifloxacin is an excellent antibiotic choice when initial antibiotics and surgery have remained ineffective.

DURATION OF ANTIBIOTICS

A common antibiotic course for orofacial infection is 7 to 10 days. Flynn and colleagues[6] hypothesized that antibiotic therapy for 4 days or less combined with appropriate surgical treatment, results in equal or better clinical outcomes, as measured by time to resolution, morbidity, selections for antibiotic-resistant strains, and expense. In this systematic review, it was found that no clinically significant difference was found at day 7 with antibiotic courses of 7 days or less with appropriately administered surgical treatment. Chardin and colleagues[15] found no difference in clinical cure rate of antibiotic therapy after surgical intervention with amoxicillin 1 g for 3 days versus the same therapy for 7 days. Lewis and colleagues[16] found similar results when comparing surgical intervention followed by 3 g of amoxicillin for 2 doses 8 hours apart with penicillin V 250 mg by mouth 4 times per day for 5 days. These studies support the emphasis on prompt and efficient surgical intervention in combination with antibiotic therapy.

COST OF ANTIBIOTICS

Consideration of the cost of antibiotics is a factor that is often overlooked during treatment of odontogenic infections. The central focus is often resolution of the infectious process with surgical treatment while providing effective and appropriate antibiotic therapy that will reduce the morbidity associated with the infection. Antibiotic cost can be compared based on the cost for a standard prescription for antibiotics of preference in oral formulations. Amoxicillin is one of the least expensive oral formulations of antibiotics. Flynn considered the retail cost for a 1-week prescription that an uninsured patient would pay for antibiotic therapy. He obtained the cost of commonly prescribed antibiotics from a pharmacy chain in the Boston area. Then, he formulated a numeric cost comparison ratio by dividing cost of the commonly prescribed medications the cost of an amoxicillin prescription. This comparison found that the cost of a 150-mg Cleocin prescription is significantly less than the 300-mg prescription with a two 150-mg capsule regimen 4 times a day being 63% of the cost of a 300-mg capsule 4 times a day[6,7] (**Table 5**).

ANTIBIOTIC RESISTANCE

A problem that has emerged regarding the effectiveness of selected antibiotic therapy for the management of odontogenic infections is antibiotic resistance. Antibiotic resistance occurs by 4 mechanisms: alteration of a drug's target site, inability of a drug to reach its target, inactivation of an antimicrobial agent, or active elimination of an antibiotic from the cell.[6,13] Alteration of the target site for an antibiotic occurs by genes allowing bacteria to synthesize peptides that prevent binding diminishing the affinity of the antibiotic. Some bacteria have bypass pathways that utilize alternate metabolic pathways when specific antibiotics are present. Antibiotics may be inactivated by

Table 5
Cost of oral antibiotics used in odontogenic infections

Antibiotic	Usual Dose (mg)	Usual Interval (h)	Wholesale Cost 2010 ($)	1-Week Retail Cost 2010 ($)	Amoxicillin Cost Ratio
Penicillins					
Amoxicillin	500	8	0.37	11.99	1.00
Penicillin V	500	6	0.74	12.29	1.03
Augmentin	875	12	5.05	51.99	4.34
Augmentin XR	2,000	12	7.38	108.99	9.09
Cephalosporins					
Cephalexin	500	6	1.23	15.19	1.27
Erythromycins					
Erythromycin	500	6	0.30	17.99	1.50
Clarithromycin	500	24	5.01	34.69	2.89
Azithromycin	250	12	7.78	120.99	10.09
Antiaerobic					
Clindamycin (generic)	150	6	1.19	31.79	2.65
Clindamycin (2T generic)	300	6	2.38	59.99	5.00
Clindamycin (generic)	300	6	3.76	87.59	7.31
Metronidazole	500	6	0.73	34.49	2.88
Other					
Vancomycin	125	6	29.10	849.99	70.89
Ciprofloxacin	500	12	5.13	13.49	1.13
Moxifloxacin (Alvelox)	400	24	16.35	138.99	11.59

Adapted from Flynn T. What are the antibiotics of choice for odontogenic infections, and how long should the treatment course last? Oral Maxillofac Surg Clin North Am 2011;23(4):531; with permission.

bacterial enzymes or the enzymes can result in neutralization. Penicillinase and beta-lactamases are examples of this mechanism. Genes presents in some bacteria produce proteins that prevent antibiotic uptake or signal for removal of the antibiotic from the cell, leading to antibiotic resistance as well.

The genes necessary to drive antibiotic resistance are acquired through 4 mechanisms: spontaneous mutation, gene transfer, bacteriophages, and mosaic genes.[4,6,13] Spontaneous mutation is considered the dominate source antibiotic resistance. Gene transfer occurs with transmissible DNA segments transfer and inserts genetic material after bacterial conjugation. Bacteriophages are viruses that infect bacteria and replicate to insert genetic material, subsequently hijacking the control of the bacteria's genetic and bacterial metabolism. Mosaic genomes are formed by bacteria incorporating fragmented DNA directly from dead members of related species. Collectively these mechanisms allow the spread of genetic material from 1 bacterial species to another and can result in the resistant strain becoming the predominate strain for the species.[6,13]

Many strides have been made to reduce the prevalence and manage antibiotic resistance. Non-antibiotics attempts mainly apply to the hospital setting. This includes reduction of colonization sites, patient isolation, decreased duration of hospital stay, and aseptic technique during intervention. Antibiotic associated attempts including limiting antibiotic therapy to as narrow of a spectrum as possible to effectively manage the offending bacteria and using a broader spectrum antibiotics only when indicated. Culture and sensitivity testing of purulent exudate aids in identifying susceptibility of bacteria to specific antibiotics. Kuriyama and colleagues[8] examined a relationship between past administration of beta-lactam antibiotics and those patients producing increased amounts of resistant bacteria with odontogenic infections. It is beneficial to the clinician and patient to be diligent in obtaining history of previous odontogenic infections to guide treatment and consideration of possible antibiotic resistance.

COMPLICATIONS OF ANTIBIOTIC THERAPY AND DRUG INTERACTIONS

Antibiotic drugs have the potential to alter the effectiveness of other drugs and interferes with the metabolism of other drugs. The cytochrome p450 system is a complex set of drug-metabolizing enzymes in the liver and gastrointestinal system that breaks down many different drugs. When antibiotics that use this metabolic pathway inhibit cytochromes that are needed for metabolism of other drugs altering, the bioavailability of one of the involved drugs. Some of these interactions can lead to some severe adverse effects.

Providers should be mindful of some of the potential adverse reactions associated with antibiotic therapy and other medications. Erythromycin and other macrolides have been found to have drug interactions with numerous drugs including statins, theophylline, warfarin, carbamazepine, triazolam/midazolam, and antiarrhythmics. Side effects of these interactions range from bleeding issues, increased sedation, confusion, and seizures to cardiac dysrhythmias and death. Metronidazole has the potential for increased bleeding with coadministration of warfarin owing a decrease in the metabolism anticoagulants. Clindamycin may destroy gut flora and prevent absorption of vitamin K, which can cause an increase in anticoagulation. Metronidazole can also affect the renal clearance of lithium and has a disulfiram effect in combination with alcohol. Fluoroquinolones have been found to interfere with theophylline metabolism and to cause seizures. These drugs have also been found to cause spontaneous tendon rupture. Fluoroquinolones should be avoided in children owing to chondrotoxicity in growing cartilage.

Antibiotic allergy information should be obtained while obtaining a patient's medical history. It is important to inquire about the nature of an allergy to access whether a true anaphylactoid allergy exist. Penicillin is a common antibiotic for which patient's report an allergy. 1% to 10% of patients develop an allergic response to penicillin during an initial course and a less than 1% chance of development of an allergic reaction exists with additional courses.[6,17] There is a possibility for cross-allergy to cephalosporins. This occurs in 10% to 15% of patients with an allergy to penicillin and often involves patients with a history of anaphylaxis.

Antibiotic-associated colitis is another possible adverse effect of antimicrobial therapy. *Clostridium difficile* is an enteric anaerobe that produces an exotoxin found in a stool assay of affected patients. Diagnosis of *C difficile* occurs after symptoms of fever, abdominal cramping, 5 or more episodes of diarrhea per day, or positive results in a stool sample. Antibiotic-associated colitis has been found to occur with clindamycin, beta-lactam/beta-lactamase inhibitor combinations, cephalosporins and other antibiotic therapy and is treated with removal of the offending antibiotic and oral metronidazole or vancomycin. If no resolution occurs, these patients should be referred as soon as possible to rule out the potential need for surgical intervention.

A patient who is taking oral contraceptive pills should be informed of the necessity to use other forms of birth control. Antibiotic therapy may kill enough the gut flora that inhibits recirculation of estrogen, which reduces the serum levels of estrogen and may allow for the patient to become pregnant. This has been found to only involve oral contraceptives, not the implantable nor injectable forms.[6,18]

SUMMARY

Odontogenic infections are a class of emergencies that may present in the outpatient setting. Management of such emergencies can occur in dental office; however, there are circumstances that warrant referral for definitive treatment. Clinicians treating orofacial infections should be able to effectively examine and assess patients, have an understanding of common microorganisms associated with an abscess, head and neck anatomy, and development and spread of an abscess. Providers choosing to engage in management should promptly provide treatment of odontogenic infections with a combination approach, involving surgical intervention and antimicrobial therapy. It is important to confirm that the patient does not have any medical condition that necessitates antibiotic prophylaxis before surgical intervention. If so, the provider should refer to the current American Heart Association guidelines for antibiotic prophylaxis regimen.

Antimicrobial therapy is complicated by the mixed flora of an abscess and varied responses of microorganisms to penicillin. Antibiotic therapy selection should be chosen according to safety, cost, consideration for a patient's medical history, effectiveness of antibiotic, and stage in abscess development. The use of clindamycin has increased in dentistry; however, multiple clinical studies comparing clindamycin to penicillin or ampicillin have found clinical success rates of 97% or higher with penicillin.[3] Penicillin continues to be the drug of choice in odontogenic infections, whereas clindamycin is an excellent alternative in patient with penicillin allergy. Seven days of antibiotic therapy has traditionally been effective; however, studies have shown that 3- to 4-day regimens should suffice in healthy patients.[6] Regardless of the empirical antibiotic choice, surgical intervention that removes the source of the infection is considered the primary treatment modality.

REFERENCES

1. Lypka M, Hammoudeh J. Dentoalveolar infections. Oral Maxillofac Surg Clin North Am 2011;23(3):415–24.
2. Sato FR, Hajala FA, Freire Filho FW, et al. Eight-year retrospective study of odontogenic origin infections in a postgraduation program on oral and maxillofacial surgery. J Oral Maxillofac Surg 2009;67:1.
3. Flynn TR, Shanti RM, Levi MH, et al. Severe odontogenic infections, part 1: prospective report. J Oral Maxillofac Surg 2006;64:1093.
4. Levi M. The microbiology of orofacial abscesses and issues in antimicrobial therapy. In: Piecuch JF, editor. Oral and maxillofacial surgery knowledge update 2001. Rosemont (IL): American Association of Oral and Maxillofacial Surgeons; 2001. p. 5–22.
5. Storoe W, Haug RH, Lillich TT. The changing face of odontogenic infections. J Oral Maxillofac Surg 2001;59:739.
6. Flynn T. What are the antibiotics of choice for odontogenic infections, and how long should the treatment course last? Oral Maxillofac Surg Clin North Am 2011;23(4):519–36.
7. Flynn TR, Halpern LR. Antibiotic selection in head and neck infections. Oral Maxillofac Surg Clin North Am 2003;15:17.
8. Kuriyama T, Nakagawa K, Karasawa T, et al. Past administration of b-lactam antibiotics and increase in the emergence of b-lactamase-producing bacteria

in patients with orofacial odontogenic infections. Oral Surg Oral Med Oral Pathol Oral Radiol Endod 2000;89:186–92.

9. Rega AJ, Aziz SR, Ziccardi VB. Microbiology and antibiotic sensitivities of head and neck space infections of odontogenic origin. J Oral Maxillofac Surg 2006; 64:1377–80.

10. Brook I. Microbiology and management of peritonsillar, retropharyngeal, and parapharyngeal abscesses. J Oral Maxillofac Surg 2004;62:1545–50.

11. Haug R. The changing microbiology of maxillofacial infections. Oral Maxillofac Surg Clin North Am 2003;15:1–15.

12. Kuriyama T, Karasawa T, Nakagawa K, et al. Bacteriologic features and antimicrobial susceptibility in isolates from orofacial odontogenic infections. Oral Surg Oral Med Oral Pathol Oral Radiol Endod 2000;90:600–8.

13. Flynn TR. Update on the antibiotic therapy of oral and maxillofacial infections. In: Piecuch JF, editor. Oral and maxillofacial surgery knowledge update 2001. Rosemont (IL): American Association of Oral and Maxillofacial Surgeons; 2001. p. 23–50.

14. Poeschl PW, Spusta L, Russmeuller G, et al. Antibiotic susceptibility and resistance of the odontogenic microbiological spectrum and its clinical impact on severe deep space head and neck infections. Oral Surg Oral Med Oral Pathol Oral Radiol Endod 2010;11:151–6.

15. Chardin H, Yasukawa K, Nouacer N, et al. Reduced susceptibility to amoxicillin of oral streptococci following amoxicillin exposure. J Med Microbiol 2009;58(Pt 8): 1092–7.

16. Lewis MA, McGowan DA, MacFarlane TW. Short course high-dosage amoxicillin in the treatment of acute dento-alveolar abscess. Br Dent J 1986;161(8):299–302.

17. Craig TJ, Mende C. Common allergic and allergic-like reactions to mediations: when the cure becomes the curse. Postgrad Med 1999;105:173–81.

18. Hersh EV. Adverse drug interactions in dental practice: interactions involving antibiotics. Part II. J Am Dent Assoc 1999;130:236–51.

Botulinum Toxin Type A
Review and Its Role in the Dental Office

Jared Miller, DDS*, Earl Clarkson, DDS

KEYWORDS

- Botox • Botulinum • Toxin • Dentist • Dental • Oral • Mouth • Face

KEY POINTS

- For the general dentist, the use of BTA confers the ability to exert control over the soft tissues surrounding the mouth to better create a harmonious smile.
- Although not technically challenging, the injection of BTA into the facial musculature requires a level of finesse to achieve the desired outcomes.
- A sound understanding of the toxin's mechanism of action and the ability to manage potential complications are also necessary, as the dentist administering BTA must be competent to the same level as other providers who have traditionally been the gatekeepers of such agents.

Once firmly secured in the armamentarium of plastic surgeons, the use of botulinum toxin type A (BTA), perhaps best-known commercially by the household name Botox, has recently begun to see a diversification in the types of practitioners employing its use. Few could argue the impact that this and other neurotoxins have had on the practice of improving facial aesthetics. Although cosmetic purposes remain the most common application, this was actually not the original indication, and still several other indications continue to emerge.

For the general dentist, BTA can be an excellent practice builder when properly utilized. Because the perioral region contributes greatly to dental aesthetics, the ability to exert control over the soft tissues surrounding the mouth equips the dentist with additional tools to create a harmonious smile.

Although not technically challenging, the injection of BTA into the facial musculature requires a level of finesse to achieve the desired outcomes. A sound understanding of the toxin's mechanism of action and the ability to manage potential complications are also a requisite, as the dentist administering BTA must be competent to the same level as other providers who have traditionally been the gatekeepers of such agents.

Department of Oral & Maxillofacial Surgery, Woodhull Medical Center, 760 Broadway, Brooklyn, NY 11206, USA
* Corresponding author.
E-mail address: jaredmillerdds@gmail.com

Dent Clin N Am 60 (2016) 509–521
http://dx.doi.org/10.1016/j.cden.2015.11.007
0011-8532/16/$ – see front matter © 2016 Elsevier Inc. All rights reserved.

MECHANISM OF ACTION

Prior to the advent of Botox and other subsequent neurotoxins used for therapeutic purposes, BTA was exclusively known as the causative agent in botulism poisoning. BTA is derived from the obligate anaerobe *Clostridium botulinum*. The earliest studied accounts of poisoning from this microbe date back to 1793, when an outbreak in Wildbad, Germany killed 6 people and affected 7 other people. The source was determined to be a contaminated batch of *Blutwurst*, or blood sausage—hence the name "botulism," after the Latin word for sausage, *botulus*. A larger outbreak in Belgium nearly a century later allowed Emile Van Ermengem to identify toxins produced by *C botulism* as the cause of botulism poisoning. This most commonly occurs when consuming food contaminated and stored under anaerobic conditions (eg, improperly canned). Per unit mass, botulinum toxin remains the most potent and lethal toxin known, with an LD50 of 1 to 3 ng/kg in people.[1]

Type A is the most potent of 8 serotypes of botulinum toxin that have been identified thus far (designated A–H, the latter being the most recently discovered in 2013).[2] Most variants cause paralysis at the neuromuscular junction by inhibiting the release of acetylcholine. Ordinarily, acetylcholine produced by the neuron remains contained in vesicles that upon depolarization of the neuron, fuse with the neuronal membrane to deposit the acetylcholine into the synaptic cleft. This process is facilitated by a complex of SNARE proteins: VAMP-2 and synaptobrevin on the vesicular surface, and syntaxin 1A and SNAP-25 on the neuronal membrane. When botulinum toxin is present, it binds to a separate class of surface proteins and becomes internalized by the neuron, subsequently cleaving the SNARE proteins that allow acetylcholine's exit into the synapse (**Fig. 1**). Owing to the storage vesicles of acetylcholine already within the motor endplate, the effect of paralysis is not manifested until 24 to 48 hours later, when these reserves are depleted. Paralysis would be permanent were it not for new axonal sprouts that are generated in 2 to 6 months, reestablishing the functional neuromuscular junction.

PREPARATION AND GENERAL CONSIDERATIONS

The first US Food and Drug Administration (FDA)-approved pharmaceutical preparations of BTA in the late 1980s were indicated for the treatment of strabismus and blepharospasm. The side effect of eliminating wrinkles in the lateral canthal region of the eye ("crow's feet") was quickly realized, and following extensive study, FDA approval for additional indications soon followed, including cervical dystonia (2000), glabellar rhytids (2002), and axillary hyperhidrosis (2004).

In the United States, BTA is available by the trade names Botox Cosmetic, Dysport, and Xeomin. All medications have similar FDA-approved indications, but Botox's *ona*botulinumtoxinA differs from Dysport's *abo*botulinumtoxinA and Xeomin's *incobo*-tulinumtoxinA primarily in regards to unit potency and nonprotein components that arise from different manufacturing processes.[3] Commercially available vials of any of the medications contain a given number of biologically active units. It is important for the clinician to realize that these units are essentially arbitrary quantities used for convenience in dosing. In general, most literature agrees on a potency equivalence of 2.5 to 3 units of Dysport to 1 unit of Botox.[4] Despite containing very similar toxins, this difference in potency can be attributed to the bacterial strain from which the toxin is sourced, the purification method, or differences in methods of testing potency.[5] For purposes of consistency, all doses in this article will refer to Botox units, with the understanding that an equivalent dose of Dysport or Xeomin would be anticipated to be equally effective.

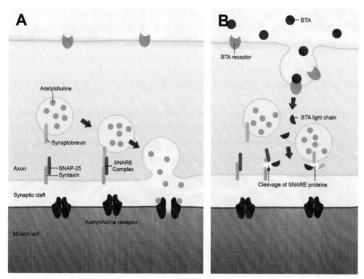

Fig. 1. Diagram depicting the action of botulinum toxin at the neuromuscular junction. (*A*) Normal acetylcholine release. Synaptobrevin and VAMP-2 (not shown) on the surface of the vesicle containing acetylcholine joins with SNAP-25 and syntaxin on the internal axonal surface. This forms a complex that allows fusion of the vesicle with the membrane to release acetylcholine into the synaptic cleft. Acetylcholine binds to its receptor on the surface of the muscle cell, opening voltage-gated sodium channels that result in membrane depolarization. (*B*) Action of botulinum toxin. BTA is internalized by the axon when bound by its receptor on the cell surface. The light chain of the toxin is taken up and cleaves the SNARE proteins before the acetylcholine vesicles can bind. The result is a lack of acetylcholine release into the synaptic cleft, and subsequent paralysis of the muscle.

All pharmaceutical preparations of BTA in the United States used from November 1979 to December 1997 came from a single 150 mg batch (dubbed 79–11) isolated by Schantz and colleagues.[6] By the time Botox Cosmetic was approved by the FDA in 2002, a newer batch (BCB 2024) had been isolated; it is from this batch that all modern Botox preparations are derived. A standard 100-unit vial of Botox contains just 4.8 ng of BTA. Because of this minuscule dose, Botox is shipped on dry ice as an empty glass vial containing a thin film of precipitate on the inside. After reconstitution with 2.5 cc preservative-free 0.9% sodium chloride for injection, it is stored under refrigeration and should be used within 24 hours. This dilution ratio allows for aspiration into 5 1 cc syringes, each containing a 0.5 cc solution of 20 units of Botox.[7]

Patients receiving BTA injections should be informed regarding the limitations of its efficacy. Because of the axonal resprouting that occurs, motor function after neurotoxin treatment begins to return after approximately 3 months. This, however, is highly variable; some patients may need to receive touch-up injections in as little as several weeks, while others can last well beyond the often-quoted 90 days before needing to repeat injections. In patients who consistently follow-up for repeat treatment, the atrophy that results from prolonged inactivity creates muscles that are less capable of forming deep rhytids, and treatment can usually be performed less frequently. Thick muscles of the face, such as the masseter, generally require less frequent injections.

Although rare, resistance to BTA has been reported. High-dose treatment with BTA over a short time span in some has been demonstrated to cause resistance to further treatment in patients being treated for cervical dystonia.[8] Some have speculated that a subclinical botulinum poisoning from contaminated food could result in antibodies against BTA in some patients.[9] In these cases, higher doses of BTA may be needed. Off-label treatment with rimabotulinumtoxinB, available commercially as Myobloc may also prove beneficial, although not in every instance. Investigation into other serotypes of botulinum toxin for treatment of these patients is underway.

Like most every intervention performed for a patient, a thorough discussion on risks, benefits, and alternatives is necessary before administering BTA. Contraindications to its use include coexisting conditions that affect neuromuscular transmission, including systemic neuromuscular disease or concomitant use of aminoglycoside or spectino-mycin antibiotics, which can potentiate BTA's effect. Pregnancy, lactation, or a known adverse reaction to any of the components in commercially available BTA are also contraindications to its use.

PERIORAL REGION
Excessive Gingival Display

For the dental practitioner, the most obvious application of BTA is in the treatment of gummy smiles, or excessive display of maxillary gingiva. Although Botox does have a role in treating a high smile line resulting from a hyperfunctional upper lip, it is important to distinguish this from other causes of gummy smiles. Short clinical crowns, for instance, would be better treated with gingivoplasty to achieve aesthetic crown lengthening. Likewise, the definitive treatment of vertical maxillary excess would necessitate maxillary impaction via a Le Fort I osteotomy. Attempts to camouflage these conditions with BTA injection would result in an unnatural appearance owing to the excessive loss of function needed to prevent gingival display.

In properly selected patients, however, BTA can have a profound impact in the treatment of high smile lines. Unfortunately, achieving a satisfactory outcome in this region is extremely technique-sensitive, as overtreatment can result in transverse elongation and dysfunctional animation of the upper lip. Novice injectors especially may wish to gradually ease into the final result by treating this area in multiple low-dose treatments over several weeks rather than in a single appointment.

In true cases of hyperfunctional upper lips, the primary contributor to excessive display of maxillary gingiva is the levator labii superioris alaeque nasi (LLSAN) muscle, which participates in the last few millimeters of upper lip elevation. This muscle is also involved in the creation of deep nasolabial folds that develop in some patients. The LLSAN originates from the superior portion of the frontal process of the maxilla near the nasal bridge, traverses inferiorly along the lateral aspect of the nose, and inserts at the nasal cartilage and the lateral upper lip. As such, its function involves dilation of the nares, and—along with the levator anguli oris, leavator labii superioris, and zygomaticus muscles—elevation of the upper lip[10] (**Fig. 2**).

For treatment of either gummy smiles or deep nasolabial folds, anywhere from 1 to 5 units of Botox may be needed for each side. The injection is placed into the LLSAN at the depth of the fold, just lateral to the piriform aperture, which can be palpated when pressing the alar–facial junction medially (**Fig. 3**). Again, it should be remembered that it is easy to overtreat this muscle, and the resultant loss of upper lip animation may be more objectionable to the patient than the original presenting complaint.

Lipstick Lines

Vertical rhytids in the upper lip, commonly referred to as lipstick lines or smoker's lines, may often be observed in aging patients, especially smokers and those with

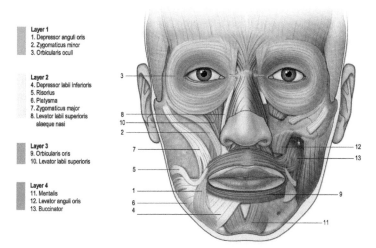

Layer 1
1. Depressor anguli oris
2. Zygomaticus minor
3. Orbicularis oculi

Layer 2
4. Depressor labii inferioris
5. Risorius
6. Platysma
7. Zygomaticus major
8. Levator labii superioris
   alaeque nasi

Layer 3
9. Orbicularis oris
10. Levator labii superioris

Layer 4
11. Mentalis
12. Levator anguli oris
13. Buccinator

Fig. 2. Muscles of facial expression, color-coded to indicate relative depths. (*From* Afifi AM, Djohan R. Anatomy of the head and neck. In: Neligan PC, ed. Plastic surgery, volume three: craniofacial, head and neck surgery. 3rd edition. London: Elsevier; 2013; with permission.)

a history of excessive sun exposure. Constant puckering action, as when smoking, whistling, or playing a wind instrument, activates the orbicularis oris muscle and contributes to the development of these wrinkles, although heredity does play a role also.

As with treating the nasolabial region, overzealous injection into the obicularis oris muscle can adversely alter a patient's ability to animate the upper lip. By the same token, completely eliminating lipstick lines is practically impossible without total paralysis of the muscle. For patients unsatisfied by merely reducing the depths of their lines, other treatment modalities may be indicated. In addition to spreading the injections over several appointments to titrate to effect, it is not unusual to concomitantly administer dermal fillers. In this manner, neurotoxin is used to relax the muscle that creates the lines initially, and filler is used to further conceal the remaining wrinkles. Although both are temporary treatments, neurotoxin prolongs the filler's effect by preventing movement of the underlying musculature.

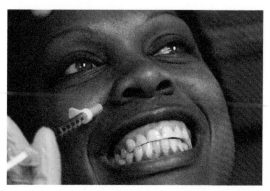

Fig. 3. Excessive gingival display is treated by injection of BTA at the depth of the nasolabial fold just lateral to the alar–facial junction.

The orbicularis oris is one of two sphincter muscles of the face, originating from the oral commissure, where fibers fuse with other perioral elevator muscles, forming the modiolus. Insertions at various subdermal layers near the midline allow movement such as pursing and protrusion of the lips, as well as closing of the mouth by drawing the lips in toward the teeth. Botox injection to treat the vertical rhytids of the upper lip is best performed by having the patient pucker his or her lips and placing 1 to 2 units in the deepest folds seen (**Fig. 4**). This usually results in 2 to 4 injection sites, depending on the patient. Because of the fineness of the wrinkles being treated, the injections are generally placed very superficially, even intradermally, as one can expect diffusion of the product up to 15 mm away from the injection site.[11]

Corners of the Mouth

Many patients may present complaining of a persistent frown, often the result of others perceiving the patient as upset or displeased. The upper face contributes much to this appearance, but in the perioral region, a subtle but impactful downturn of the corners of the mouth is the result of the depressor anguli oris muscle. This muscle is shaped like an inverted fan, with the broad end originating from the inferior border of the mandible and the insertion into the modiolus. Paralysis of the muscle allows the perioral elevator muscles, especially levator anguli oris and zygomaticus major, to function unopposed. The resultant change is slight but noticeable for many patients.

Special care must be taken to isolate the depressor anguli oris when injecting neurotoxin. Placement of the needle too far inferiorly can affect the marginal mandibular branch of the facial nerve as it courses anteriorly; consequently, the site of injection should remain at least 1 cm above the inferior border of the mandible. Anterior injection will affect the depressor labii inferioris, which, if paralyzed, may result in incompetence of the lower lip, an asymmetric smile, and food impaction in the lower anterior vestibule of the mouth. Guided by these boundaries, the depressor anguli oris is isolated by having the patient drop his or her lower lip in an effort to display the mandibular incisors. A Botox injection of 2 to 5 units (bilaterally) into the belly of the muscle is appropriate to achieve subtle elevation of the corners of the mouth.

Chin Dimpling

The paired mentalis muscles originate from the parasymphyseal region of the mandible and course inferomedially to insert into the dermis of the chin. With elevation

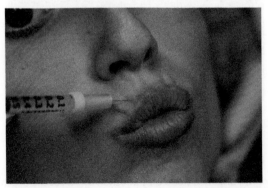

Fig. 4. Asking the patient to pucker his or her lips highlights the deepest folds of lipstick lines.

of the lower lip, as occurs during speech or chewing, some patients may exhibit dimpling of the chin that bears resemblance to an orange peel, hence the term for this appearance, peau d'orange. Unlike persistent rhytids such as crow's feet or glabellar 11s, which are formed by years of muscle action, chin dimpling is often first noticed by people observing the patient during activity such as speech. As such, many patients may not notice dimpling unless they observe it in a mirror or are told by somebody. Nonetheless, it can easily be treated by BTA injection in patients who find its presence unsightly or distracting.

Injecting a total of 2 to 5 units of Botox throughout the chin in the areas of greatest dimpling is usually sufficient. Care should be taken to keep the injection superficial (closest to the dermal insertion of the mentalis muscles, not the origin), as even minor overtreatment can negatively affect phonation of consonants that require drawing the bottom lip upward, such as B, M, or P sounds. Lateral injection can also affect the depressor labii inferioris muscle, which is to be avoided. Often, obtaining the desired cosmesis requires at least some compromise of function, although many patients will be accepting of this trade-off. As with other perioral muscles, multiple lower-dose treatments may be best until an acceptable balance is met.

Masseter Treatments

Although not a perioral muscle per se, the masseter muscle plays a central role in oral function and will be considered here. As a muscle of mastication, it has considerably more bulk than the previously discussed muscles of facial expression. It is composed of 2 heads that fuse near their insertion to facilitate a common function. The larger superficial head originates from the anterior two-thirds of the zygomatic arch (ie, the inferior surface of the zygomatic bone) and courses posteriorly to insert on the lateral mandibular ramus and angle. The smaller deep head originates from the posterior one-third of the zygomatic arch at the medial and inferior surfaces. Owing to its more posterior origin, it courses in a straighter superior–inferior direction to insert slightly higher on the lateral ramus than the superficial head. Together, they function to elevate and protrude the mandible, with some involvement in lateral excursive movements. Noteworthy structures passing superficial to the masseter include the parotid gland and duct, transverse facial artery, and branches of the facial nerve.

Masseter treatments serve a dual indication; in addition to cosmetic treatment of hypertrophic muscles, using BTA to reduce the strength of the masseter can also serve to treat myofascial pain or temporomandibular joint dysfunction secondary to bruxism. In Asian populations especially (though not exclusively), the procedure is used to slim the face; one study demonstrated a mean reduction in masseter thickness by up to 2.9 mm 3 months postoperatively.[12] Regardless of the reason for treatment, the masseter is unique in that the goal of treatment is to reduce bulk and not eliminate undesirable rhytids. As such, the eventual atrophy that BTA induces will necessitate less frequent redosing than needed for other muscles. For these patients, recall every 4 to 6 months is typical.

Because of its increased bulk relative to other facial muscles, treating the masseter requires a much higher dose of BTA. By having the patient clench his or her teeth, the most prominent areas of hypertrophy are identified and treated first (a surgical marking pen is helpful with this) (**Fig. 5**). Multiple sites of injection per side are typical, with 5 to 10 units per site being a good starting dose, although some patients may require as much as 100 units for bilateral treatment. Follow-up evaluation after several weeks will reveal if additional units are needed.

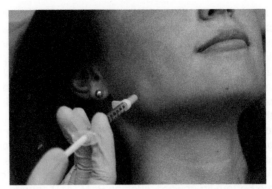

Fig. 5. The masseter is treated in the areas of greatest hypertrophy. Injections for this muscle are typically deeper than used in other areas of the face.

PERIORBITAL AND MIDFACIAL REGIONS
Jelly Roll

With advancing age, an unaesthetic bulging or laxity of the soft tissue beneath the orbit creates an appearance that many patients seek to have corrected. It is important to understand that this phenomenon can be due to a variety of etiologies, and a correct diagnosis is critical in order to avoid unnecessary treatment that is potentially irreversible. For the lower eyelid, distinguishing hypertrophy of the orbicularis oculi muscles from prolapse of the infraorbital fat pads is a skill that every practitioner performing BTA injections must possess.

The orbital septum is a membranous barrier that forms the anterior boundary of the orbit and is essentially a continuation of the periosteum peripheral to the orbital rims. This septum lies deep to the orbicularis oculi muscle. With age, the septum weakens and allows prolapse of the infraorbital fat pads, which can lead to a bulge (known as steatoblepharon) that many patients find bothersome. Because these fat pads are easily susceptible to fluid and gravitational shifting, they often create eyelid bags or dark circles that lend a fatigued appearance. However, a similar bulge can be created by hypertrophic orbicularis oculi muscles and is most evident when a patient smiles with the eyes or squints. This is primarily the result of the orbital portion of the muscle, which functions to voluntarily and forcefully contract the palpebral fissure (in contrast, the palpebral portion of the muscle lightly closes the eyes involuntarily, as in blinking).

To distinguish 1 subciliary bulge from the other, the practitioner can first observe the appearance and disappearance of bulges during animation, a strong indicator of orbicularis hypertrophy. Fat prolapse, conversely, can be made more evident by retropulsion of the globe, which is performed by gently pressing the globe inward with the patient's eyes closed; the lower fat pads should become more pronounced. The same effect can be elicited by having the patient gaze upwards with an open mouth. If the bulge is caused by fat prolapse, a blepharoplasty can be performed to excise the fat and excess skin in the lower lid.

For obicularis hypertrophy, BTA injection can help relieve the excessive closing force applied by the muscle. The cosmetic benefit from this is twofold; the subciliary bulge is reduced, and the eye is allowed to remain open more easily, creating a more awake appearance. A pretarsal injection of 1 to 2 units of Botox approximately 3 mm inferior to the ciliary margin and in the pupillary midline is usually sufficient. Care must be taken, however, to prevent injecting too deeply, as the skin of the eyelids is some of the thinnest on the body. Iatrogenic dry eye resulting from an inability to spread the tear film across the corneal surface is a potential complication. Patients with a pre-existing compromised ability to close the lower lids should avoid treatment; previous blepharoplasty, laser resurfacing, or excessive laxity of the lower lid skin can be problematic.

Crow's Feet

Treating the lateral canthal region to eliminate crow's feet remains one of the most popular BTA treatments. The lateral portion of the orbicularis oculi, where the concentric rings of muscle contract in a superior–inferior direction, creates a fan-shaped pattern of horizontal rhytids that converge at the lateral aspect of the eye. Excessive muscle activity can accentuate and deepen these folds, and in such patients, BTA can yield a profound influence on maintaining a youthful aesthetic. Wrinkling of the skin independent of muscle activity occurs with advancing age, however, and BTA may prove to be of little benefit in these cases.

Treatment of crow's feet demands extremely superficial injections. Because of the abundance of large, superficial vasculature in this region, ecchymosis and hematomas can easily occur with needle insertion. As with treating lipstick lines of the upper lip, intradermal injection can allow diffusion of BTA to the target muscle. However, this same effect that works to the practitioner's advantage can also have devastating complications when neurotoxin is injected too close to the orbit. To avoid paralysis of the extraocular muscles or ptosis of the eyelid, maintaining a distance of at least 10 to 15 mm from the bony orbital rim is paramount (**Fig. 6**). Novice injectors may be wise to measure and mark the skin prior to injecting. In the event that eyelid ptosis does occur, an emergency treatment of apraclonidine HCl (Iopidine) ophthalmic drops or 2.5% phenylephrine serves as an alpha adrenergic agonist to stimulate the autonomically innervated Mueller muscle, which is involved in the minor elevation of the eyelid that occurs with subconscious blinking. Unfortunately, the effect of these drugs is short-lived, and their usefulness is limited to mitigating embarrassing social situations. In a worst-case scenario, a patient may be unresponsive to this treatment and may simply have to wait for the neurotoxin's influence to wear off, although the ptosis effect often does not last as long as the desired outcome.

Injections are ideally placed in a semilunar pattern that follows the fan-shaped rhytids; 10 units of Botox spread over 3 to 4 injection sites are typical. In patients who have a particularly long lateral extension of rhytids that extend over the zygoma, a second row of injections following a concentric pattern to the first may be needed, but at a

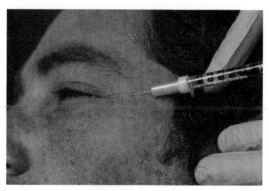

Fig. 6. Treating crow's feet requires superficial injections that parallel the lateral orbital rim at a distance of 10 to 15 mm.

lower dose of 1 to 2 units per site. Care must be taken when injecting at the inferior-most site, as downward diffusion of neurotoxin can have unwanted effects on lip elevators. A low dose of 1 to 2 units for this area is prudent.

Nasal Treatment

In some individuals, horizontal rhytids across the nasal dorsum are formed during frowning or squinting. These bunny lines can be the result of a portion of hyperactive nasalis muscle, a thin band that originates from the maxilla on either side of the nose and inserts medially into the nasal cartilage. As the primary compressor of the nares, contraction of this muscle can form rhytids perpendicular to the direction of its pull. When the procerus muscle is also recruited, as happens in some patients, the lines can be accentuated to the point of forming fissures that span the intercanthal distance. In this latter situation, Botox is used to treat the area in approximately 4 evenly spaced injections of 2 units, strategically placed in the areas of strongest contracture (**Fig. 7**). When pure nasalis action is observed, the injections remain more lateral, but the dose is unchanged. Occasionally, a patient who exhibits hyperactivity of only one of the muscles discussed here will unconsciously recruit the other following treatment, warranting additional injections later on.

Infrequently, patients may present with a distracting flare of the nares that occurs with inspiratory effort. The effect is most often noticed by others who are observing the patient when speaking. The result stems from hyperactive dilator naris muscles of the lateral ala. These small muscles, actually a component of the paired nasalis muscles, originate from the maxilla and lesser alar cartilage with cutaneous insertions. Superficial injection of 2 to 4 units of Botox into each ala eliminates flaring.

UPPER FACE
Frown Lines

The 11, perhaps the most commonly requested region for BTA treatment, is the manifestation of hyperactive or chronic brow furrowing by the procerus, corrugator supercili, and medial orbicularis oculi muscles. Often presenting as 2 vertical lines between the eyebrows (though 1 line or 3 lines can be seen as well), glabellar rhytids respond well to treatment and can have a dramatic effect on the facial appearance of a patient. Indeed, treatment of these frown lines is the only on-label cosmetic indication for Dysport and Xeomin, and along with crow's feet, 1 of 2 on-label cosmetic indications for Botox.[13–15]

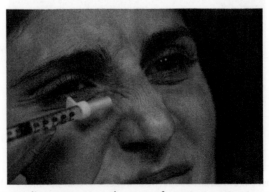

Fig. 7. Hyperactive nasalis treatment at the area of greatest contracture.

The anatomy of the glabellar musculature involves the overlapping and blending of several muscles. The procerus, extending from the nasal bone and cartilage to its insertion into the skin of the forehead, spreads laterally as its fibers run in a superior direction. Activation of this muscle causes wrinkling of the overlying skin, as discussed earlier. At the medial aspect of the superior orbital rim originates the corrugator supercilii muscle, which approximately follows the contour of the rim as it runs laterally to insert into the skin at the middle of the eyebrow. This muscle assists in furrowing the brow, drawing the eyebrow inferomedially. These 2 muscles, in conjunction with the medial and superior portions of orbicularis oculi, are the primary targets when treating frown lines.

In most cases, 20 to 30 units of Botox evenly spread across the offending muscles are sufficient, although patients with especially hypertrophic muscles or deep frown lines may need as much as double this amount. In the common presentation of 2 fissures (the 11), a single 5-unit centrally placed injection into the bulk of the procerus muscle is performed, followed by 5 units into each corrugator supercilii and each superior orbicularis oculi (**Fig. 8**). When the procerus rhytids are more varied and multiple ridges are noted, the central 5-unit injection is spread evenly across them. Isolation of the injection sites can be aided by having the patient deliberately frown, although some patients may need to see a mirror in order to do so reliably (ie, without recruitment of the frontalis muscle). The corrugator supercilii can be highlighted by manipulating the muscle with upward pressure into the soft tissue overlying the superior orbital rim. Owing to the proximity of the supraorbital and supratrochlear vessels in this region, aspiration prior to injection is a prudent maneuver.[16] As with other periorbital injections, maintaining a distance of 10 to 15 mm away from the orbital rim reduces the risk of unwanted muscle paralysis.

Forehead Wrinkles

The frontalis muscle is a broad, thin quadrilateral muscle with vertical fibers spanning the forehead. It originates from the galea aponeurotica of the scalp and inserts into the fibers of the various brow muscles previously discussed. Because of its large surface area but thin bulk, treatment of frontalis rhytids involves multiple low-dose injections of BTA in a manner similar to that of a field block with local anesthetic. The 10 to 15 mm diffusion of neurotoxin from the injection site means that typical treatment allows injection points to be placed 20 to 30 mm apart. Botox doses are usually 2 to 5 units per injection, with the higher end of this range being

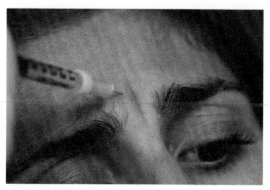

Fig. 8. In this patient, a single midline rhytid is seen on animation. Bilateral injection into the bulk of the procerus on either side is used for treatment in such cases.

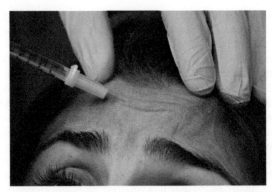

Fig. 9. Frontalis treatment with multiple diffuse injections. Care is taken to include rhytids near the hairline.

reserved for patients with particularly thick skin or musculature. Less neurotoxin (2–3 units) can be used when less paralysis is desired, as this will produce a softening of rhytids without an outright loss of expressive capability. Generally, these doses amount to anywhere from 10 to 30 units of Botox across the forehead, depending on the desired result. During injection, assessment of the ideal needle placement is done by having the patient animate his or her forehead. Using the nondominant hand to stabilize the position minimizes the depressor effect of orbicularis oculi (**Fig. 9**).

In some patients, but especially in women, there exists a subconscious habitual elevation of the brow as a compensatory effort to hide excess upper eyelid skin (dermatochalasis) or an otherwise low brow line. When these patients are treated for frontal rhytids, they may likely find difficulty in maintaining their typical brow posture, which often becomes apparent when they apply eye shadow. Preoperatively, patients seeking frontalis treatment should be evaluated closely for such posturing and be educated on this possible change. Sparing the inferolateral-most injection sites may minimize the brow ptosis in patients who cannot accommodate this loss of function; a downside to this approach is the potential for V-shaped brows that many patients may find unattractive. If this occurs, balance can be restored with 1 unit injected into the spared region.

SUMMARY

With an ever-growing number of practitioners incorporating the use of BTA in their practice, dentists and other doctors who treat the maxillofacial region are able to provide a valuable service to their patients in becoming educated in its use. Few interventions have had such an impact as neurotoxin treatment while still maintaining a relatively approachable barrier to entry into the practice. The key to success is not necessarily the doctor's background training, but quality experience and a sound understanding of the pearls and pitfalls of BTA.

REFERENCES

1. Horowitz BZ. Botulinum toxin. Crit Care Clin 2005;21(4):825–39.
2. Barash JR, Arnon SS. A novel strain of *Clostridium botulinum* that produces type B and type H botulinum toxins. J Infect Dis 2014;209(2):183–91.

3. Nestor MS, Ablon GR. Duration of action of abobotulinumtoxinA and onabotuli-numtoxinA: a randomized, double-blind study using a contralateral frontalis model. J Clin Aesthet Dermatol 2011;4(9):43–9.
4. Niamtu J. Cosmetic facial surgery. St Louis (MO): Mosby; 2010.
5. Nigam PK, Nigam A. Botulinum toxin. Indian J Dermatol 2010;55(1):8–14.
6. Schantz EJ, Johnson EA. Properties and use of botulinum toxin and other micro-bial neurotoxins in medicine. Microbiol Rev 1992;56(1):80–99.
7. BOTOX Cosmetic (onabotulinumtoxinA) for injection, for intramuscular use [Package insert]. Irvine, CA: Allergan, Inc; 2014.
8. Sadick NS, Herman AR. Comparison of botulinum toxins A and B in the aesthetic treatment of facial rhytides. Dermatol Surg 2003;29:340–7.
9. Niamtu J. Complications in Fillers and Botox. Oral Maxillofac Surg Clin North Am 2009;21:13–21.
10. Norton NS. Netter's head and neck anatomy for dentistry. 2nd edition. Philadel-phia: Elsevier; 2012.
11. Haggerty CJ, Laughlin RM. Atlas of operative oral and maxillofacial surgery. Ames (IA): John Wiley & Sons; 2015.
12. Park NY, Ahn KY, Jung DS. Botulinum toxing type A treatment for contouring of the lower face. Dermatol Surg 2003;29(5):477–83.
13. BOTOX® Cosmetic (onabotulinumtoxinA) official site. Welcome! Irvine (CA): Allergan, Inc; 2015. Available at: http://www.botoxcosmetic.com/. Accessed August 1, 2015.
14. Dysport® for temporary improvement of moderate to severe frown lines. Lausanne (Switzerland): Galderma Laboratories, L.P.; 2015. Available at: http://www.dysportusa.com/. Accessed August 1, 2015.
15. XEOMIN® (incobotulinumtoxinA) for injection, for intramuscular use. Raleigh (NC): Merz North America; 2015. Available at: http://www.xeominaesthetic.com/. Ac-cessed August 1, 2015.
16. Guttenberg SA. Cosmesis of the mouth, face and jaws. Chichester (United Kingdom): Wiley-Blackwell; 2012. Special thanks to Rinil Patel DDS, Joshua Weiler DDS, Lynda Asadourian, and Saidah Jack-Glidden.

Medication for Gravid and Nursing Dental Patients

Avichai Stern, DDS*, Jonathan Elmore, DDS

KEYWORDS

• Dentistry • Pregnancy • Nursing • Drugs • Medications • Lactating • Risk

KEY POINTS

• There is a new labeling system for the safety of medications in pregnant and lactating patients.
• Available data related to the safe use of medications in pregnant and lactating patients are constantly changing.
• The benefits of using a medication must always be weighed against its risks for that patient.

The topics the authors address in this article are in many ways both broad and narrow. The broadness of this topic is clear when one considers the intersection of 2 of the more complex areas in medicine: pharmacology and obstetrics. At the same time when considered in the format of a review article, one can only hope to provide a snapshot of information, which will inevitably change over time. The information provided here is for reference only and the authors suggest consultation with the patients' obstetrician (or pediatrician for breastfeeding patients) for up-to-date and patient-specific information on a case-by-case basis.

The effect of a medication on a developing fetus depends on many factors. One medication may have a variety of different adverse effects depending on fetal development at the time it is administered. Other considerations include molecular weight of a drug and whether it is lipid or water soluble. Maternal factors, such as altered gastric absorption, may also play a roll.

There are very few known teratogenic medications, and most contraindications to the use of medicaments in gravid patients are relative contraindications only. In other words, rarely is it necessary to prescribe an alternative medication for pregnant patients. The establishment of teratogenicity depends on the meeting of several criteria. Review of these criteria is irrelevant for this article. The reader may refer to Buhimschi and Weiner[1] "Medications in Pregnancy and Lactation: Part 1" for more information. It

The Brooklyn Hospital Center, 121 DeKalb Avenue, Brooklyn, NY 11201, USA
* Corresponding author.
E-mail address: avistern.dds@gmail.com

Dent Clin N Am 60 (2016) 523–531
http://dx.doi.org/10.1016/j.cden.2015.11.008
0011-8532/16/$ – see front matter © 2016 Elsevier Inc. All rights reserved.

is important to realize, however, that one of the reasons that there are so few established teratogens is that it is difficult to prove for a particular drug that all criteria have been met for teratogenicity.

The publication of this article coincides with a new labeling system recently instituted by the Food and Drug Administration (FDA). Doctors *and patients* are both familiar with the grading system instituted by the FDA in 1979 for indicating drug safety in pregnant patients (**Table 1**).

There are several problems with this labeling scheme (**Box 1**). Firstly it oversimplifies the decision-making process for prescribing medications to pregnant patients. By narrowly defining medications within the framework of this system, many practitioners feel limited to prescribing medications in the A and B categories only. Indication for use of a category C drugs often triggers a medical clearance request to the obstetrician often delaying care of patients.

Secondly, when viewed through a medical-legal lens, this system provides easy fodder for plaintiff's attorneys to clearly present to a jury supposed evidence of a dentist's deviation from the standard of care.

Finally, assignment of a medication to a category often becomes a lifetime sentence, as said assignment is seldom updated when new evidence becomes available. This point becomes clear when considering the X designation assigned to triazolam, which has been considered safe for use during pregnancy since the 1990s.

Fortunately, the FDA has recently set forth new guidelines for pregnancy and lactation labeling of medications.[2,3] This new labeling scheme went into effect on June 30, 2015 and includes sections for both pregnancy and lactation as well as the new

Table 1
Previous FDA drug labeling for pregnancy

Category	Description
A	Adequate, well-controlled studies in pregnant women have not shown an increased risk of fetal abnormalities to the fetus in any trimester of pregnancy.
B	Animal studies have revealed no evidence of harm to the fetus; however, there are no adequate and well-controlled studies in pregnant women. *OR* Animal studies have shown an adverse effect, but adequate and well-controlled studies in pregnant women have failed to demonstrate a risk to the fetus in any trimester.
C	Animal studies have shown an adverse effect, and there are no adequate and well-controlled studies in pregnant women. *OR* No animal studies have been conducted, and there are no adequate and well-controlled studies in pregnant women.
D	Adequate well-controlled or observational studies in pregnant women have demonstrated a risk to the fetus. However, the benefits of therapy may outweigh the potential risk. For example, the drug may be acceptable if needed in a life-threatening situation or serious disease for which safer drugs cannot be used or are ineffective.
X	Adequate well-controlled or observational studies in animals or pregnant women have demonstrated positive evidence of fetal abnormalities or risks. The use of the product is contraindicated in women who are or may become pregnant.

From FDA use-in-pregnancy ratings. Available at: http://www.perinatology.com/exposures/Drugs/FDACategories.htm. Accessed July 29, 2015; with permission.

| Box 1 |
Problems with grading system
Delay of care when category C drugs are indicated
Rigidity of existing system limiting to dentists medical-legally
Lack of updating based on latest evidence

category of women and men of reproductive potential. The new labeling scheme will eliminate the long-standing A-B-C-D-X grading system. The pregnancy label, which also includes labor and delivery, will always include a risk summary subsection. A subsection entitled clinical considerations, data, and pregnancy exposure registry will be included when relevant information is available. When the clinical considerations subsection is required, further subsections, such as disease-associated maternal and/or embryo/fetal risk, dose adjustments during pregnancy and the postpartum period, maternal adverse reactions, fetal/neonatal adverse reactions, and labor or delivery, will be included when information is available. The pregnancy exposure registry is a voluntary collection of data collected by physicians and/or pregnant patients who are taking certain medications during pregnancy.[4] The lactation label will include information such as the amount of the drug in breast milk and any potential risk for the child.

- Pregnancy
  - Risk summary: always included
  - Clinical considerations: when data available
    - Disease-associated maternal and/or embryo/fetal risk
    - Dose adjustments during pregnancy and the postpartum period
    - Maternal adverse reactions
    - Fetal/neonatal adverse reactions
    - Labor and delivery
  - Pregnancy exposure registry: when data available
  - Data: when available
    - Human data
    - Animal data
- Lactation
  - Risk summary: always included, must include a risk-benefit statement unless the drug is contraindicated
    - Presence of drug in human milk when drug is absorbed systemically
    - Effects of drug on the breastfed child when drug is absorbed systemically
    - Effects of drug on milk production when drug is absorbed systemically
- Men and women of reproductive age
  - Only when indicated

Although the new rules took effect on June 30, 2015, implementation will take place over a 3- to 5-year period with a total estimated cost of about $78 million. The goal of this significant change in drug labeling as described by the FDA is to "facilitate informed prescribing and safe and effective product use."[2] This change brings drug labeling for pregnancy and lactation into the twenty-first century and directly addresses the primary issues related to the grading system. Clinical decisions can be made based on information directly on the drug insert. Additionally, this construct encourages the practitioner to make decisions based on updated evidence that may not have made it to print on the drug packaging. This change will, over time, diminish the delay of care related to unnecessary obstetric and pediatric consultations.

The new labeling rule also directly impacts an area that affects all dental practitioners. Many obstetricians recommend that no epinephrine be used in conjunction with local anesthetics during pregnancy. Once this recommendation is made, the dentist's options for anesthetizing are limited. Some practitioners turn to mepivacaine, which is the same class C category as epinephrine. Alternatively, one may consider lidocaine without an epinephrine additive, which often results in less than adequate anesthesia. The new labeling allows for the unproven possibility of teratogenicity of a medication while also allowing the practitioner to weigh the risks and benefits of the drug for that particular patient. This change frees the dental practitioner to use lidocaine with epinephrine during pregnancy after a risk-benefit analysis and to discuss with patients without the need to tether that decision to an obstetric consultation.

Another area impacted by the labeling change is pain management. Opioid analgesics are commonly prescribed during pregnancy for pain; however, they are currently classified as class C by the FDA, hobbling dental practitioners as with epinephrine. The new labeling rule will allow the dentists more latitude with opioid prescriptions when considering the latest literature in a risk-benefits discussion. Although there is an increased risk of neural tube defects with peri-conception use of some opioids (codeine, hydrocodone, and oxycodone) by about 2%,[5] opioid use during the second trimester is generally considered safe. Caution should be taken during the third trimester because of a risk of newborn opioid dependence. Opioid use can be safely used during the third trimester; however, the obstetrician should be involved so that the newborn can be assessed for dependence after birth.

To summarize, with the activation of a new medication-labeling scheme for pregnant and lactating patients, the FDA has put the decision-making onus back on the individual practitioner. It is always the dentist's responsibility to be up to date with the constantly changing evidence related to medications and pregnancy. Finally, when considering any medication in any scenario, one must continue to weigh the benefit of using the medication against all possible risks to patients before administering or prescribing it (**Table 2**).

PHARMACOLOGY IN LACTATING PATIENTS

The benefits of breastfeeding have been well documented in the literature and are supported by both the American Academy of Pediatrics (AAP) and the World Health Organization as the gold standard for infant nutrition. The AAP recommends exclusive breastfeeding (with the addition of vitamin D) for the first 6 months but encourages breastfeeding to the length of 12 months or an age that is acceptable for mother and child. During the nursing period, however, mothers may encounter circumstances necessitating the need for pharmacologic intervention. As a dentist, it is important to have a knowledge of the effects of the medication given as well as the possible effects the medication will have on the nursing infant. Often times, mothers are given recommendations to postpone breastfeeding while taking medications. This course of action may not be needed. This section aims to review some of the common medications given by dentists and also how these medications may affect the lactating mother and the nursing child.

PHARMACOKINETICS

When a nursing mother is taking medications, the substance is able to incorporate into the breast milk by diffusion or active transport. Some characteristics of the drug can

Table 2 Drugs in pregnancy		Previous Classification	Comments[6]
Local anesthetics	Lidocaine	B	No known risks
	Mepivacaine	C	No known risks
	Bupivacaine	C	No known risks
	Benzocaine	C	No known risks
	Epinephrine	C	Reports of fetal malformations with intravenous doses; no documented risk when used in association with a local anesthetic
Antibiotics	Amoxicillin	B	None
	Penicillin	B	None
	Amoxicillin and clavulanate potassium (Augmentin)	B	None
	Clindamycin	B	None
	Azithromycin	B	None
	Metronidazole (Flagyl)	B	Fetal carcinogen in mammals; no proven risk in humans; contraindicated for use in first trimester as per manufacturer
Analgesics	Ibuprofen	B	• Associated with ductus arteriosus constriction when used during first trimester • Associated with pulmonary hypertension when used in the third trimester
	Acetaminophen	B	Frequent use may be associated with fetal abnormality
	Opioids (oxycodone, hydrocodone, codeine)	C	• First trimester use: low risk of neural tube defects • Third trimester use: risk of fetal dependence and newborn respiratory depression
Anxiolytics	Diazepam (Valium)	D	Associated with craniofacial and thoracic abnormalities first/ second trimester;
	Triazolam	X	No known association with fetal abnormalities
	Midazolam	D	Use near birth associated with adverse neonatal neurobehavior
Steroids	Dexamethasone	Not applicable	Low risk of oral clefts during first trimester
	Triamcinolone	C	First trimester risk of oral clefts; continued use may restrict fetal growth
	Prednisone	Not applicable	Low risk of oral clefts during first trimester
Muscle relaxant	Cyclobenzaprine	B	—

Data from Van Hoover C, Briggs GG, Freeman RK, et al. Drugs in pregnancy and lactation: a reference guide to fetal and neonatal risk. 6th Edition. Journal of Midwifery & Women's Health 2203;48:294.

determine how easily this process occurs. Some characteristics include the amount of protein binding by the drug, the drug's ability to ionize, the drug size, and its lipid solubility.[7] The drug's ability to bind tightly to plasma proteins decreases the amount of drug that will enter breast milk. The pKa and pH of the plasma and the breast milk play an important role in the ion trapping phenomenon. Lipophilic drugs are more likely to accumulate in milk. When it comes to the molecular weight of a drug, there is an inverse relationship of molecular weight to the ease at which the drug is transported into breast milk.

DRUG SAFETY MEASUREMENTS

In order to estimate the amount of drug that the infant is exposed to, the milk to plasma (M/P) ratio was created. One important fact to remember about this ratio is that it does not take into account the clearance and bioavailability of the drug to the infant. This ratio also depends on the time between consumption and measurement of levels in the mother and infant. The M/P of a drug is calculated by dividing the drug level in the milk by the drug level in the plasma. It has been accepted that an M/P ratio of a drug less than 1 is usually safe to breastfeed.[7]

An alternate calculation for the safety of a drug for a nursing mother is the relative infant dose (RID). This calculation uses a theoretic infant dose, which is adjusted for the weight of the child, and compares it with the maternal weight-adjusted dose. When the RID is less than 10% of the maternal dose, the medication is considered safe to use during breastfeeding.[7]

Other factors that contribute to infant exposure are listed in **Box 2**.

LOCAL ANESTHETICS

Local anesthetics used during dental procedures are generally maintained in a localized region because of the common practice of use with vasoconstrictors. These medications will eventually enter the general circulation by either diffusion or direct injection into the vasculature. The most common local anesthetic used in the dental office is lidocaine 2% with epinephrine 1:100,000. No studies were found addressing the presence of lidocaine in breast milk following a dental procedure. Based on studies involving postpartum use of lidocaine and measurements of the levels in breast milk, the FDA stated that lidocaine was compatible with breastfeeding. When evaluating the use of epinephrine separately, limited studies have also been performed, and caution is advised because of the possible effects on milk production. The safety of mepivacaine hydrochloride (Carbocaine), articaine, and bupivacaine are unknown.

Box 2
Factors contributing to infant exposure to a drug

Initial dose taken by the mother

The dosing interval taken by the mother

The elimination half-life

Number of feeds by the infant

Proximity of feeding time to the ingestion of the drug

Amount of milk consumed at feeding

COMMON ANTIBIOTICS

Of the penicillin drug class, amoxicillin and ampicillin have been approved by the AAP to be compatible with breastfeeding. Penicillins incorporate into breast milk in small doses. After intramuscular dosing of 100,000 IU, the M/P ratio varied from 0.03 to 0.13.[7] Oral administration of penicillins has been shown to be lower. Overall, breast-feeding should not be stopped while taking penicillins.

Cephalosporins have a similar profile to penicillin drugs in regard to presence in breast milk. These drugs are found in low concentrations and are considered compatible with breastfeeding.

First-generation cephalosporins were found to be undetectable in breast milk. No significant studies have been performed on second-generation cephalosporins, but no adverse effects have been reported by nursing mothers taking the drug. Third-generation cephalosporins have been observed to be at lower levels in breast milk than first- and second-generation cephalosporins. For example, a 100-mg oral dose of cefixime was undetectable in milk after 1 to 6 hours.[8]

Metronidazole has been shown to cause carcinogenesis in rodents but has not been shown to cause similar outcomes in humans. The AAP considers its effects on nursing infants as unknown but urges caution.

The macrolides (erythromycin, clarithromycin, azithromycin), based on the low levels transferred in breast milk, do not support the need for stopping breastfeeding. When a macrolide is needed, the AAP recommends the use of erythromycin.

TRIMETHOPRIM/SULFAMETHOXAZOLE

This drug is excreted in breast milk in small amounts. It is recommended that care be taken when giving the drug to neonates with hyperbilirubinemia. The FDA states that the drug is contraindicated during the first 2 months. The AAP approves trimethoprim/sulfamethoxazole for use in lactating women.

PAIN MANAGEMENT

Analgesics are another common class of drugs given after dental procedures. Nonsteroidal antiinflammatory drugs (NSAIDs) are often the first-line drugs given to patients for pain management. The reviews have shown that most drugs in this class are safe. The safety of the drugs commonly used by dentists was reviewed and charted based on the estimated RID from studies (**Table 3**).[9]

PARACETAMOL (ACETAMINOPHEN)

Only about 0.04% to 0.23% of the maternal dose is excreted in breast milk. There has been one reportable adverse effect of the drug on nursing infants, which was a rash that resolved in 24 hours after stopping the drug.[7] The AAP considers this drug compatible with breastfeeding.

OPIOIDS

Codeine use has received mixed recommendations. Normal doses of codeine given to lactating women have been seen to reach high concentration levels of the active metabolite, morphine, in breastfeeding infants. Some infants possess the ability to rapidly metabolize the drug causing high levels in the blood. Some are more sensitive to the drug in neonatal periods.[10] When given at lower levels (<240 mg/d), codeine has been shown to be present in breast milk in small amounts. Hydrocodone has also

Table 3
Compatibility of NSAIDs in a breastfeeding mother

Drug	RID (%)	Safety Recommendation	Notes
Aspirin	9–21	Potential toxicity	Give with caution; should be given at low doses (<150 mg/d); consider alternate choice if possible
Celecoxib	0.3	Usually compatible	—
Diclofenac	1	Usually compatible	—
Ibuprofen	0.6	Usually compatible	—
Indomethacin	0.4	Usually compatible	—
Ketorolac	0.2–0.4	Usually compatible	Black box warning that it is contraindicated because of potential adverse effects
Naproxen	1–3	Usually compatible	—

Adapted from Bloor M, Paech M. Nonsteroidal antiinflammatory drugs during pregnancy and the initiation of lactation. Anesth Analg 2013;116(5):1069; with permission.

been shown to reach as high as 9% of the maternal dose. Therefore, caution is advised when giving codeine or hydrocodone in the nursing infant.

Hydromorphone seems to be tolerated well by infants and is preferable over codeine and hydrocodone use.[11] Other narcotics, like oxycodone and meperidine, are not recommended for the use in nursing infants because of the relatively high amounts found in human milk.

ANXIOLYTICS

Previous statements by the AAP categorized anxiolytics' effects in nursing patients as "unknown but may be of concern."[11] Few long-term studies have been completed regarding the effects of the drugs on the nursing infant. Because of the long half-life of some of the drugs in this class and the immature metabolism and excretion of infants, these drugs could potentially accumulate to high levels. The risks versus the benefits of this drug use should be evaluated before administration to a nursing mother. It may also be beneficial for the mother to waste the breast milk produced, while taking these medications, until the drug has been cleared from her system.

SUMMARY

Many of the common drugs used by dentists have been found to be safe for breast-feeding women. Before prescribing any drug to a nursing mother, the dentist should consider some of the following questions:

- Is this drug absolutely necessary for the treatment of this patient?
- Is this drug the safest option for this patient? (eg, acetaminophen versus aspirin)
- What are the chances of this drug reaching high concentration levels in the infant and potentially causing problems?
- Is it necessary to plan dosing around the feeding schedule to minimize infant exposure to the medications?
- Should the mother be encouraged to discard her breast milk for a certain amount of time before returning to feeding?

Consideration of these questions can lead to both the effective and safe treatment of both the nursing mother and the infant. Consultation with the treating physician may also be indicated if needed.

REFERENCES

1. Buhimschi C, Weiner C. Medications in pregnancy and lactation part 1. Teratology. Obstet Gynecol 2009;113(1):166–88.
2. Available at: https://s3.amazonaws.com/public-inspection.federalregister.gov/2014–28241.pdf. Accessed July 29, 2015.
3. Available at: http://www.fda.gov/drugs/developmentapprovalprocess/developmentresources/labeling/ucm093307.htm. Accessed July 29, 2015.
4. Available at: http://www.fda.gov/ScienceResearch/SpecialTopics/WomensHealthResearch/ucm251314.htm. Accessed July 29, 2015.
5. Yazdy MM, Mitchell AA, Tinker SC, et al. Periconceptional use of opioids and the risk of neural tube defects. Obstet Gynecol 2013;122(4):838–44.
6. Van Hoover C, Briggs GG, Freeman RK, et al. Drugs in pregnancy and lactation: a reference guide to fetal and neonatal risk. 6th Edition. Journal of Midwifery & Women's Health 2003;48:294. http://dx.doi.org/10.1016/S1526-9523(03)00148-X.
7. Bar-Oz B, Bulkowstein M, Benyamini L, et al. Use of antibiotic and analgesic drugs during lactation. Drug Saf 2003;26(13):925–35.
8. American Academy of Pediatrics. The transfer of drugs and other chemicals into human milk. Pediatrics 2001;108:776–89.
9. Bloor M, Paech M. Nonsteroidal anti-inflammatory drugs during pregnancy and the initiation of lactation. Anesth Analg 2013;116(5):1063–75.
10. Anderson PO, Manoguerra AS, Valdes V. A review of adverse reactions in infants from medications in breast milk. Clin Pediatr (Phila) 2015. [Epub ahead of print].
11. Sachs HC. The transfer of drugs and therapeutics into human breast milk: an update on selected topics. Pediatrics 2013;132(3):e796–809.

Medications to Assist in Tobacco Cessation for Dental Patients

Joshua M. Levy, DMD[a], Shelly Abramowicz, DMD, MPH[b],*

KEYWORDS

- Smoking cessation • Nicotine replacement therapy • Nicotine patch • Nicotine gum

KEY POINTS

- Smoking is the leading cause of preventable illness in the United States and accounts for approximately 20% of deaths.
- Nicotine replacement therapy (NRT), buproprion, and varenicline are first-line pharmacologic therapies to assist with smoking cessation.
- Varenicline and combination NRT are more effective than single NRT or buproprion for smoking cessation.
- Combinations of varenicline with NRT, buproprion with NRT, and varenicline with buproprion have proved to be efficacious for users who have failed monotherapy.

INTRODUCTION

According to a US Centers for Disease Control and Prevention report published in 2014, 17.8% of adults in the United States currently smoke cigarettes.[1] Smoking is the leading cause of preventable illness in the United States and accounts for approximately 20% of deaths. There are 16 million Americans living with smoking-related diseases such as cancers, cardiovascular diseases, and respiratory diseases.[2,3] Smoking has been shown to decrease life expectancy by approximately 10 years.[2] In 2010, 68% of adult smokers wished to quit smoking, whereas 52% had made an attempt to quit in the past year.[4] Many smokers try to quit without assistance and only 3% to 6% are successful 1 year later without assistance.[5,6]

Disclosure: The authors have nothing to disclose.
[a] Division of Oral and Maxillofacial Surgery, Department of Surgery, Emory University School of Medicine, 1365 Clifton Road, Suite 2300, Building B, Atlanta, GA 30322, USA; [b] Division of Oral and Maxillofacial Surgery, Department of Surgery, Children's Healthcare of Atlanta, Emory University School of Medicine, 1365 Clifton Road, Northeast, Suite 2300 Building B, Atlanta, GA 30322, USA
* Corresponding author.
E-mail address: sabram5@emory.edu

This article reviews the current therapies available to encourage and assist patients with smoking cessation. It covers the 5 As (ask, advise, assess, assist, arrange) algorithm of counseling, pharmacotherapy, behavioral therapy, and combination therapy for smoking cessation.

FIVE A'S

Because such a significant percentage of the population smokes, dentists play an important role in identifying smokers and assisting them in their quitting efforts. The 5 As is an algorithm recommended by the US Department of Health and Human Services for clinicians to use to help their patients quit.[6,7]

Ask

At each visit, it is important to ask about the patient's tobacco use.[6] For those who use tobacco, a thorough history should be taken that includes the amount, products used, and previous attempts to quit.

Advise

The US Department of Health and Human Services recommends that patients be advised to quit at each clinical encounter.[7] There is evidence that brief clinician advice can increase quit rates by 1% to 3%.[6,8]

Assess

At each visit, dentists should assess whether the patient is ready to quit at that moment.

Assist

For the patients who are ready to quit, the clinician should provide resources and information on treatment to help the patient quit.[7] It is important to review whether the patient has previously attempted to quit and what methods have been used. It is also important to help patients address any barriers to quitting that they may have.[6]

Arrange

For those patients who are willing to quit, it is important to arrange follow-up contact within 1 week in order to prevent relapse. The follow-up should provide reinforcement for the patient and assess the response to pharmacotherapy as well as any side effects the patient may experience.[6] For those that are unwilling to quit, it is important to ask, advise, and assess at the next clinical visit, because this should be completed at every clinical visit.[7]

PHARMACOTHERAPY

Tobacco products contain the highly addictive substance nicotine, which causes dopamine release and leads to physical dependence and tolerance. After long-term use, patients may smoke to control withdrawal symptoms rather than for its positive effects.[3] Common nicotine withdrawal symptoms include increased appetite, weight gain, dysphoria, insomnia, irritability, anxiety, restlessness, and difficulty concentrating.[9]

Nicotine replacement therapy (NRT), buproprion, and varenicline are first-line pharmacologic therapies to assist with smoking cessation recommended by the US Department of Health and Human Services.[7,10] **Table 1** summarizes the dosing and side effects of these medications.

Table 1
First-line pharmacologic agents for smoking cessation

Drug	Dosing	Side Effects
Nicotine patch	Half a pack per day: • 21 mg patch/day for 6 weeks • 14 mg patch/day for the next 2 weeks • 7mg patch/day for the next 2 weeks Half a pack per day or <45 kg (99lbs): • 14mg patch/day for 6 weeks • 7mg patch/day for the next 2 weeks	• Headache • Nausea and vomiting • Diarrhea • Abdominal pain • Skin sensitivity and irritation • Vivid dreams • Insomnia
Nicotine gum	>25 cigarettes per day: • 4-mg dose <25 cigarettes per day: • 2-mg dose • 1 piece of gum every 1–2 h for 6 wk • Tapered to 1 piece every 2–4 h then every 4–8 h over the next 6 wk	• Headache • Nausea and vomiting • Diarrhea • Abdominal pain • Oral mucosa irritation and ulceration • Temporomandibular joint disease
Nicotine lozenge	Smokes within 30 min of waking: • 4-mg lozenge Smokes after 30 min of waking: • 2-mg lozenge • 1 lozenge every 1–2 h for first 6 wk • Tapered to 1 piece every 2–4 h then every 4–8 h over the next 6 wk	• Headache • Nausea and vomiting • Diarrhea • Abdominal pain • Oral mucosa irritation and ulceration
Nicotine inhaler	• 6–16 cartridges per day for first 6–12 wk • Tapered gradually over the next 6–12 wk	• Headache • Nausea and vomiting • Diarrhea • Abdominal pain • Local irritation to oropharynx
Nicotine nasal spray	1–2 sprays per hour for 3 mo	• Headache • Nausea and vomiting • Diarrhea • Abdominal pain • Nasal and pharyngeal irritation
Buproprion	• Begin 1 wk before quit date • 150 mg/d for first 3 d • 150 mg twice a day after first 3 d	• Insomnia • Dry mouth • Nausea • Headache • Seizures • Neuropsychiatric symptoms
Varenicline	• Begin one week before quit date • 0.5mg/day for first 3 days • 0.5mg twice/day for days 4–7 • 1mg twice/day for 11 weeks	• Nausea • Insomnia • Headache • Abnormal dreams • Neuropsychiatric symptoms • Cardiovascular events in patients with known cardiovascular disease

Nicotine Replacement Therapy

The goal of NRT is to facilitate the smoking cessation process by providing smokers with a certain amount of nicotine in order to reduce withdrawal symptoms and the desire to smoke.[3] Many different forms of NRT are available. Their use depends mainly on patient preference. The side effects common to all forms of NRT are headache, nausea, vomiting, diarrhea, and abdominal pain.[10]

The transdermal nicotine patch is an over-the-counter medication that produces a constant level of nicotine over 24 hours, although it takes several hours to reach its peak level. The patch has the advantage of high patient compliance. However, the user cannot control the nicotine dose in order to respond to cravings.[10] Patients who smoke more than half a pack per day start with a dose of one 21-mg patch per day for 6 weeks followed by one 14-mg patch per day for 2 weeks, then one 7-mg patch per day for 2 weeks. Those who smoke less than half a pack per day or weigh less than 45 kg (99 lbs) start with a dose of 14 mg/d for 6 weeks, then 7 mg/d for 2 weeks.[10] The most common side effect with the transdermal nicotine patch is local skin sensitivity and irritation. This irritation is often mild and rarely causes the patient to stop using the patch.[3] It can be avoided by having the patient rotate the site of patch placement daily.[10] Vivid dreams and insomnia have also been reported in patients who wear the patch overnight. These side effects can be avoided by having the patient remove the patch at night.[10]

Nicotine gum is an over-the-counter chewing gum that releases nicotine, which is absorbed through the oral mucosa. Peak nicotine blood levels occur 20 minutes after the gum is first chewed. The gum should be chewed until the nicotine taste begins to develop and then it should be held against the buccal mucosa until the taste disappears. This process is then repeated for 30 minutes. Patients who smoke more than 25 cigarettes per day should use the 4-mg dose and those who smoke less than 25 cigarettes per day should use the 2-mg dose. For the first 6 weeks, patients should chew 1 piece of gum every 1 to 2 hours, with at least 9 pieces per day. Over the next 6 weeks this should be tapered to every 2 to 4 hours and then every 4 to 8 hours. Acidic beverages should be avoided 15 minutes before using nicotine gum because the acidity of the oral pH causes the nicotine to ionize and reduces absorption. Side effects are mainly caused by overzealous chewing, which can cause nicotine to be released in amounts greater than the maximum that can be absorbed by the oral mucosa, leading to the nicotine being swallowed.[10] Swallowing nicotine leads to gastrointestinal symptoms such as nausea, vomiting, and abdominal pain. Local irritation by nicotine can lead to irritation and oral ulcers. In addition, excessive chewing can worsen myofacial pain and temporomandibular joint dysfunction (TMD); therefore, nicotine gum should be avoided in patients with TMD.[3]

Nicotine lozenges are an over-the-counter NRT that have a similar mechanism of action to the nicotine gum, but they do not need to be chewed. The lozenge is placed in the mouth and dissolves over 30 minutes. For smokers who smoke within 30 minutes of waking, the 4-mg lozenge dose should be used, whereas those who smoke after 30 minutes of waking should use the 2-mg dose. Smoking within 30 minutes of waking is used as a measure of the degree of nicotine dependence. Just as with the gum, the lozenge should be used every 1 to 2 hours for the first 6 weeks and then tapered for the following 6 weeks. The lozenges may cause local irritation and oral ulcers. Because the lozenge is not chewed, it is a better alternative for smokers with TMD.[10]

The nicotine inhaler is a prescription NRT. It has a mouthpiece and a cartridge that causes nicotine vapor to be released, deposited in the oropharynx, and absorbed though the oral mucosa. About 6 to 16 cartridges should be used per day for the first 6 to 12 weeks and then tapered gradually over the next 6 to 12 weeks. The main side effect of the nicotine inhaler is local irritation in addition to the side effects seen with all forms of NRT.[10]

The nicotine nasal spray is a prescription-only NRT that delivers aqueous nicotine to the nasal mucosa. The spray reaches peak concentration in about 10 minutes. Either 1 or 2 sprays per hour are recommended for 3 months. Nasal and pharyngeal irritation is a common side effect and often limits its use.[10]

Combination NRT combines the long-acting basal effect of the transdermal patch to control baseline withdrawal symptoms with the short-acting effects of the gum, lozenge, inhaler, or nasal spray to control breakthrough cravings.[10] A meta-analysis comparing different forms of NRT found that they are all equally effective. The same study found that combination NRT is more effective than any single NRT.[3]

Buproprion

Buproprion has been approved for use in depression since 1985. In 1997 it was approved by the US Food and Drug Administration (FDA) as a sustained-release form to assist with smoking cessation.[3] It was the first non-nicotine medication to be approved for smoking cessation.[7] Buproprion is thought to cause central nervous system dopaminergic and noradrenergic release.[10] It also may have nicotinic acetylcholinergic antagonistic properties. It functions to relieve withdrawal symptoms and reduce cravings by blocking the effects of nicotine.[3] A 2014 meta-analysis found that patients taking buproprion for smoking cessation had a 1.62-times greater chance of successful cessation after 1 year.[11]

The sustained-release form is started approximately 1 week before the user's quit date to allow the drug to reach steady state levels, which takes about 5 days. The dose is 150 mg/d for 3 days then 150 mg twice per day every day thereafter. For patients who cannot tolerate the side effects of 150 mg twice per day, 150 mg/d may be used. The drug should be continued for 12 weeks.[10]

The common side effects associated with buproprion are insomnia, dry mouth, nausea, and headache.[3,10] Cessation of treatment occurs in 7% to 12% of users because of undesirable side effects.[3] Buproprion reduces the seizure threshold and seizures have been reported in 0.1% of users. Thus, buproprion should be avoided in patients with a history of seizures or those with a predisposition to seizures, such as those with anorexia nervosa or bulimia nervosa. In addition, buproprion should be avoided in patients on monoamine oxidase inhibitors.[10]

In 2009, the FDA issued a warning that sustained-release buproprion may be associated with serious neuropsychiatric symptoms, such as suicidal ideation, suicide attempts, depressed mood, hostility, and agitation. This warning was in response to 29 reports of suicidal behavior and 46 reports of suicidal ideation from 1997 to 2007.[3] The clinician should follow up with the patient 1 week after beginning treatment to monitor for adverse effects. The patient should be told to stop the drug if any of these symptoms develop.[10]

Varenicline

Varenicline was approved by the FDA for smoking cessation in 2006.[7] Varenicline is a nicotine receptor partial agonist that causes the release of some dopamine to mitigate withdrawal symptoms while occupying nicotine receptor sites to reduce the positive effects of smoking.[12] A 2013 meta-analysis comparing varenicline with placebo found that patients taking varenicline had a 2.88-times greater chance of quitting compared with those taking placebo.[3]

Because it takes 1 week for varenicline levels to reach steady state, patients should be taking the medication 1 week before smoking cessation. Varenicline should be administered at a dose of 0.5 mg/d for 3 days followed by 0.5 mg twice per day for 4 days followed by 1 mg twice per day for the rest of the course.[13] The total drug course should be 12 weeks.[10]

The most common side effect of varenicline is nausea, which has an approximately 30% incidence.[13] Titrating the drug and reducing the dose can reduce the incidence of nausea.[3] Other common side effects include insomnia, headache, and abnormal dreams.[10] Drug discontinuation rates because of undesirable side effects range from 0.6% to 7.6%.[3] Neuropsychiatric effects and cardiovascular effects are important safety concerns of varenicline.

In 2008, the FDA required a boxed warning on the packaging informing users and clinicians of an increased possibility of neuropsychiatric effects, including behavior change, suicidal ideation, depression, and agitation.[3] Although the evidence concerning the neuropsychiatric effects of varenicline is inconclusive it is important that a careful psychiatric history be taken in all patients before initiating therapy, and varenicline should be avoided in those with an unstable psychiatric history or with previous suicidal ideation. Follow-up is recommended with patients on varenicline to assess for any neuropsychiatric symptoms.[10]

In 2011 the FDA issued a Drug Safety Communication that varenicline may increase the incidence of cardiovascular events in patients with known cardiovascular disease.[3] This warning was based on a trial that showed that patients with known cardiovascular disease treated with varenicline had increased incidence of nonfatal myocardial infarctions and increased need for coronary revascularization, although the results of the trial were not statistically significant.[10,14] Varenicline is not contraindicated in patients with stable cardiovascular disease but it is important to monitor these patients for any new or worsening cardiovascular signs or symptoms.[10]

In 2013 a meta-analysis compared the efficacy of single NRT, combination NRT, buproprion, and varenicline. It concluded that single NRT and buproprion are comparable with placebo in assisting with smoking cessation. All types of NRT are equally effective, whereas combination NRT is superior to single NRT and to buproprion. Varenicline may be similar in efficacy to combination NRT and superior to both single NRT and buproprion.[3]

NONPHARMACOLOGIC THERAPY

Although pharmacologic therapy has been shown to be effective for smoking cessation, the combination of pharmacologic therapy and behavioral therapy has been shown to be more effective than either form of therapy individually.[6,15] For patients who are willing to quit, it is recommended that the maximum behavioral therapy acceptable to the patient be used.[6] For most patients this includes brief counseling by a health care provider during office visits.[16] A study found that clinician counseling by oral health professionals incorporating an oral examination in their counseling significantly improved smoking cessation rates among their patients.[17] In addition to brief physician counseling, clinicians can provide resources to their patients about behavioral therapy and group therapy to assist with smoking cessation.[16] Clinicians can also inform their patients about a free telephone counseling service in the United States called 1-800-QUIT-NOW. This service provides free counseling to tobacco users as well as providing them with numerous resources to help with the quitting process.[18]

TREATMENT RESISTANCE

Although pharmacologic therapy significantly increases the rate of smoking cessation, some users fail to quit. For these patients it is important to first inquire about their medication to use to find out whether there was proper medication adherence. For those who cannot tolerate the side effects of the medications, it is recommended to either reduce the dose or switch to an alternate therapy.[10]

Patients who fail to quit with a trial of first-line therapy should try adding another first-line agent. Combinations of varenicline with NRT, buproprion with NRT, and varenicline with buproprion have proved to be efficacious for users who have failed monotherapy. Although drug combinations can be more efficacious, they can also have increased side effects. Nortriptyline, a tricyclic antidepressant, can also be used alone or in combination with NRT when first-line agents have been ineffective.[3,10] The side effects associated with nortriptyline include dry mouth, constipation, and drowsiness.[3]

RELAPSE

Many smokers who attempt to quit relapse and require multiple attempts before successfully quitting. Patients who relapse often do so because of inadequate control of withdrawal symptoms, medication side effects, or inadequate behavioral support.[6] For those who relapse because of inadequate control of withdrawal symptoms, clinicians can increase the dose of the medication or switch medications. For medication side effects, clinicians can reduce the dose or change medications. For those who relapse, it is important to increase behavioral therapy. Smokers who have had multiple relapses should be referred to a smoking cessation program for more intensive behavioral therapy. If a medication was previously helpful for a patient, the same medication should be restarted and can be supplemented with another pharmacologic aid and additional behavioral therapy.[3]

SUMMARY

- Smoking is the leading cause of preventable illness in the United States and accounts for approximately 20% of deaths.
- The 5 As is an algorithm recommended by the US Department of Health and Human Services for clinicians to use to help their patients quit.
- NRT, buproprion, and varenicline are first-line pharmacologic therapies to assist with smoking cessation.
- Varenicline and combination NRT are more effective than single NRT or buproprion for smoking cessation.
- The combination of pharmacologic therapy and behavioral therapy is more effective than either individual form of therapy.
- Combinations of varenicline with NRT, buproprion with NRT, and varenicline with buproprion have proved to be efficacious for users who have failed monotherapy.
- Smokers who have had multiple relapses should be referred to a smoking cessation program for more intensive behavioral therapy.

REFERENCES

1. Jamal A, Agaku IT, O'Connor E, et al, Centers for Disease Control and Prevention. Current cigarette smoking among adults—United States, 2005–2013. MMWR Morb Mortal Wkly Rep 2014;63(47):1108–12.
2. US Department of Health and Human Services. The health consequences of smoking—50 years of progress: a report of the surgeon general. Atlanta (GA): US Department of Health and Human Services; Centers for Disease Control and Prevention; National Center for Chronic Disease Prevention and Health Promotion; Office on Smoking and Health; 2014.

3. Cahill K, Stevens S, Perera R, et al. Pharmacological interventions for smoking cessation: an overview and network meta-analysis. Cochrane Database Syst Rev 2013;(5):CD009329.

4. Centers for Disease Control and Prevention (CDC). Quitting smoking among adults–United States, 2001–2010. MMWR Morb Mortal Wkly Rep 2011;60(44): 1513–9.

5. Rigotti NA. Strategies to help a smoker who is struggling to quit. JAMA 2012;308: 1573.

6. Rigotti NA, Rennard SI, Daughton DM. Overview of smoking cessation management in adults. In: Post TW, editor. UpToDate. Waltham (MA): UpToDate; Accessed July 3, 2015. Available at: http://www.uptodate.com/contents/overview-of-smoking-cessation-management-in-adults?source=search_result&search=Overview+of+smoking+cessation+management+in+adults&selectedTitle=1~150.

7. Fiore MC, Jaen CR, Baker TB, et al. Treating tobacco use and dependence: 2008 update. Rockville, MD: US Department of Health and Human Services; 2008.

8. Lancaster T, Stead L. Physician advice for smoking cessation. Cochrane Database Syst Rev 2004;(4):CD000165.

9. Rigotti NA, Rennard SI, Daughton DM. Benefits and risks of smoking cessation. In: Post TW, editor. UpToDate. Waltham (MA): UpToDate; Available at: http://www.uptodate.com/contents/benefits-and-risks-of-smoking-cessation?source=search_result&search=Benefits+and+risks+of+smoking+cessation&selectedTitle=1~150. Accessed July 3, 2015.

10. Rennard SI, Rigotti NA, Daughton DM. Pharmacotherapy for smoking cessation in adults. In: Post TW, editor. UpToDate. Waltham (MA): UpToDate; Available at: http://www.uptodate.com/contents/pharmacotherapy-for-smoking-cessation-in-adults?source=search_result&search=Pharmacotherapy+for+smoking+cessation+in+adults&selectedTitle=1~150. Accessed July 3, 2015.

11. Hughes JR, Stead LF, Hartmann-Boyce J, et al. Antidepressants for smoking cessation. Cochrane Database Syst Rev 2014;(1):CD000031.

12. Hays JT, Ebbert JO. Varenicline for tobacco dependence. N Engl J Med 2008; 359:2018.

13. Available at: www.pfizer.com/files/products/uspi_chantix.pdf. Accessed July 5, 2014.

14. Rigotti NA, Pipe AL, Benowitz NL, et al. Efficacy and safety of varenicline for smoking cessation in patients with cardiovascular disease: a randomized trial. Circulation 2010;121:221.

15. Stead LF, Lancaster T. Combined pharmacotherapy and behavioural interventions for smoking cessation. Cochrane Database Syst Rev 2012;(10):CD008286.

16. Park ER. Behavioral approaches to smoking cessation. In: Post TW, editor. UpToDate. Waltham (MA): UpToDate; Available at: http://www.uptodate.com/contents/behavioral-approaches-to-smoking-cessation?source=search_result&search=Behavioral+approaches+to+smoking+cessation&selectedTitle=1~150. Accessed July 10, 2015.

17. Carr AB, Ebbert J. Interventions for tobacco cessation in the dental setting. Cochrane Database Syst Rev 2012;(6):CD005084.

18. Center for Disease Control and Prevention. Quitting smoking. Available at: http://www.cdc.gov/tobacco/data_statistics/fact_sheets/cessation/quitting/. Accessed July 10, 2015.

Index

Note: Page numbers of article titles are in **boldface** type.

Dent Clin N Am 60 (2016) 541–549
http://dx.doi.org/10.1016/S0011-8532(16)30008-8
0011-8532/16/$ – see front matter © 2016 Elsevier Inc. All rights reserved.

Printed and bound by CPI Group (UK) Ltd, Croydon, CR0 4YY

03/10/2024

01040392-0010